Evidence-Based Medical Consultation

Evidence-Based Medical Consultation

Daniel I. Steinberg, MD
Assistant Professor of Medicine
Albert Einstein College of Medicine of Yeshiva University
Associate Program Director
Internal Medicine Residency Training Program
Beth Israel Medical Center
New York, New York

Jennifer S. Myers, MD
Assistant Professor of Clinical Medicine
Division of General Internal Medicine
University of Pennsylvania School of Medicine
Hospital of the University of Pennsylvania
Philadelphia, Pennsylvania

C. Komal Jaipaul, MD
Assistant Professor of Clinical Medicine
Division of General Internal Medicine
University of Pennsylvania School of Medicine
Hospital of the University of Pennsylvania
Philadelphia, Pennsylvania

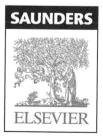

SAUNDERS

ELSEVIER

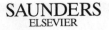

1600 John F. Kennedy Blvd.
Ste 1800
Philadelphia, PA 19103-2899

EVIDENCE-BASED MEDICAL CONSULTATION   ISBN: 978-1-4160-2213-8
Copyright © 2007 by Saunders, an imprint of Elsevier Inc.

Notice

Knowledge and best practice in this field are constantly changing. As new research
and experience broaden our knowledge, changes in practice, treatment and drug
therapy may become necessary or appropriate. Readers are advised to check the
most current information provided (i) on procedures featured or (ii) by the
manufacturer of each product to be administered, to verify the recommended dose
or formula, the method and duration of administration, and contraindications. It is
the responsibility of the practitioner, relying on their own experience and knowledge
of the patient, to make diagnoses, to determine dosages and the best treatment for
each individual patient, and to take all appropriate safety precautions. To the fullest
extent of the law, neither the Publisher nor the Editors assume any liability for any
injury and/or damage to persons or property arising out of or related to any use of
the material contained in this book.

The Publisher

Library of Congress Cataloging-in-Publication Data
Evidence based medical consultation / [edited by] Daniel Steinberg,
Jennifer S. Myers, Chitra Komal Jaipaul. — 1st ed.
    p.; cm.
    Includes bibliographical references and index.
    ISBN 978-1-4160-2213-8
  1. Medical consultation. 2. Evidence-based medicine. I. Steinberg,
Daniel, 1969- II. Myers, Jennifer S. III. Jaipaul, Chitra Komal.
    [DNLM: 1. Evidence-Based Medicine. 2. Research—methods. WB 102
E9288 2007]
R727.8.E95 2007
616—dc22
                                                              2007019320

Acquisitions Editor: Rolla Couchman
Editorial Assistant: John Ingram
Senior Production Manager: David Saltzberg
Design Direction: Steve Stave

Working together to grow
libraries in developing countries
www.elsevier.com | www.bookaid.org | www.sabre.org

ELSEVIER   BOOK AID International   Sabre Foundation

Printed in United States of America

Last digit is the print number: 9 8 7 6 5 4 3 2 1

Dedication

There is something to learn from every patient. This is the premise upon which we, the editors, approached the writing of this book. Medical consultation is an area of hospital medicine that may seem routine to some, yet overly broad to others. Still others find medical consultation to be unsettling because of a perceived lack of a focused evidence base on which to practice. Our personal experiences in performing medical consultations have presented numerous opportunities to use the principles of evidence-based medicine to make sound clinical decisions. In contrast, gaps in the literature where uncertainties lie are also often identified, forcing us to rely on sound judgment and experience for decision making. Both scenarios provide valuable teaching moments, which can enhance the education of students, residents, or faculty members.

We would like to dedicate this book to all of the past, current, and future internal medicine residents at the Hospital of the University of Pennsylvania. Their energy and intelligence have made us better doctors, learners, and teachers. We hope that you, the reader, are able to use the material in this book to both improve patient care during your medical consultations and to instill the skills of lifelong learning in your students.

Sincerely,
The Editors,

Daniel I. Steinberg, MD
Jennifer S. Myers, MD
C. Komal Jaipaul, MD

Contents

Introduction

Many clinical questions faced by internal medicine consultants on surgical or other non-medical services are distinct from those faced in general inpatient medicine. For some of these questions, there is a paucity or clear lack of medical research to guide practice. For others, there is abundant literature to guide practice but often no single reference summarizing the existing evidence. Some physicians practice medical consultation infrequently, making the command of this unique body of knowledge even more difficult. While summaries of evidence in medical consultation are increasing,[1,2] there is no single resource that concisely provides evidence-based answers to common medical consultation questions. Searching for the latest information is challenging, as new information can appear in any number of journals or in the guidelines of various organizations.

The hospitalist movement has created a renewed interest in perioperative medicine through interventions designed to improve the quality of care for hospitalized surgical patients.[3,4] Some hospitalists and hospitalist groups have also chosen consultative medicine as an area of clinical and academic focus. Internal medicine residents are required to have experiences in general medical consultation during their training,[5] and in academic centers hospitalists often provide these experiences. As hospitalists and medical educators, the editors perceived a need for a concise, evidence-based reference to serve our colleagues who practice medical consultation.

With this book we hope to provide clinicians with a pocket reference that addresses these challenges and improves

[1]Basaviah P, Frost S. Update in Hospital Medicine. Ann Intern Med 2006;145:685-691.

[2]Smetana GW, Cohn SL, Lawrence VA. Update in perioperative medicine. Ann Intern Med 2004;140:452-461.

[3]Huddleston JM, Long KH. Medical and Surgical Co management after Elective Hip and Knee Arthroplasty: A Randomized, Controlled Trial. Ann Intern Med 2004;141:28-38.

[4]Roy A, Heckman MG, Roy V. Associations between the hospitalist model of care and quality-of-care-related outcomes in patients undergoing hip fracture surgery. Mayo Clin Proc 2006;81(1):28-31.

[5]Program Requirements for Residency Education in Internal Medicine. Available at http://www.acgme.org/acWebsite/downloads/RRC_progReq/140pr703_u704.pdf. Accessed May 14, 2007.

medical practice at the point of care. Within each chapter, topics are organized as focused clinical questions. We attempt to bridge the gap between narrative reviews, which leave readers curious about how information was obtained, and systematic reviews, which can be too complex to read and apply in real time. Each question is accompanied by a clear description of the literature search strategy, allowing the reader to immediately see how, where, and when the authors formulated the answer. We made our search strategies transparent so that clinicians could easily query the medical search engines and update the searches over time as literature expands. All references are graded with a level of evidence rating, as described below:

I. Systematic Review/Meta-analysis
II. Randomized Controlled Trial
III. Observational Studies: Cohort Trial, either prospective or retrospective, Case-Control Studies, which are by definition retrospective
IV. Clinical Practice Guidelines
V. Expert Opinion, Narrative Review
VI. Case Series or Case Report

Several other strategies are used consistently throughout the text. By providing and interpreting confidence intervals, the authors give readers not only the point estimates of effect, but also the best and worst case scenarios for estimates of effect—information that is not immediately available from the P values alone. When diagnostic studies are discussed, Bayesian theory and likelihood ratios are discussed to allow readers to form patient-specific estimates of post-test probability. Because guidance is required for many questions in medical consultation that have yet to be rigorously studied, we have employed approaches to help the reader identify and manage areas of uncertainty.

We hope that this reference will provide medical consultants with the tools and information needed to optimize care for their patients and with a method for self-learning that will enable them to continue to update their knowledge base in years to come.

Daniel I. Steinberg, MD
Jennifer S. Myers, MD
C. Komal Jaipaul, MD
Spring 2007

Contributors

Kathryn E. Ackerman, MD, MPH
Clinical Fellow
Department of Endocrinology, Diabetes and Hypertension
Brigham and Women's Hospital
Boston, Massachusetts

Nadia Ahmad, MD
Department of Medicine
Hospital of the University of Pennsylvania
Philadelphia, Pennsylvania

Helen Azzam, MD
Fellow
Department of Internal Medicine, Infectious Diseases
Hospital of the University of Pennsylvania
University of Pennsylvania
Philadelphia, Pennsylvania
Academic Hospitalist
Internal Medicine
Lankenau Hospital
Wynnewood, Pennsylvania

Aba Barden-Maja, MD, MS
Assistant Professor of Clinical Medicine
Department of Medicine
University of Pennsylvania
Assistant Professor of Clinical Medicine
Department of Internal Medicine
University of Pennsylvania Health Systems
Philadelphia, Pennsylvania

Daniel C. R. Chen, MD, MSc
Assistant Professor of Medicine
Department of Internal Medicine
Boston Medical Center
Boston University School of Medicine
Boston, Massachusetts

Melissa Reimel Cognetti, MD
Department of Internal Medicine
University of Pennsylvania
Philadelphia, Pennsylvania

Gary Crooks, MD
Ruth & Raymond G. Perelman Associate Professor
of Medicine
Department of Internal Medicine
Unioversity of Pennsylvania School of Medicine
Attending Physician
Hospital of the University of Pennsylvania
Philadelphia, Pennsylvania

Colleen M. Crumlish, MD
Instructor
Department of Medicine
Harvard Medical School
Associate Physician
Department of Medicine
Brigham and Women's Hospital
Boston, Massachusetts

C. Jessica Dine, MD
Fellow
Department of Internal Medicine
Division of Pulmonary and Critical Care
University of Pennsylvania
Philadelphia, Pennsylvania

John Evans, MD
Fellow
Division of Cardiovascular Medicine
Oregon Health and Science University
Portland, Oregon

Jason S. Fritz, MD
Fellow
Division of Pulmonary, Critical Care and Sleep Medicine
University Hospitals Case Medical Center
Case Western Reserve University School of Medicine
Cleveland, Ohio

Robert R. Gaiser, MD
Associate Professor
Department of Anesthesiology and Critical Care
University of Pennsylvania
Attending Anesthesiologist
Department of Anesthesiology and Critical Care
Hospital of the University of Pennsylvania
Philadelphia, Pennsylvania

Lee Goldberg, MD, MPH
Associate Professor of Medicine
Department of Cardiovascular Medicine
University of Pennsylvania School of Medicine
Associate Medical Director, Heart Failure/Transplant
Program
Medical Director, Heart Failure/Transplant Ambulatory
Care Center
Medical Dire

Todd E. H. Hecht, MD
Assistant Professor of Clinical Medicine
Department of Medicine
Hospital of the University of Pennsylvania
University of Pennsylvania School of Medicine
Philadelphia, Pennsylvania

David Horowitz, MD
Medical Director
Department of Clinical Effectiveness and Quality
Improvement
Chief Medical Officer
Penn Home Care Services
University of Pennsylvania Health System
Assistant Professor of Clinical Medicine
Department of Medicine
University of Pennsylvania
Philadelphia, Pennsylvania

C. Komal Jaipaul, MD
Assistant Professor of Clinical Medicine
Division of General Internal Medicine
University of Pennsylvania School of Medicine
Hospital of the University of Pennsylvania
Philadelphia, Pennsylvania

Laura M. Kosseim, MD
Assistant Professor of Clinical Medicine
Department of General Internal Medicine
University of Pennsylvania Health System
Philadelphia, Pennsylvania

Susan Krekun, MD
Assistant Professor of Clinical Medicine
Department of General Internal Medicine
University of Pennsylvania Health System
Hospitalist
Department of Medicine
Hospital of the University of Pennsylvania
Philadelphia, Pennsylvania

Deborah H. Kwon, MD
Cardiology Fellow
Cardiovascular Medicine
Cleveland Clinic Foundation
Cleveland, Ohio

Anita C. Lee, MD
Assistant Professor of Clinical Medicine
Department of Medicine
University of Pennsylvania
Attending Physician
Department of Internal Medicine
Penn Presbyterian Medical Center
Philadelphia, Pennsylvania

Ingi Lee, MD
Fellow
Division of Infectious Diseases
Department of Internal Medicine
Hospital of the University of Pennsylvania
Philadelphia, Pennsylvania

Mary K. McHugh, MD
Instructor of Anesthesia
Department of Anesthesia
University of Pennsylvania
Philadelphia, Pennsylvania

Jennifer S. Myers, MD
Assistant Professor of Clinical Medicine
Division of General Internal Medicine
University of Pennsylvania School of Medicine
Hospital of the University of Pennsylvania
Philadelphia, Pennsylvania

Matthew L. Ortman, MD
Fellow
Department of Cardiology
Thomas Jefferson University Hospital
Philadelphia, Pennsylvania

Sean Pierre Pickering, MD
Hospitalist
Penn Hospital Care Physicians
Division of Internal Medicine
Department of General Internal Medicine
Hospital of the University of Pennsylvania
Philadelphia, Pennsylvania

Atif Qasim, MD
Chief Resident
Department of Medicine
University of Pennsylvania
Philadelphia, Pennsylvania

Jodi Savitz, MD
Assistant Professor of Clinical Medicine
Department of Internal Medicine
University of Pennsylvania
Philadelphia, Pennsylvania

Daniel I. Steinberg, MD
Assistant Professor of Medicine
Albert Einstein College of Medicine of Yeshiva University
Associate Program Director
Internal Medicine Residency Training Program
Beth Israel Medical Center
New York, New York

Kendal Williams, MD, MPH
Assistant Clinical Professor
Department of Medicine
University of Pennsylvania
Director
Center for Evidence-based Practice
Hospital of the University of Pennsylvania
Hospitalist Division
University of Pennsylvania Health System
Philadelphia, Pennsylvania

Preoperative Evaluation of the Healthy Patient

Ingi Lee and Anita C. Lee

1. Are preoperative electrocardiograms able to predict adverse events in asymptomatic, healthy patients undergoing noncardiac surgery? What electrocardiographic abnormalities are associated with cardiac morbidity and mortality?

Search Date: May 2005

Search Strategy: PubMed, search of preoperative AND (electrocardiogram OR ECG OR EKG). Limited to human, all adults 19+ years, and English language; 866 citations retrieved. Titles and abstracts scanned, with relevant citations selected. Bibliographies of all relevant citations, ACC/AHA guidelines, and references from questions 2-9 reviewed.

YOUNG HEALTHY INDIVIDUALS

There is no evidence that preoperative electrocardiograms in young, healthy individuals can predict perioperative cardiovascular events (Table 1-1). This finding is echoed by the American College of Cardiology and American Heart Association (ACC/AHA); their guidelines do not support the use of screening electrocardiograms in asymptomatic patients (class III).[1] The staging systems for heart failure and the updated (2005) ACC/AHA classification of therapeutic recommendations are provided in Tables 1-2 and 1-3.

OLDER INDIVIDUALS

There is an association between age and an increased likelihood of electrocardiographic abnormalities and of coronary artery disease. Given this association and the

Table 1-1. Summary of Utility of Routine Preoperative Testing

Test	Target Cases	Utility of Test
Preoperative electrocardiogram	In patients undergoing noncardiac surgery	May be useful in men > 45 and women > 55 years old with ≥ 2 atherosclerotic risk factors Goal: detect recent undiagnosed myocardial infarction, nonsinus rhythm or premature atrial contractions, and frequent ventricular ectopy
Preoperative chest radiograph	In otherwise healthy patients undergoing noncardiopulmonary surgery	May be useful in patients > 59 years old
Preoperative urinalysis	In clean-wound procedures	No evidence to support preoperative urinalysis
Preoperative potassium level	In patients undergoing cardiac or noncardiac surgery	No evidence to support preoperative use in healthy patients; may be useful for patients with cardiac disease or undergoing cardiac or vascular surgery
Preoperative glucose level determination	In otherwise healthy, asymptomatic patients	No evidence to support use

Preoperative liver function tests	In patients with no history or physical examination results to suggest liver disease	No evidence to support use
Preoperative renal function tests	In otherwise healthy patients	May be useful in patients > 49 years old and those undergoing major surgery
Preoperative tests of hemostasis	In patients with no history or physical examination results to suggest coagulopathy	No evidence to support use
Preoperative hemoglobin level determination	In otherwise healthy patients	May be useful in patients with preexisting anemia or those undergoing surgery associated with significant blood loss

Table 1-2. Classifications of Heart Failure

ACC/AHA Stage		NYHA Functional Class	
Stage	Description	Class	Description
A	Patients are at high risk for HF because of the presence of conditions that are strongly associated with the development of HF (e.g., systemic hypertension, coronary artery disease, diabetes mellitus, history of cardiotoxic drug therapy or alcohol abuse, personal history of rheumatic fever, family history of cardiomyopathy). Patients have no identified structural or functional abnormalities of the pericardium, myocardium, or cardiac valves and have never shown signs or symptoms of HF.	—	There is no functional class comparable to stage A.
B	Patients have developed structural heart disease that is strongly associated with the development of HF (e.g., left ventricular hypertrophy or fibrosis, left ventricular dilatation or hypocontractility, asymptomatic valvular heart disease, previous myocardial infarction), but they have never shown signs or symptoms of HF.	I (mild)	Patients have no limitation of physical activity. Ordinary physical activity does not cause undue fatigue, palpitation, or dyspnea.
C	Patients have current or prior symptoms of HF associated with underlying structural heart disease (e.g., dyspnea or fatigue due to left ventricular systolic dysfunction, currently asymptomatic but undergoing treatment for prior symptoms of HF).	II (mild)	Patients have slight limitation of physical activity. They are comfortable at rest, but ordinary physical activity causes fatigue, palpitation, or dyspnea.

	III (moderate)	Patients have marked limitation of physical activity. They are comfortable at rest, but less than ordinary activity causes fatigue, palpitation, or dyspnea.
	IV (severe)	Patients are unable to carry out any physical activity without discomfort. They have symptoms of cardiac insufficiency at rest, and any physical activity increases the discomfort.
D	Patients have advanced structural heart disease and marked symptoms of HF at rest despite maximal medical therapy and those who require specialized interventions (e.g., frequently hospitalized for HF or cannot be safely discharged from the hospital, awaiting heart transplantation, receiving continuous intravenous support for symptom relief supported with a mechanical circulatory assist device, treated in a hospice setting).	

ACC, American College of Cardiology; AHA, American Heart Association; HF, heart failure; NYHA, New York Heart Association.
Adapted from Hunt SA, Abraham WT, Chin MH, et al: ACC/AHA 2005 guideline update for the diagnosis and management of chronic heart failure in the adult: A report of the American College of Cardiology/American Heart Association Task Force on Practice Guidelines (Writing Committee to Update the 2001 Guidelines for the Evaluation and Management of Heart Failure): Developed in collaboration with the American College of Chest Physicians and the International Society for Heart and Lung Transplantation: Endorsed by the Heart Rhythm Society: Circulation 2005;112:154-253; Heart Failure Society of America. Available at http://www.abouthf.org/questions_stages.htm/ Accessed March 19, 2007.

Table 1-3. ACC/AHA Classifications of Recommendations for Therapy

Class	Recommendations
Class I	Conditions have evidence that a given procedure or therapy is beneficial, useful, or effective. Benefits of the recommendation outweigh risks, and the procedure or treatment should be performed or administered.
Class II	Conditions have conflicting evidence or divergence of opinion about the usefulness or efficacy of a procedure or therapy.
Class IIa	Weight of evidence or opinion is in favor of usefulness or efficacy. Benefits outweigh risks, and it is reasonable to perform or administer treatment.
Class IIb	Usefulness or efficacy is less well established by evidence or opinion. Benefits are equal to or greater than risks, and the procedure or treatment may be considered.
Class III	Conditions have evidence or general agreement that a procedure or therapy is not useful or effective and, in some cases, may be harmful. Risks are equal to or greater than benefits. The procedure or treatment should not be performed or administered.

ACC, American College of Cardiology; AHA, American Heart Association; Adapted from Hunt SA, Abraham WT, Chin MH, et al: ACC/AHA 2005 guideline update for the diagnosis and management of chronic heart failure in the adult: A report of the American College of Cardiology/American Heart Association Task Force on Practice Guidelines (Writing Committee to Update the 2001 Guidelines for the Evaluation and Management of Heart Failure): Developed in collaboration with the American College of Chest Physicians and the International Society for Heart and Lung Transplantation: Endorsed by the Heart Rhythm Society. Circulation 2005;112:154-253.

morbidity and mortality of perioperative cardiac events, many experts have recommended obtaining preoperative electrocardiograms for older patients who may be at greater risk for occult heart disease.[2-5] The ACC/AHA guidelines, however, do not recommend for or against preoperative electrocardiograms in this particular population; they state that there is conflicting evidence regarding routine 12-lead electrocardiograms in asymptomatic men older than 45 years and women older than 55 years with two or more atherosclerotic risk factors (class IIb).[1]

PREOPERATIVE ELECTROCARDIOGRAPHIC ABNORMALITIES

Abnormal preoperative electrocardiograms are common and increase with age. Liu and colleagues[6] performed a prospective, observational study of patients older than 69 years who were undergoing noncardiac surgery and found that 75.2% had at least one electrocardiographic abnormality. However, the incidence of adverse cardiac events is minimal in healthy patients with abnormal electrocardiograms. Gold and coworkers[2] retrospectively reviewed the records of 751 patients undergoing ambulatory noncardiac surgery. The patients were between the ages of 14 and 88 years, and 91.3% were classified as having American Society of Anesthesiologists (ASA) physical status levels of P1 or P2 (Table 1-4).[2] Although 42.7% had baseline electrocardiographic abnormalities, only 12 patients (1.6%) had adverse cardiovascular events (defined as hypotension, arrhythmias, intraoperative electrocardiographic abnormalities, or chest pain).[2] Six of the patients with adverse events (five of whom were older than 59 years) had abnormal preoperative electrocardiograms.[2] Turnbull and Buck[7] performed a retrospective study of 1010 otherwise healthy patients who underwent cholecystectomy. Four of the 101 patients

Table 1-4. ASA Physical Status Classification System

Status Level	Description
P1	Normal healthy patient
P2	Patient with mild systemic disease
P3	Patient with severe systemic disease
P4	Patient with severe systemic disease that is a constant threat to life
P5	Moribund patient who is not expected to survive without the operation
P6	Declared brain-dead patient whose organs are being removed for donor purposes

Adapted from the American Society of Anesthesiologists (ASA). Available at http://www.asahq.org/clinical/physicalstatus.htm/ Accessed March 19, 2007.

who had preoperative electrocardiographic abnormalities suffered cardiac complications.[7] No preoperative decisions were changed because of electrocardiographic abnormalities.[7] Similar results have been shown in older patients. Liu and colleagues[6] found that in patients older than 69 years, electrocardiographic abnormalities did not predict which patients were at an increased risk for postoperative cardiac complications (odds ratio [OR] = 0.63; 95% CI: 0.28 to 1.40; $P = .26$).

Myocardial infarction within the past 6 months has been associated with adverse perioperative cardiac morbidity and mortality.[8] Because patients are not always aware that they have had a myocardial infarction, screening electrocardiograms may be used in an attempt to detect previous myocardial infarction in unsuspecting patients. However, less than 0.05% of myocardial infarctions occurring within the past 6 months are "silent" (i.e., detected only by Q waves on electrocardiograms).[3] Goldman and coworkers[8] also identified two arrhythmias (i.e., nonsinus rhythms or premature atrial contractions and ventricular ectopy, defined as more than 5 premature ventricular beats per minute) that are associated with adverse cardiac events.

The goal of preoperative electrocardiograms is to identify high-risk patients (i.e., those with unsuspected recent myocardial infarction, nonsinus rhythm or premature atrial contractions, and frequent ventricular ectopy) to alter their preoperative management through closer perioperative monitoring, the addition of beta blockers, or in some instances, postponement of elective surgery.

2. Is there evidence to support the use of routine preoperative chest radiography in healthy patients undergoing noncardiopulmonary surgery?

Search Date: May 2005

Search Strategy: *PubMed, search of preoperative AND (CXR or chest radiograph). Limited to human, all adults 19+ years, and English language; 82 citations retrieved. Titles and abstracts scanned, with relevant citations selected. Bibliographies of all relevant citations and references from questions 1 and 3-9 reviewed.*

Abnormalities seen on the chest radiograph are common and increase with age. The incidence varies per study but is on average 10% when all routine chest radiographs are considered.[9] The incidence of abnormalities (i.e., cardiomegaly, pulmonary congestion, chronic obstructive pulmonary disease, infiltrates or atelectasis, nodules, pleural effusions, hilar lymphadenopathy, and aortic aneurysms) rises to as high as 53% when limited to patients older than 59 years.[10]

ASSOCIATION OF CLINICAL CHARACTERISTICS AND CHEST X-RAY ABNORMALITIES

Two studies investigated whether certain clinical characteristics could predict abnormalities on chest radiography. Rucker and colleagues[11] screened 905 surgical patients to determine whether the following were possible predictive risk factors for abnormalities detected by chest radiography: age older than 60 years; a history of malignancy, cardiac, or pulmonary disease; smoking; occupational exposures; recent thoracic surgery; and signs, symptoms, or physical examination consistent with chest disease. Twenty-two percent of patients with identifiable risk factors had abnormalities seen on chest radiographs.[11] Only 1 of the 368 patients who had no risk factors had an abnormality identified on the chest radiograph (i.e., elevated hemidiaphragm).[11] Velanovich[12] found that patients with the following risk factors had a higher incidence of abnormalities seen on chest radiographs: age older than 60 years, ASA physical status levels P3 or P4, and a history of respiratory or peripheral vascular disease.

UTILITY OF ROUTINE CHEST X-RAY ABNORMALITIES IN CLINICAL DECISION MAKING

The utility of routine screening chest radiography in clinical decision-making is unclear. A study by the Royal College of Radiologists followed 10,619 patients undergoing nonacute, noncardiopulmonary surgery and determined that chest radiography neither altered the decision to operate (96.2% of patients with normal chest radiographs and 92% of patients with abnormal chest radiographs proceeded to surgery) nor the choice of anesthetic (96.7% of patients with normal chest radiographs and 96.1% of patients with abnormalities seen on chest radiographs underwent inhalation anesthesia).[13] The study also questioned the utility of a screening chest radiograph as a baseline for patients who subsequently developed perioperative pulmonary complications.[13] They calculated that up to 90% of patients undergoing surgery would require chest radiographs to ensure that there was a baseline available if postoperative complications developed.[13] The authors acknowledged that their study was not designed to answer this particular question. However, their calculation led them to question the risk-benefit ratio in this situation.[13] A meta-analysis by Archer and coworkers[9] similarly found that only 0.1% (95% CI: 0% to 0.6%) of screening chest radiographs had unexpected findings affecting clinical management, including performing additional studies or postponing surgery. In contrast, Mendelson and associates[14] determined that there was a role for screening chest radiography. They reviewed the records of 369 consecutive patients admitted to the general surgery service.[14] A single radiologist reviewed the postoperative chest radiographs and determined which chest radiographs had mild to moderate findings (i.e., blunting of costophrenic angles, subsegmental atelectasis, elevated hemidiaphragm, cardiomegaly or congested heart failure, air trapping, subcutaneous emphysema, or a lung mass) requiring a baseline radiograph for comparison.[14] The radiologist believed that 33 patients (9%) had postoperative findings on their chest radiographs requiring baseline comparisons.[14] After comparing the baseline and postoperative chest radiographs, a third of the findings were found to be unchanged.[14]

CONCLUSION

The evidence suggests that there is no role for routine preoperative chest radiography in healthy patients younger than 60 years. In this patient population, clinical history and physical examination findings should guide whether a chest radiograph is warranted. However, chest abnormalities and perioperative complications increase with age, especially in patients older than 59 years,[4,11,12] and it appears reasonable to obtain preoperative chest radiographs in these otherwise healthy older patients (Table 1-1).

3. Does a preoperative urinalysis in healthy patients prevent post-operative infections in clean-wound procedures?

Search Date: May 2005

Search Strategy: PubMed, search of preoperative AND urinalysis. Limited to human, all adults 19+ years, and English language; 38 citations retrieved. Titles and abstracts scanned, with relevant citations selected. Bibliographies of all relevant citations and references from questions 1-2 and 4-9 reviewed.

Preoperative urinalysis is often performed to detect a silent infection that could result in postoperative wound infection. Lawrence and Kroenke[15] researched this hypothesis in a retrospective study of 200 patients who underwent clean-wound, orthopedic, nonprosthetic knee procedures.[15] Screening urinalysis results were abnormal in 15% of cases.[15] Of the 19 patients who were diagnosed with pyuria, only 5 were treated with antibiotics.[15] Postoperative wound infections were rare, and there was no statistical difference in the incidence rates for those with normal or abnormal preoperative urinalysis results. A follow-up economic evaluation showed that $1.5 million would need to be spent on urinalysis to prevent one wound infection.[16] No evidence supports preoperative urinalysis (Table 1-1).

4. Is there evidence to support measurement of potassium as part of the routine preoperative evaluation in patients undergoing cardiac/noncardiac surgery?

Search Date: May 2005

Search Strategy: PubMed, search of preoperative AND potassium. Limited to human, all adults 19+ years, and English language; 240 citations retrieved. Titles and abstracts scanned, with relevant citations selected. Bibliographies of all relevant citations and references from questions 1-3 and 5-9 reviewed.

Preoperative potassium levels are often checked for abnormalities that could result in cardiac arrhythmias. Several studies have evaluated whether an association between hypokalemia and perioperative complications actually exists.

HYPOKALEMIA IN NONCARDIAC SURGERY

Vitez and associates[17] evaluated 150 patients undergoing noncardiac surgery and determined that chronic hypokalemia (defined as potassium level between 2.6 and 3.4 mEq/L) did not statistically increase the risk of perioperative arrhythmias ($P = .8$).

HYPOKALEMIA IN HIGH-RISK SURGERY

Hirsch and colleagues[18] conducted a study of 447 higher-risk patients who were undergoing major cardiac or vascular surgery. Forty-three percent of patients were hypokalemic (i.e., potassium < 3.6 mEq/L), and 9% were found to have potassium levels equal to 3 mEq/L. Despite the common finding of hypokalemia in this high-risk population, the incidence of arrhythmias was unrelated to preoperative potassium levels. In contrast, Wahr and coworkers[19] conducted a multicenter, observational study of 2402 patients undergoing coronary artery bypass grafting. In this high-risk population, a potassium level less than 3.5 mmol/L was predictive of perioperative (OR = 2.2; 95% CI: 1.2 to 4) and intraoperative (OR = 2; 95% CI: 1 to 3.6) arrhythmia, as well as postoperative atrial fibrillation and flutter (OR = 1.7; 95% CI: 1 to 2.7), even after correcting for age, sex, and history of arrhythmia.[19] However, for intraoperative arrhythmia and postoperative atrial fibrillation and flutter, the confidence interval includes 1.

EMPIRIC POTASSIUM SUPPLEMENTATION IN NORMOKALEMIA

No studies have evaluated whether correcting hypokalemia alters the occurrence of perioperative or other arrhythmias. A randomized, double-blind study by Zehender and coworkers[20] evaluated 232 normokalemic patients with ventricular arrhythmias and assigned them to a placebo group or a potassium and magnesium replacement group. Repletion was associated with a 17% reduction in premature ventricular beats ($P = .001$).[20] Although similar studies in hypokalemic patients have not been done, Wahr and associates[19] argue for active therapy in patients undergoing cardiac surgery because of the low risk and economic burden of potassium repletion.

CONCLUSION

There is no evidence supporting preoperative potassium blood work for healthy patients undergoing noncardiac surgery. There are conflicting data regarding hypokalemia and its association with arrhythmias in higher-risk patients (i.e., with underlying cardiac disease or undergoing cardiac or vascular surgery). Potassium levels should be considered only as part of the screening evaluation in this high-risk population (Table 1-1).

5. Is there evidence to support obtaining glucose levels as part of the preoperative evaluation in asymptomatic patients?

Search Date: May 2005

Search Strategy: PubMed, search of preoperative AND glucose. Limited to human, all adults 19+ years, and English language; 538 citations retrieved. Titles and abstracts scanned, with relevant citations selected. Bibliographies of all relevant citations and references from questions 1-4 and 6-9 reviewed.

The blood concentration of glucose is often measured during the preoperative evaluation to detect previously undiagnosed diabetes mellitus. This practice stems from initial evidence in the literature suggesting an increased perioperative cardiac risk for patients with diabetes mellitus.[21] However, subsequent studies have demonstrated that the relationship of diabetes or asymptomatic hyperglycemia to surgical morbidity and mortality is ambiguous. A retrospective study by Hjortup and coworkers[22] found that diabetics did not experience increased cardiac and noncardiac postoperative complications. Other retrospective studies, however, have found that diabetes is a risk factor for postoperative adverse events in patients undergoing vascular operations[23] or coronary artery bypass grafting.[24] A study by Lee and colleagues[25] conducted a prospective cohort study of 4315 patients who

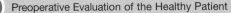

were 50 years or older and undergoing elective non-cardiac surgery. They demonstrated that only diabetic patients undergoing insulin treatment were at risk for postoperative cardiac events.[25]

INCIDENCE OF PREVIOUSLY UNDIAGNOSED HYPERGLYCEMIA

During routine blood work, approximately 1.8% to 5.5% of patients without a previous diagnosis of hyperglycemia are found to have elevated glucose levels.[4] The prevalence of hyperglycemia and diabetes mellitus increases with age. Twenty-three percent of patients older than 60 years are found to have abnormal glucose values.[26] However, the number of asymptomatic patients older than 60 years who have hyperglycemia is not clear.

TREATMENT OF INCIDENTALLY DIAGNOSED PREOPERATIVE HYPERGLYCEMIA

Although asymptomatic hyperglycemia may be detected incidentally with preoperative laboratory work, physician intervention in response to the abnormal value is usually minimal. Narr and colleagues[27] reviewed 3782 asymptomatic, healthy patients undergoing elective surgery. Seventy patients had abnormal screening glucose levels, and only one eventually required treatment with insulin.[27] Turnbull and Buck[7] assessed 2570 healthy patients undergoing cholecystectomy and found that 8 had hyperglycemia. Hyperglycemia was clinically significant (occurring after total parenteral nutrition was initiated) in only 1 of these 8 patients.[7]

CONCLUSION

Although the frequency of hyperglycemia does increase with age, the association of asymptomatic hyperglycemia or diabetes to surgical morbidity and mortality is not well elucidated. There is no evidence to recommend routine preoperative glucose screening (Table 1-1).

6. Is there evidence that preoperative liver function test results affect surgical morbidity or mortality in patients with no history or physical examination findings to suggest liver disease?

Search Date: May 2005

Search Strategy: PubMed, search of preoperative AND (transaminase or liver function or AST or ALT). Limited to human, all adults 19+ years, and English language; 1229 citations retrieved. Titles and abstracts scanned, with relevant citations selected. Bibliographies of all relevant citations reviewed and references from questions 1-5 and 7-9 reviewed.

Severe liver disease resulting from viral or alcoholic hepatitis, biliary obstruction, or malignancy has been associated with significant surgical morbidity and mortality.[28] Physicians can often identify patients with severe liver disease by obtaining a complete history and performing a thorough physical examination. The association between mild elevations in transaminase levels and perioperative adverse events, however, is unclear.

Unexpected liver function abnormalities occur in 0.1% to 3.3% of patients undergoing elective surgery.[27,29,30] Sanders and associates[29] reviewed 101 admissions of patients who were undergoing elective total hip replacement and found that one case of hepatitis had not been previously diagnosed.[29] One patient in the study population developed postoperative hepatitis, but this patient had normal results for preoperative liver function studies.

Given that abnormal liver function test results rarely occur for healthy patients undergoing elective surgery and that there is no defined relationship between mild transaminase elevations and perioperative morbidity and mortality, there is no evidence to support routine preoperative liver function testing (Table 1-1).

7. Is there evidence that preoperative test results of renal function in healthy patients predict postoperative cardiac and noncardiac complications?

Search Date: May 2005

Search Strategy: PubMed, search of preoperative AND creatinine. Limited to human, all adults 19+ years, and English language; 798 citations retrieved. Titles and abstracts scanned, with relevant citations selected. Bibliographies of all relevant citations and references from questions 1-6 and 8-9 reviewed.

INCIDENCE OF ASYMPTOMATIC AZOTEMIA

Renal function is often checked preoperatively to isolate patients who have asymptomatic underlying renal insufficiency. Abnormal blood urea nitrogen (BUN) or creatinine (Cr) levels are found in 0.2% to 2.4% of patients undergoing preoperative screening,[7,29,31,32] and the prevalence of asymptomatic azotemia increases with age. Velanovich[26] determined that in patients 46 to 60 years old, the incidence is 9.8%, and in patients older than 60 years, the incidence is 22.2%. Velanovich[12] identified the following risk factors associated with elevated creatinine levels: patients in ASA physical status level greater than P3, coronary artery disease and other heart disease, peripheral vascular disease, underlying renal disease, hypertension, and diabetes mellitus.

ASSOCIATION BETWEEN RENAL INSUFFICIENCY AND PERIOPERATIVE COMPLICATIONS

There is evidence to suggest that renal insufficiency may be associated with increased perioperative complications. A review of 28 studies by Novis and colleagues[33] repeatedly found that elevated preoperative levels of Cr or BUN, or both, were risk factors for postoperative renal dysfunction in vascular, cardiac, general, and biliary surgery patients. They were unable to specify a particular BUN or Cr level at which complications occurred because each study used a different value to define renal failure[33] Lee and coworkers[25] evaluated 4315 patients, who were 50 years old or older and undergoing elective noncardiac surgery, to determine risk factors associated with postoperative cardiac complications. Their revised cardiac risk index included a serum Cr > 2 mg/dL as an independent cardiac risk factor.[25] A study by Anderson and colleagues[34] evaluated 834 patients undergoing cardiac valve surgery at Veterans Affairs Medical Centers. Patients with baseline Cr levels between 1.5 and 3 mg/dL had greater 30-day mortality rates ($P = .023$), postoperative bleeding ($P = .023$), respiratory complications ($P = .02$), and cardiac complications

($P = .002$).[34] Lok and associates[35] followed 26,506 patients undergoing coronary artery bypass surgery and compared mortality rates in the following groups: normal renal function (Cr < 1.4 mg/dL), mild renal insufficiency (Cr = 1.4 to 2 mg/dL), and moderate to severe renal insufficiency (Cr > 2 mg/dL). Renal insufficiency was a significant predictor of 30-day (OR = 3.1; 95% CI: 2 to 4.7) and 1-year mortality (OR = 3.4; 95% CI: 2.5 to 4.8) for patients with moderate to severe renal insufficiency.[35]

A prospective study by Hou and colleagues[36] observed 2216 consecutive medical and surgical admissions and found that there was a high risk of mortality associated with renal failure. This study determined that approximately one third of patients who developed acute renal failure (defined as specific increase in Cr, which depended on the patient's baseline Cr level) died as inpatient.[36] Although patients who developed oliguria and those who had an increase in the Cr > 3 mg/dL were at risk for inpatient mortality, admission serum Cr levels were not predictive of mortality.[36] A study by Turnbull and Buck[7] also did not find an association between baseline creatinine levels and postoperative complications. This study evaluated 2570 patients undergoing elective cholecystectomy and found that only 2 patients had significantly elevated Cr levels (1.8 and 3.2 mg/dL). There was no evidence that these abnormal Cr values altered clinical management or resulted in complications.[7]

CONCLUSION

There are no official recommendations regarding the utility of renal function as part of the preoperative evaluation. However, given that the incidence of renal insufficiency is common in patients 50 years old or older, that renal insufficiency may be associated with perioperative cardiac and noncardiac complications, and that medications often are adjusted for renal impairment, it appears reasonable to check renal function in older patients and those undergoing major surgery (Table 1-1).

8. Is there evidence to support the routine preoperative use of tests of hemostasis to prevent postoperative bleeding complications?

Search Date: May 2005

Search Strategy: *PubMed, search of preoperative AND (bleeding time OR protime OR partial thromboplastin OR PT OR PTT). Limited to human, all adults 19+ years, and English language; 347 citations retrieved. Titles and abstracts scanned, with relevant citations selected. Bibliographies of all relevant citations and references from questions 1-7 and 9 reviewed.*

The tests of hemostasis include those assessing coagulation factors (i.e., prothrombin time [PT] and partial thromboplastin time [PTT]); platelet count; and platelet function (i.e., bleeding time). These tests are performed as part of the preoperative evaluation to identify patients at risk for postoperative hemorrhage and to intervene with treatments to minimize this bleeding risk.

INCIDENCE OF ABNORMAL COAGULATION RESULTS

Unexpected abnormalities of the tests of hemostasis are relatively uncommon, particularly in otherwise healthy patients who have a low risk of bleeding based on the history and physical examination findings.[31,37-41] Bushick and coworkers[37] evaluated 829 consecutive patients undergoing elective orthopedic surgery and found that 0.3% had abnormal PT results and 0.9% had abnormal PTT results requiring clinical intervention. Eisenberg and colleagues[42] evaluated 750 patients on the surgical service and found that 25 of 139 patients with a history or physical examination findings suggesting possible bleeding diathesis had abnormal values, compared with 13 of 480 patients with no history or physical examination findings indicating a bleeding risk.

ASSOCIATION BETWEEN ABNORMAL COAGULATION RESULTS AND PERIOPERATIVE HEMORRHAGE

The association between abnormal coagulation test results and postoperative hemorrhage is unclear. Suchman and Muslin[38] performed a prospective study of patients undergoing invasive diagnostic or therapeutic procedures during 1 year at a large university hospital and found that prolonged PTT was a modest predictor of bleeding complications in high-risk patients (i.e., patients with known coagulopathy; potential factor deficiency, such as patients with liver disease, malabsorption, or malnutrition; trauma; or hemorrhage) but not in low-risk patients; the positive likelihood ratio in the high-risk group was 1.74, compared with 0.58 in the low-risk group. Similar to the results found with coagulation studies, bleeding time has also been found to be a poor indicator of postoperative hemorrhage.[43-45] Gewirtz and colleagues[45,46] performed a literature search and a retrospective study, and they found that there was no significant correlation between abnormal bleeding time and bleeding risk, concluding that a bleeding time should not be part of the preoperative evaluation. Other studies have yielded similar conclusions. A prospective study by Houry and associates[47] evaluated 3242 general surgery patients and found that there was no difference in rates of postoperative hemorrhage for patients with or without abnormal test results for markers of hemostasis. In this study, bleeding disorders were treated only when patients had concomitant histories consistent with coagulopathy.[47] Similarly, a review by Eckman and coworkers[41] concluded that performing routine tests of hemostasis was not clinically useful. There was a contradictory conclusion by Schramm and associates,[48] who performed a retrospective study of 1211 neurosurgical patients and found that a prolonged PTT was associated with a potential bleeding risk (OR = 23.83; 95% CI: 3.79 to 150; P = .0007). However, they determined that most of the cases of elevated PTT were predictable with a thorough history and physical examination.[48]

CONCLUSION

The literature demonstrates that routine tests of hemostasis in otherwise healthy individuals are not indicated given that unexpected abnormalities are uncommon and that there is no clear association between these abnormalities and the risk for bleeding complications. Some authorities have suggested that the best screening test to evaluate for postoperative hemorrhage is a complete history and physical examination, which should include the family history of any bleeding diathesis and a thorough medical history that seeks information about obstetric history, previous transfusions, and the use of medications associated with increased bleeding risk, such as warfarin, aspirin, and clopidogrel.[4,44,49,50]

The data suggest that these tests should be performed only if the patient has a history or physical examination findings that suggest coagulopathy (Table 1-1).

9. Is there evidence that hemoglobin levels affect surgical morbidity and mortality? When should preoperative hemoglobin screening be performed?

Search Date: May 2005

Search Strategy: *PubMed, search of preoperative AND hemoglobin. Limited to human, all adults 19+ years, and English language; 756 citations retrieved. Titles and abstracts scanned, with relevant citations selected. Bibliographies of all relevant citations and references from questions 1-8 reviewed.*

The prevalence of anemia depends on the hemoglobin level used to define anemia. Mild abnormalities are common. As many as 9% of ambulatory surgical patients are found to have unexpected hemoglobin abnormalities when hemoglobin levels less than 14 g/dL for men and less than 12.5 g/dL for women are used.[51] However, severe, asymptomatic anemia is less common. Kaplan and associates[31] determined that 1% of elective surgical patients have unexpected hemoglobin levels of less than 10 g/dL.

Certain patients seem to be at higher risk for asymptomatic anemia. Velanovich[12] determined that anemia occurred more often in the following patient populations: patients older than 60 years, patients in ASA physical status level P3 or P4, and patients with kidney disease, cancer, or diabetes mellitus.

RISKS ASSOCIATED WITH PERIOPERATIVE ANEMIA

Significant blood loss after major surgery is common, and evidence suggests that in the postoperative period, lower hemoglobin levels are associated with increased morbidity and mortality. A retrospective cohort study by Carson and associates[52] followed 1958 consecutive patients who underwent surgery (excluding very minor procedures and open heart operations) but refused transfusion for religious reasons. They found that the 30-day mortality rate was 1.3% for patients with preoperative hemoglobin levels of 12 g/dL or higher, compared with 33.3% for patients with preoperative hemoglobin levels less than 6 g/dL.[52] A case-control study of 125 surgery patients found that mortality was inversely associated with hemoglobin.[53] This study also concluded that the amount of blood lost during surgery was associated with mortality.[53] Mortality rates were 8% for patients who lost less than 500 mL of blood and 43% for patients who lost more than 2000 mL of blood.[53] A study by Faris and coworkers[54] found that in orthopedic surgery patients, preoperative hemoglobin levels correlated with perioperative transfusions. Those with hemoglobin levels between 10 and 13 g/dL had twice the risk of requiring transfusion of those with hemoglobin levels greater than 13 g/dL.[54] Not all studies, however, reached the same conclusion. A study by Velanovich[26] did not find that preoperative hemoglobin levels were predictive of postoperative complications in patients undergoing elective surgery on the general, vascular, thoracic, and head and neck services.

CONCLUSION

Although no official guidelines exist, the literature suggests that significant preexisting anemia and procedures associated with pronounced blood loss are associated with postoperative morbidity and mortality. It appears reasonable to obtain screening hemoglobin levels for high-risk patients or those undergoing surgery associated with significant blood loss (Table 1-1).

10.   Does the evidence support the use of preoperative autologous blood donation?

Search Date: November 2005

Search Strategy: *PubMed, search of preoperative AND (preoperative autologous donation or autologous blood donation or PAD). Limited to human, English language, and adults >19. Titles and abstracts scanned, with relevant citations selected; 332 citations retrieved. Bibliographies of all relevant citations reviewed.*

Review of citations from UpToDate on "controversial areas in preoperative autologous blood donation" and "preoperative autologous blood donation" also performed. References from question 2 also reviewed.

Blood loss is a common problem in many operations. Orthopedic and spinal operations often have the highest average blood loss for elective surgery, and for this reason, they have been the most studied models for blood transfusions, preoperative epoetin alfa treatment, and surgical blood-conservation techniques. The average blood loss in unilateral total hip replacement (THR) and unilateral total knee replacement (TKR) operations, for example, are 4.07 and 3.85 g/dL, respectively.[55] The preoperative hemoglobin level is the most powerful predictor of the risk of requiring a transfusion[56] and mortality.[57]

ADVANTAGES TO PAD

Allogeneic or autologous (i.e., preoperative autologous donation [PAD]) blood transfusion has been the standard treatment for blood loss, along with some use of other blood-conserving procedures, including acute normovolemic intraoperative hemodilution. The main risk of allogeneic blood transfusion remains clerical: administrative error and transfusion of ABO-incompatible blood.[58] Starting in the 1980s with public concern about transfusion-transmitted infections, PAD gained popularity as a strategy to decrease the risk of infection and to decrease transfusion reactions with allogeneic blood transfusion. This risk, however, has become increasingly less likely as better tests have put the risk of transmission of human immunodeficiency virus (HIV) per unit of blood at 2 cases per 1,000,000 transfusions to 1 case per 1,800,000 transfusions and the risk of transmission of hepatitis C at 1 case per 100,000 to 1,600,000 transfusions.[55,59] Despite the low incidence of transfusion-transmitted infection, the public perception is that blood supplies are not safe,[55] with 50% to 75% of patients opting for PAD when it is offered.[56] PAD is mandated by many states to be offered to patients undergoing surgery with anticipated blood loss of more than 2 g.[58]

Other advantages to PAD include possibly decreasing wound infections and volume overload compared with allogeneic transfusion. In a U.S. prospective study of

9482 THR and TKR patients, 57% of the THR patients and 39% of the TKR patients received transfused blood perioperatively. One third of patients had preoperative hemoglobin levels of less than 13 g/dL. Two thirds of the blood transfusions were autologous, and one third were allogeneic. Patients receiving allogeneic blood transfusion were more likely to have fluid overload and a slightly increased rate of postoperative infections (7% versus 3% in the PAD and no transfusion groups, respectively; $P < .001$). Those receiving allogeneic blood had an increased length of stay compared with PAD patients (6.2 days versus 5.2 days, $P < .001$).[60] Almost one half of the autologous units were not used and subsequently discarded.

Another study of 3945 patients in Europe found similar results. Seventy-five percent of patients undergoing elective joint replacement surgery required blood transfusion, and allogeneic blood conferred an increased risk of wound infection (4.1% versus 1% for PAD, $P < .001$).[61] There may also be a slight increased risk of postoperative bacterial infection with allogeneic blood transfusion, but a meta-analysis of these data was inconclusive.[59]

DISADVANTAGES TO PAD
One of the major drawbacks to PAD is cost. PAD is no more cost-effective than postoperative blood salvage or acute normovolemic intraoperative hemodilution.[62] Given the relative safety of allogeneic blood and waste of unused PAD blood, the cost-effectiveness ratios ranged from $235,000 to more than $23 million per quality-adjusted year of life saved, and an allogeneic blood cost of $68 increasing to $4783 per unit of autologous blood added very little health benefit.[63] This has been shown in many studies involving elective operations, including orthopedic procedures, radical retropubic prostatectomy, and gynecologic operations.[64-66] In studies of orthopedic patients, PAD was not useful in patients with hemoglobin levels greater than 13 g/dL; only 8% of these patients needed PAD, and two thirds of the PAD was wasted.[67] The phlebotomy from PAD in itself increases the likelihood of postoperative transfusion becoming a self-fulfilling prophecy. PAD has the same potential complications from bacterial contamination and clerical errors as allogeneic transfusions, and the risk

with banked PAD is therefore similar to that with the use of allogeneic blood.[68]

CONCLUSIONS ON PAD

In conclusion, PAD was more popular at a time of worry about transmission-related infections, but as the blood supply has become safer, cost has become a major issue because of the expense of acquiring autologous blood and because of discarding unused blood. Typically, PAD is not useful in patients with preoperative hemoglobin levels of more than 13 g/dL and is itself a risk factor for postoperative transfusion. It may decrease postoperative infections and fluid overload and decrease the length of hospital stay marginally. PAD may have a role in patients with hemoglobin levels of more than 13 g/dL undergoing operations with an anticipated blood loss of at least 2 g. In these cases, patients typically donate blood weekly for 1 or 2 weeks up to at least 72 hours before surgery.[68]

11. Is there evidence to support the use of epoetin alfa to increase hemoglobin before elective surgery?

Search Date: July 2005

Search Strategy: PubMed, search of preoperative AND (epogen or erythropoietin). Limited to human and English language; 228 citations retrieved. Titles and abstracts scanned with relevant citations selected. Bibliographies of all relevant citations reviewed. Review of citations from UpToDate on "controversial areas in preoperative autologous blood donation." Review of Epogen and Procrit prescribing information.

Concerns about the safety and cost of allogeneic transfusion and PAD led to the study of using epoetin alfa preoperatively for blood conservation. Bloodless care was investigated for reasons of religion, such as Jehovah's Witnesses who do not accept transfused blood; short supply; and autoantibody formation. Erythropoietin is a glycoprotein synthesized in the kidney in response to tissue hypoxia, which is responsive to the hematocrit level. Epoetin alfa (Epogen, Procrit) is a genetically engineered form that is most effective when given subcutaneously, allowing for sustained plasma levels and a longer half-life than the intravenous form.[57] Epoetin alfa was initially studied to improve the endogenous response to PAD.[58] Without epoetin alfa, the endogenous response to 1 unit of blood donated each week for 4 weeks is about 2 or 3 units over the 4 weeks. With epoetin alfa given weekly, the response is about 2 to 5 units.[58] Epoetin alfa is dose responsive, and the response is not age or sex related. Studies concluded that although epoetin alfa did increase preoperative red blood cell production, there was no clinical benefit in nonanemic patients (defined as a hematocrit > 39).[69] In a randomized, controlled trial, patients undergoing orthopedic surgery with hemoglobin levels between 10 and 13 g/dL were treated preoperatively with epoetin alfa or with standard care.[70] Although Epogen-treated patients had higher hemoglobin values from the day of surgery until discharge (14.3 g/dL down to about 11.9 g/dL versus 12.3 g/dL down to about 10.4 g/dL), there was no significant effect on postoperative recovery. However, time to ambulation was shorter, as was time to discharge (10.2 versus 12.9 days, $P < .0001$) in the group of patients who received epoetin alfa preoperatively.[70] Transfusion requirements were diminished in the epoetin alfa group, with 12% versus 46% of patients needing transfusion. The study did not comment on long-term mortality or morbidity rates.

Another randomized, controlled trial found that among patients with baseline hemoglobin levels of 10 to 13 g/dL who were undergoing elective orthopedic surgery, epoetin alfa–treated patients received fewer allogeneic blood transfusions than those not treated with epoetin alfa (16% versus 45%).[71] Epoetin alfa was given as 300 IU/kg for 15 consecutive days, given 10 days before, on the day of, and for 4 days after surgery. When epoetin alfa was compared with PAD for orthopedic operations, the preoperative hemoglobin level was higher in the epoetin arm (average of 13.8 versus 11.1 g/dL). In the epoetin group, 12.9% received a blood transfusion; 71% of the PAD group received autologous blood, with an additional 12.9% receiving allogeneic blood.[72] Based on this study, epoetin was approved for preoperative use in anemic patients (hemoglobin levels > 10 g/dL but < 13 g/dL) undergoing elective, noncardiac, nonvascular surgery to reduce the need for allogeneic blood transfusions in patients with significant anticipated blood loss.[71,73-75] Patients with hemoglobin levels greater than 13 g/dL did not benefit from epoetin alfa treatment. There were not enough patients with hemoglobin levels less than 10 g/dL to determine whether epoetin therapy would be useful in this population.

Subsequent dosing regimens were studied, and comparable results were found with weekly dosing of 600 IU/kg subcutaneously each week at 21, 14, 7, and 0 days before surgery and daily 300 IU/kg subcutaneously dosing 14 days before surgery or 10 days before plus 4 days after surgery. As an example of efficacy, a case report described a Jehovah's Witness patient who was given epoetin (200 units/kg) daily for 14 days. The hematocrit increased from 25 to 39 over 2 weeks.[69] A meta-analysis of the cost-effectiveness of epoetin concluded that epoetin does decrease the exposure to allogeneic blood donation, but that the cost per life year was 66 million Canadian dollars.[59] The study also concluded that the life-years gained per patient were minimal. Epoetin given subcutaneously weekly for 4 weeks is more cost-effective than when given daily for 14 days, and the subcutaneous route is preferable physiologically and economically to the intravenous route.

The evidence suggests that although epoetin alfa does increase hemoglobin levels alone and in the setting of PAD, it may not significantly affect mortality. It is economically not cost-effective but may be preferable to patients instead of allogeneic blood transfusion. Epoetin alfa is indicated for patients with moderate anemia (defined as a hemoglobin level of 10 to 13 g/dL) who are undergoing elective surgery with an estimated blood loss of 2 liters or more and who decline PAD. It is likely that patients with hemoglobin levels below 10 g/dL would also benefit, but there are few randomized, controlled trials in the literature to evaluate this idea. However, case reports of Jehovah's Witness patients suggest it is useful.[69,77] Epoetin alfa, if used, should be given at a dose of 600 IU/kg subcutaneously weekly at 21, 14, 7, and 0 days before surgery, if time allows. If not, an equally effective alternate dose is daily 300 IU/kg subcutaneously dosing 14 days before surgery or 10 days before plus 4 days after surgery. It should be supplemented with oral iron (equivalent of iron sulfate) at 325 mg three times each day.[77]

12. Is there evidence to support the cessation or continuation of the following medications perioperatively: aspirin, NSAIDs, antihypertensive drugs, and herbal medications?

Search Date: July 2005

Search Strategy: PubMed, search of (preoperative or perioperative or surgery) AND (aspirin or antihypertensive or herbal medicine or nsaids) AND (stop or withdrawal). Limited to human and English language; 379 citations retrieved. Titles and abstracts scanned, with relevant citations selected. PubMed, to 2005, search of (NSAIDs half-lives); 30 citations retrieved. Titles and abstracts scanned, with relevant citations selected. Bibliographies of all relevant citations reviewed. ASA website reviewed.

Medication management is an important and challenging aspect of perioperative care. In the perioperative period, the patient is exposed to many medications in a brief but intense time. The risk of adverse drug reactions increases exponentially with the number of medications taken by a patient. Routine medications can cause more damage in the perioperative period because of drug interactions and changes in hemodynamics and renal function.[78] Postoperative complications are more likely in patients taking multiple medications (especially cardiovascular and central nervous system medications) and in patients in whom medications were stopped for more than 24 hours.[79] There are few prospective data on medication management, especially of herbal supplements, and much of the information about the cessation or continuation of medications is based on manufacturer's recommendations, consensus, anecdotes, and presumed pharmacokinetics of the drug in question.[80] The risk and benefit of stopping or continuing medications depend on the individual risk-benefit profile for that medication. Typically, if a medication is to be stopped, it should be stopped 5 half-lives before surgery.

ASPIRIN

Aspirin inhibits platelet cyclooxygenase with irreversible platelet dysfunction. It takes 7 to 10 days to renew platelets, and the traditional recommendation is to stop aspirin 7 to 10 days before surgery. In a study of healthy volunteers, bleeding time normalized in 96 hours, and platelet function normalized in 144 hours after discontinuation of aspirin at both doses of 75 mg and 325 mg.[81] A survey of anesthesiology program directors revealed that most stop aspirin before surgery in a variable time course.[82] The AHA perioperative guidelines do not comment on aspirin cessation or continuation in their discussion of perioperative medical therapy.[1] A meta-analysis of patients receiving aspirin for secondary cardiac prevention reviewed 41 studies from 1970 to October 2004.[83] Overall, the bleeding risk ranged from 0% (dermatologic and cataract surgery) to 7.5% (transurethral resection of the prostate), with an average increased frequency of bleeding risk of 1.5 in patients in whom aspirin was continued perioperatively. Spinal anesthesia, cataract surgery, dermatologic procedures, oral surgery, breast biopsy, and peritoneal dialysis catheter placement[84] seem to be safely performed in patients remaining on aspirin. Orthopedic studies were conflicting in their results. One study demonstrated increased transfusions of packed red blood cells, but two others did not.[83] Tonsil, urologic, and vascular surgery all resulted in an increased rate of bleeding in patients receiving aspirin. The patients undergoing urologic surgery also required more blood transfusions. The three studies reviewed vascular operations (carotid endarterectomy and femoral bypass) and found an increased bleeding risk of 1.4 over baseline in patients who continue aspirin, but the studies did not comment on the increased need for blood transfusion.

The clinical significance of increased bleeding time and platelet dysfunction due to aspirin remains unclear. In the studies in which an increased rate of bleeding was observed, there was generally no increased severity of bleeding (i.e., management was the same whether the patient was on aspirin or not). Although continuing aspirin did not increase the need for blood transfusion, in patients who continued aspirin and required blood transfusions, the amount of blood transfused was increased.

The number of transfusions was increased in patients undergoing coronary artery bypass who were continued on aspirin, but the length of hospital stay was unchanged. The transfusion requirements were typically increased only in patients who had discontinued aspirin within 2 days of cardiac surgery.[85] Only neurosurgery and urologic operations may have had a higher level of bleeding.

The main risk of withdrawing aspirin is a potential increase in cardiovascular events. Aspirin has been shown to decrease the risk of myocardial infarction by one third and decrease the risk of death in secondary prevention by one sixth.[83] In three retrospective studies, up to 10.2% of acute myocardial infarctions occurred within 8.5 days after discontinuing aspirin. In the majority of these cases, aspirin was withdrawn before surgery.[83] A prospective cohort study followed 1358 patients admitted for acute coronary syndromes for 30 days.[86] Of the 1358 patients, 355 were prior users of aspirin (defined as chronic use for at least 3 weeks before admission), and 73 (5%) were recent withdrawers (defined as stopping aspirin within the 3 weeks before admission). The withdrawers had stopped aspirin on average 12 days before admission. Forty-seven of these patients were told specifically to stop aspirin before a variety of elective operations, including vascular (30 patients), coronary artery bypass grafting, orthopedic, eye, pacemaker, prostatectomy, and skin procedures. In a multivariate analysis, discontinuing aspirin in patients admitted with acute coronary syndrome was an *independent* predictor of mortality at 30 days ($P = .03$; CI: 2.05 [1.08 to 3.89]). For these patients, there was a twofold increase in death compared with prior users, possibly an acute rebound effect with coronary thrombosis. Others have also cited an increased risk of cardiovascular events with the preoperative withdrawal of aspirin.[87-89]

Discontinuation of aspirin remains a controversial subject. It appears safe to continue aspirin in minor procedures, such as dermatologic, cataract, oral, and dental procedures. Neurosurgery and urologic operations may have a significantly increased bleeding, and aspirin should be discontinued at least 5 days before these operations. For patients who are on aspirin for secondary prevention, the risks and benefits of discontinuing aspirin must be evaluated on an individual basis.

Patients on aspirin usually have tolerated vascular surgery without significantly increased bleeding and may benefit from continuation of aspirin for other operations.[83] Discontinuation of aspirin should not be a routine, absolute requirement before elective surgery.

NSAIDS

Nonsteroidal anti-inflammatory drugs (NSAIDs) reversibly inhibit platelet cyclooxygenase. Traditionally, patients are instructed to stop these medications 7 days before surgery. There are no prospective studies on the bleeding risk with NSAIDs. Discontinuation of the medication depends on the type of NSAID. Longer-acting NSAIDs, such as naproxen (half-life of 12 to 17 hours), take about 3 days to clear, whereas shorter-acting ones, such as ibuprofen (half-life of 2 to 5 hours), take only 1 day to eliminate.[80] A small, prospective study of volunteers taking ibuprofen (600 mg three times each day) demonstrated that platelet function normalized 24 hours after cessation of ibuprofen as measured by a platelet function analyzer.[90] A retrospective study of patients undergoing hip replacement revealed more bleeding complications (mostly gastrointestinal bleeding) in patients maintained on NSAIDs but no difference in mortality.[91] Bleeding complications and hypotension were more frequent in patients using NSAIDs with half-lives longer than 6 hours. Perhaps more worrisome is the additive effects of NSAIDs and possible hypotension with anesthesia or surgery causing renal dysfunction. However, there is no evidence for or against this.

NSAIDs should be discontinued based on the half-life of the individual drug. NSAIDs with half-lives of less than 6 hours (e.g., diclofenac, ibuprofen, indomethacin, ketoprofen, mefenamic acid) can be discontinued one day before surgery. NSAIDs with longer half-lives (e.g., ketorolac, meloxicam, nabumetone, naproxen, oxaprozin, piroxicam, sulindac) should be discontinued at least 3 days before surgery.[92] In patients with renal dysfunction, it may be prudent to stop NSAIDs a few days earlier because they usually are not urgent medications. Liver disease may also cause a decrease in NSAID metabolism (especially ibuprofen, piroxicam, diclofenac, nabumetone, and sulindac[92]) and necessitate earlier withdrawal.

ANTIHYPERTENSIVES

Preoperative antihypertensive medication management is also controversial, with little evidence to support any decision made by the clinician. Most antihypertensive drugs are given up to and including the day of surgery. Some experts believe that a mildly elevated blood pressure is acceptable and preferable to causing autonomic instability or volume depletion[80] in the setting of anesthesia, which itself can cause hypotension on induction. There is consensus that beta blockers should be continued. Observational data suggest an increased risk of infarction and death in vascular patients in whom beta blockers were discontinued postoperatively.[93] The effects of beta blockers in the prevention of postoperative cardiac complications are well known. Clonidine is continued because of well-described rebound hypertension on its withdrawal, and calcium channel blockers usually are continued. There is a lack of consensus about diuretics. In the survey of anesthesiology program directors, most withheld diuretics for 1 day before surgery to decrease the risk of hypokalemia or avoid intravascular volume depletion.[82] Similarly, opinions on the discontinuation of angiotensin-converting enzyme (ACE) inhibitors and angiotensin receptor blockers (ARBs) vary, with some experts continuing ACE inhibitors or ARBs.[94] There may be some evidence from two studies that ACE inhibitors cause a significant decrease in blood pressure with anesthesia induction. Some physicians therefore stop ACE inhibitors or ARBs for 24 hours before surgery or for one dose of the medication, but most continue this medication.[79] Recommendations for perioperative use of aspirin, NSAIDs, and antihypertensive drugs are summarized in Table 1-5.

HERBAL MEDICINES

The physician must take a comprehensive medication history, asking specifically about over-the-counter drugs, herbal medications, and dietary supplements. Herbal medications are often not spontaneously reported by patients. In a questionnaire of 2560 patients undergoing noncardiac elective surgery in 2001, 39.2% reported using alternative medications, with 26% using herbal medications. Forty-four percent did not consult a physician before starting the medication, and 56.4% did not report herbal medication use to the anesthesiologist.

Table 1-5. **Perioperative Use of Aspirin, NSAIDs, and Antihypertensives**

Medication	Discontinue Preoperatively	Time to Discontinue before Surgery
Aspirin		
Low-bleeding-risk operations*	No	N/A
High-bleeding-risk operations[†]	Yes	5-7 days
Vascular operations	No	N/A
NSAIDs		
Short half life, < 6 hours[‡]	Yes	1-2 days
Long half life, > 6 hours[§]	Yes	3 days
Antihypertensives		
Beta blockers	No	N/A
Clonidine	No	N/A
Calcium channel blockers	No	N/A
Diuretics	Maybe	1 day
ACE-I/ARBs	Maybe	1 day

*Spinal anesthesia, cataract surgery, dermatologic procedures, oral and dental operations, breast biopsy, and peritoneal dialysis catheter placement.
[†]Neurosurgery and urologic operations.
[‡]Diclofenac, ibuprofen, indomethacin, ketoprofen, and mefenamic acid.
[§]Ketorolac, meloxicam, nabumetone, naproxen, oxaprozin, piroxicam, and sulindac.
ACE-I, angiotensin-converting enzyme inhibitor; ARBs, angiotensin receptor blockers; N/A, not applicable; NSAIDs, nonsteroidal anti-inflammatory drugs;

About one third of the patients discontinued their herbal medications within 7 days of surgery.[95] At least 17% of the patients reported using herbal supplements that can cause bleeding or cardiovascular side effects.

Another hospital survey from 2000 found similar results. Approximately one third of patients being evaluated for elective surgery were taking herbal medications, and 70% did not disclose this to their physician during routine preoperative assessment.[96] Another problem is that 20% of patients are not able to properly identify the herb they are taking.[97] Herbal medications are especially problematic. Because of their classification as dietary supplements, no U.S. Food and Drug Administration (FDA) approval is needed, and product labels may not necessarily be accurate.

About 20,000 different single-herb and combination-herb nutraceuticals are sold in the United States.[98]

There are no randomized trials comparing stopping or continuing herbal medications perioperatively, and the ASA does not have a specific guideline. However, in their patient and physician information handouts, they do implicitly recommend stopping herbal medications about 2 to 3 weeks before surgery.[99] Most of the information about herbal medicines is based on case reports and known pharmacokinetics of the herbs. Ang-Lee and coworkers[97] identified the eight most common herbs that posed the greatest impact on care. These eight medications account for more than 50% of the 1500 to 1800 single-herb preparations sold in the United States. They are briefly described here and summarized in Table 1-6:

- Echinacea is used in the treatment of upper respiratory infections and may have an immunostimulatory and then immunosuppressive action. The pharmacokinetics has not been studied. Possible side effects include liver toxicity, anaphylaxis, and poor wound healing. It should be stopped as far in advance of surgery as possible.

Table 1-6. Perioperative Use of Herbal Medication

Herbal Medication	Indication	Half-life	Time to Discontinue before Surgery
Echinacea	Upper respiratory infection	Unknown	As soon as possible
Ephedra	Energy booster	5 hours	24 hours
Garlic	Coronary artery disease, hyperlipidemia	Unknown	7 days
Ginkgo	Vertigo, memory loss	3-10 hours	3 days to 3 weeks
Ginseng	Stress	0.8-7.4 hours	7 days
Kava	Anxiolytic	9 hours	7 days
St. John's wort	Depression	43 hours	5 days
Valerian	Depression	Unknown	Taper over several weeks

- Ephedra is used to increase energy. Its physiologic effect is to increase blood pressure and heart rate by beta 1 and beta 2 activity. It has a half-life of 5 hours, and the side effects include hypertension, tachyphylaxis, and arrhythmias. Ang-Lee and colleagues[97] recommend discontinuing ephedra 24 hours before surgery.
- Garlic is used to decrease the risk of coronary heart disease and decrease hypercholesterolemia. It inhibits platelet aggregation, perhaps irreversibly, and may potentiate other platelet inhibitors. Its half-life is unknown. It should be stopped 7 days before surgery.
- Ginkgo is used to treat a variety of conditions, including vertigo, altitude sickness, and memory loss. The terpenoids and glycosides in gingko alter vasoregulation, may be antioxidants, and may modulate neurotransmitter and receptor activity and may inhibit platelet-activating factor. It has a half-life of 3 to 10 hours. There are case reports of spontaneous intracranial hemorrhage and a case report of postoperative bleeding after a laparoscopic cholecystectomy that were attributed to gingko. It should be stopped 36 hours before surgery.
- Ginseng is thought to protect the body from stress. Its mechanism is unclear, but it may behave as a steroid hormone. It can decrease glucose levels and inhibit platelet aggregation, possibly irreversibly. Conversely, it also interacts with warfarin to decrease its anticoagulation effects or INR levels. With a half-life of 0.8 to 7.4 hours and a main side effect of bleeding, it should be stopped 7 days before surgery.
- Kava is an anxiolytic and sedative, and it works as a γ-aminobutyric acid (GABA)–inhibitory neurotransmitter with a half-life of 9 hours. Its main side effect is sedation, and it should be stopped 7 days before surgery.
- St. John's wort is used for depression and inhibits serotonin, norepinephrine, and dopamine. It has a half-life of up to 43 hours for one of its components. Main side effects include interaction as a cytochrome P450 inducer. It can double the metabolic activity of certain medications, including cyclosporine, NSAIDs, Coumadin, calcium channel blockers, and selective

serotonin reuptake inhibitors. It should be stopped at least 5 days before surgery.

- Valerian is used for depression. It works as a GABA-inhibitory transmitter and has a short half-life. Main side effects include a benzodiazepine-like acute withdrawal syndrome. Because of the withdrawal syndrome, it should be tapered over several weeks before surgery, but if surgery is imminent, it may be prudent to continue the medication through surgery.

Many herbal medications are thought to inhibit platelet aggregation, inhibit clotting, or interfere with warfarin. For lack of literature on their effects, the best approach is to stop taking them 2 to 3 weeks before surgery. These herbal medications are listed in Table 1-7.

CONCLUSION

In conclusion, the perioperative management of medications is complex and often not based on controlled trials. For aspirin, it is reasonable to stop the medication at least 5 days before elective operations that are associated with a high risk for bleeding, such as neurosurgery or urologic surgery. For procedures with a low risk of bleeding, including oral, cataract, and dermatologic operations, aspirin can likely be safely continued perioperatively. If aspirin is being used for secondary prevention of coronary artery disease, the risk of stopping it and the associated increased risk of cardiovascular events may outweigh the benefit of decreasing bleeding and transfusion risk. NSAIDs can be stopped 1 to 3 days before surgery without increased bleeding, depending on the half-life of the drug. Ibuprofen, which has a short

---

Table 1-7. **Herbal Medication That May Inhibit Platelet Aggregation, Inhibit Clotting, or Interfere with Warfarin**

Bilberry	Bromelain	Chamomile	Dandelion root
Danshen	Don quoi	Feverfew	Fish oil
Flax seed oil	Ginger	Grape seed extract	Horse chestnut

Adapted from Mercado DL, Petty BG: Perioperative medication management. Med Clin North Am 2003;87:41-57; Ang-Lee MK, Moss J, Yuan CS: Herbal medicines and perioperative care [review]. JAMA 2001;286:208-216; Kaye AD, Kucera I, Sabar R: Perioperative anesthesia clinical considerations of alternative medicines [review]. Anesthesiol Clin North Am 2004;22:125-139.

half-life, can be stopped 1 day before surgery, and naproxen, which has a half-life longer than 6 hours, should be stopped 3 days before surgery. There is ongoing debate about antihypertensives; the general consensus is to continue beta blockers, clonidine, and calcium channel blockers and to withhold diuretics and consider withholding ACE inhibitors or ARBs to prevent further intraoperative hypotension at the time of anesthetic induction and to prevent renal insufficiency. Although pharmacokinetics of specific herbs may help to establish a time for stopping herbal medications preoperatively, the easiest and safest plan is to discontinue herbal medications 2 to 3 weeks before surgery.

REFERENCES

1. American College of Cardiology/American Heart Association: ACC/AHA guideline update for perioperative cardiovascular evaluation for noncardiac surgery—Executive summary. J Am Coll Cardiol 2002;39:542-553. IV

2. Gold BS, Young ML, Kinman JL, et al: The utility of preoperative electrocardiograms in the ambulatory surgical patient. Arch Intern Med 1992;152:301-305. III

3. Goldberger AL, O'Konski M: Utility of the routine electrocardiogram before surgery and on general hospital admission: Critical review and new guidelines. Ann Intern Med 1986;105:552-557. V

4. Macpherson DS: Preoperative laboratory testing: Should any tests be "routine" before surgery? Med Clin North Am 1993;77:289-308. V

5. Jones T, Isaacson JH: Preoperative screening: What tests are necessary? Cleve Clin J Med 1995;62:374-378. V

6. Liu LL, Dzankic S, Leung JM: Preoperative electrocardiogram abnormalities do not predict postoperative cardiac complications in geriatric surgical patients. J Am Geriatr Soc 2002;50:1186-1191. III

7. Turnbull JM, Buck C: The value of preoperative screening investigations in otherwise healthy individuals. Arch Intern Med 1987;147:1101-1105. III

8. Goldman L, Caldera DL, Nussbaum SR, et al: Multifactorial index of cardiac risk in non-cardiac surgical procedures. N Engl J Med 1977;297:845-850. III

9. Archer C, Levy AR, McGregor M: Value of routine preoperative chest x-rays: A meta-analysis. Can J Anaesth 1993;40:1022-1027. I

10. Boghosian SG, Mooradian AD: Usefulness of routine preoperative chest roentgenograms in the elderly patients. J Am Geriatr Soc 1987;35:142-146. III

11. Rucker L, Frye E, Staten M: Usefulness of screening chest roentgenograms in preoperative patients. JAMA 1983;250:3209-3211. III

12. Velanovich V: Preoperative laboratory screening based on age, gender, and concomitant medical diseases. Surgery 1994;115:56-61. III

13. Royal College of Radiologists: Preoperative chest radiology. National Study by the Royal College of Radiologists. Lancet 1979;2:83-86. III

14. Mendelson DS, Khilnani N, Wagner LD, et al: Preoperative chest radiography: Value as a baseline examination for comparison. Radiology 1987;165:341-343. III

15. Lawrence VA, Kroenke K: The unproven utility of preoperative urinalysis. Arch Intern Med 1988;148:1370-1373. III

16. Lawrence VA, Gafni A, Gross M: The unproven utility of the preoperative urinalysis: Economic evaluation. J Clin Epidemiol 1989;42:1185-1192. III

17. Vitez TS, Soper LE, Wong KC, et al: Chronic hypokalemia and intraoperative dysrhythmias. Anesthesiology 1985;63:130-133. III

18. Hirsch IA, Tomlinson DL, Slogoff S, et al: The overstated risk of preoperative hypokalemia. Anesth Analg 1988;67:131-136. III

19. Wahr JA, Parks R, Boisvert D, et al: Preoperative serum potassium levels and perioperative outcomes in cardiac surgery patients. JAMA 1999;281:2203-2210. III

20. Zehender M, Meinertz T, Faber T, et al: Antiarrhythmic effects of increasing the daily intake of magnesium and potassium in patients with frequent ventricular arrhythmias. J Am Coll Cardiol 1997;29:1028-1034. II

21. Kahn O, Wagner W, Bessman AN: Mortality of diabetic patients treated surgically for lower limb infection and/or gangrene. Diabetes 1974;23:287-292. III

22. Hjortup A, Sorensen C, Dyremose E, et al: Influence of diabetes mellitus on operative risk. Br J Surg 1985;72:783-785. III

23. Eagle KA, Coley CM, Newell JB, et al: Combining clinical and thallium data optimizes preoperative assessment of cardiac risk before major vascular surgery. Ann Intern Med 1989;110:859-866. III

24. Higgins TL, Estafanous FG, Loop FD, et al: Stratification of morbidity and morality outcome by preoperative risk

factors in coronary artery bypass patients. A clinical severity score. JAMA 1992;267:2344-2348. **III**

25. Lee TGH, Marcantonio ER, Mangione CM, et al: Derivation and prospective validation of a simple index for prediction of cardiac risk of major noncardiac surgery. Circulation 1999;100:1043-1049. **III**

26. Velanovich V: The value of routine preoperative laboratory testing in predicting postoperative complications: A multivariate analysis. Surgery 1991;109:236-243. **III**

27. Narr BJ, Hansen TR, Warner MA: Preoperative laboratory screening in healthy Mayo patients: Cost-effective elimination of tests and unchanged outcomes. Mayo Clin Proc 1991;66:155-159. **III**

28. Powell-Jackson P, Greenway B, Williams R: Adverse effects of exploratory laparotomy in patients with unsuspected liver disease. Br J Surg 1982;69:449-451. **III**

29. Sanders DP, McKinney FW, Harris WH: Clinical evaluation and cost effectiveness of preoperative laboratory assessment on patients undergoing total hip arthroplasty. Orthopedics 1989;12:1449-1453. **III**

30. Schemel WH: Unexpected hepatic dysfunction found by multiple laboratory screening. Anesth Analg 1976;55:810-812. **III**

31. Kaplan EG, Sheiner LB, Boeckmann AJ, et al: The usefulness of preoperative laboratory screening. JAMA 1985;253:3576-3581. **III**

32. Macpherson DS, Snow R, Lofgren RP: Preoperative screening: Value of previous tests. Ann Intern Med 1990;113:969-973. **III**

33. Novis BK, Roizen MF, Aronson S, et al: Association of preoperative risk factors with postoperative renal failure. Anesth Analg 1994;78:143-149. **III**

34. Anderson RJ, O'Brien M, MaWhinney S, et al: Mild renal failure is associated with adverse outcome after cardiac valve surgery. Am J Kidney Dis 2000;35:1127-1134.

35. Lok CE, Austin PC, Wang H, et al: Impact of renal insufficiency on short- and long-term outcomes after cardiac surgery. Am Heart J 2004;148:430-438. **III**

36. Hou SH, Bushinsky DA, Wish JB, et al: Hospital-acquired renal insufficiency: A prospective study. Am J Med 1983;74:243-248. **III**

37. Bushick JB, Eisenberg JM, Kinman J, et al: Pursuit of abnormal coagulation screening tests generates modest

hidden preoperative costs. J Gen Intern M 1989;4: 493-497. [III]

38. Suchman AL, Mushlin AI: How well does the activated partial thromboplastin time predict postoperative hemorrhage? JAMA 1986;256:750-753. [III]

39. Rohrer MJ, Michelotti MC, Nahrwold DL: A prospective evaluation of the efficacy of preoperative coagulation testing. Ann Surg 1988;208:554-557. [III]

40. Erban SB, Kinman JL, Schwartz JS: Routine use of the prothrombin and partial thromboplastin times. JAMA 1989;262:2428-2342. [III]

41. Eckman MH, Erban JK, Singh SK, et al: Screening for the risk for bleeding or thrombosis. Ann Intern Med 2003;138:W15-W24. [V]

42. Eisenberg JM, Clarke JR, Sussman SA: Prothrombin and partial thromboplastin times as preoperative screening tests. Arch Surg 1982;177:48-51. [III]

43. Rodgers RP, Levin J: A critical reappraisal of the bleeding time. Semin Thromb Hemost 1990;16:1-20. [I]

44. Peterson P, Hayes TE, Arkin CF, et al: The preoperative bleeding time test lacks clinical benefit: College of American Pathologists' and American Society of Clinical Pathologists' position article. Arch Surg 1998; 133:134-139. [V]

45. Gewirtz AS, Kottke-Marchant K, Miller ML: The preoperative bleeding time test: Assessing its clinical usefulness. Cleve Clin J Med 1995;62:379-382. [V]

46. Gewirtz AS, Miller ML, Keys TF: The clinical usefulness of the preoperative bleeding time. Arch Pathol Lab Med 1996;120:353-356. [III]

47. Houry S, Georgac C, Hay JM., et al: A prospective multicenter evaluation of preoperative hemostatic screening tests. Am J Surg 1995;109:19-23. [III]

48. Schramm B, Leslie K, Myles PS, et al: Coagulation studies in preoperative neurosurgical patients. Anaesth Intensive Care 2001;29:388-392. [III]

49. Rapaport SI: Preoperative hemostatic evaluation: Which tests, if any? Blood 1983;61:229-236. [V]

50. Borzotta AP, Keeling MM: Value of the preoperative history as an indicator of hemostatic disorders. Ann Surg 1984;200:648-652. [III]

51. Johnson JH, Kenn-Ioli S, Butler TA: Are routine preoperative laboratory screening tests necessary to evaluate ambulatory surgical patients? Surgery 1988;104:639-645. [III]

52. Carson JL, Duff A, Poses RM, et al: Effect of anaemia and cardiovascular disease on surgical mortality and morbidity. Lancet 1996;348:1055-1060. III

53. Carson JL, Poses RM, Spence RK, et al: Severity of anaemia and operative mortality and morbidity. Lancet 1988;1:727-729. III

54. Faris PM, Spence RK, Larholt KM, et al: The predictive power of baseline hemoglobin for transfusion risk in surgery patients. Orthopedics 1999;22(Suppl):135-140. III

55. Keating EM: Preoperative evaluation and methods to reduce blood use in orthopedic surgery. Anesth Clin North Am 2005;23:305-313, vi-vii. V

56. Keating EM, Meding JB: Perioperative blood management practices in elective orthopaedic surgery. J Am Acad Orthop Surg 2002;10:393-400. V

57. Goodnough LT, Monk TG, Andriole GL: Erythropoietin therapy. N Engl J Med 1997;336:933-938. V

58. Goodnough LT, Shander A, Spence R: Bloodless medicine: Clinical care without allogeneic blood transfusion. Transfusion 2003;43:668-676. V

59. Coyle D, Lee KM, Fergusson DA, Laupacis A: Economic analysis of erythropoietin use in orthopaedic surgery. Transfus Med 1999;9:21-30. I

60. Bierbaum BE, Callaghan JJ, Galante JO, et al: An analysis of blood management in patients having a total hip or knee arthroplasty. J Bone Joint Surg Am 1999;81:2-10. III

61. Rosencher N, Kerkkamp HE, Macheras G, et al: Orthopedic Surgery Transfusion Hemoglobin European Overview (OSTHEO) study: Blood management in elective knee and hip arthroplasty in Europe. Transfusion 2003;43:459-469. III

62. Goodnough LT, Despotis GJ, Merkel K, Monk TG: A randomized trial comparing acute normovolemic hemodilution and preoperative autologous blood donation in total hip arthroplasty. Transfusion 2000;40:1054-1057. II

63. Etchason J, Petz L, Keeler E, et al: The cost effectiveness of preoperative autologous blood donations. N Engl J Med 1995;332:719-724. III

64. Billote DB, Glisson SN, Green D, Wixson RL: A prospective, randomized study of preoperative autologous donation for hip replacement surgery. J Bone Joint Surg Am 2002;84:1299-1304. II

65. Morioka M, Yamamoto T, Furukawa Y, et al: Efficacy of preoperative donation of autologous blood in patients

undergoing radical retropubic prostatectomy. Int J Urol 2002;9:210-214. III

66. Horowitz NS, Gibb RK, Menegakis NE, et al: Utility and cost-effectiveness of preoperative autologous blood donation in gynecologic and gynecologic oncology patients. Obstet Gynecol 2002;99(Pt 1):771-776. III

67. Keating EM, Meding JB, Faris PM, Ritter MA: Predictors of transfusion risk in elective knee surgery. Clin Orthop 1998;(357):50-59. III

68. Goodnough LT: Autologous blood donation. Critical Care 2004;8(Suppl 2):S49-S52. V

69. Holt RL, Martin TD, Hess PJ, et al: Jehovah's Witnesses requiring complex urgent cardiothoracic surgery. Ann Thorac Surg 2004;78:695-697. VI

70. Goodnough LT, Price TH, Friedman KD, et al: A phase III trial of recombinant human erythropoietin therapy in nonanemic orthopedic patients subjected to aggressive removal of blood for autologous use: Dose, response, toxicity, and efficacy. Transfusion 1994; 34:66-71. II

71. Weber EW, Slappendel R, Hemon Y, et al: Effects of epoetin alfa on blood transfusions and postoperative recovery in orthopaedic surgery: The European Epoetin Alfa Surgery Trial (EEST). Eur J Anaesthesiol 2005;22:249-257. II

72. de Andrade JR, Jove M, Landon G, et al: Baseline hemoglobin as a predictor of risk of transfusion and response to epoetin alfa in orthopedic surgery patients. Am J Orthop 1996;25:533-542. II

73. Stowell CP, Chandler H, Jove M, et al: An open-label, randomized study to compare the safety and efficacy of perioperative epoetin alfa with preoperative autologous blood donation in total joint arthroplasty. Orthopedics 1999;22(Suppl):s105-s112. II

74. Epoetin drug information available at http://www. epogen.com/pdf/epogen_pi.pdf Accessed April 2007.

75. Goldberg MA, McCutchen JW, Jove M, et al: A safety and efficacy comparison study of two dosing regimens of epoetin alfa in patients undergoing major orthopedic surgery. Am J Orthop 1996;25:544-552. II

76. Faris PM, Ritter MA, Abels RI: The effects of recombinant human erythropoietin on perioperative transfusion requirements in patients having a major orthopaedic operation. J Bone joint Surg Am 1996;78:62-72. II

77. Carson JL, Noveck H, Berlin JA, Gould SA: Mortality and morbidity in patients with very low postoperative Hb levels who decline blood transfusion. Transfusion 2002;42:812-818. III

78. Spell NO 3rd:Stopping and restarting medications in the perioperative period. Med Clin North Am 2001;85: 1117-1128. V

79. Pass SE, Simpson RW: Discontinuation and reinstitution of medications during the perioperative period. Am J Health Syst Pharm 2004;61:899-912. V

80. Mercado DL, Petty BG: Perioperative medication management. Med Clin North Am 2003;87:41-57. V

81. Cahill RA, McGreal GT, Crowe BH, et al: Duration of increased bleeding tendency after cessation of aspirin therapy. J Am Coll Surg 2005;200:564-573. II

82. Kroenke K, Gooby-Toedt D, Jackson JL: Chronic medications in the perioperative period. South Med J 1998; 91:358-364. III

83. Burger W, Chemnitius JM, Kneissl GD, Rucker G: Low-dose aspirin for secondary cardiovascular prevention—Cardiovascular risks after its perioperative withdrawal versus bleeding risks with its continuation—Review and meta-analysis. J Intern Med 2005;257:399-414. I

84. Shpitz B, Plotkin E, Spindel Z, et al: Should aspirin therapy be withheld before insertion and/or removal of a permanent peritoneal dialysis catheter? Am Surg 2002;68:762-764. III

85. Weightman WM, Gibbs NM, Weidmann CR, et al: The effect of preoperative aspirin-free interval on red blood cell transfusion requirements in cardiac surgical patients. J Cardiothorac Vasc Anesth 2002;16:54-58. III

86. Collet JP, Montalescot G, Blanchet B, et al: Impact of prior use or recent withdrawal of oral antiplatelet agents on acute coronary syndromes. Circulation 2004;110:2361-2367. III

87. Mak S, Amoroso P: Stop those anti-platelet drugs before surgery! BJU Int 2003;91:593-594. V

88. Dudderidge T, Arya M, Young J, Davies A: Stop those anti-platelet drugs before surgery! [Comment on BJU Int 2003;91:593-594.] BJU Int 2003;92:654-655. V

89. Alexandrou K, Matthews PN: Stop those anti-platelet drugs before surgery! [Comment on BJU Int 2003;91:593-594.] BJU Int 2003;92:655. V

90. Goldenberg NA, Jacobson L, Manco-Johnson MJ: Duration of platelet dysfunction after a 7-day course of ibuprofen [brief communication]. Ann Intern Med 2005;142: 506-509. III

91. Connelly CS, Panush RS: Should nonsteroidal anti-inflammatory drugs be stopped before elective surgery? Arch Intern Med 1991;151:1963-1966. III

92. Davies NM, Skjodt NM: Choosing the right nonsteroidal anti-inflammatory drug for the right patient. Clin Pharmacokinet 2000;38:377-392. V

93. Shammash JB, Trost JC, Gold JM, et al: Perioperative beta-blocker withdrawal and mortality in vascular surgical patients. Am Heart J 2001;141:148-153. III

94. Cygan R, Waitzkin H: Stopping and restarting medications in the perioperative period. J Gen Intern Med 1987; 2:270-283. V

95. Leung JM, Dzankic S, Manku K, Yuan S: The prevalence and predictors of the use of alternative medicine in presurgical patients in five California hospitals. Anesth Analg 2001;93:1062-1068. III

96. Kaye AD, Clarke RC, Sabar R, et al: Herbal medicines: Current trends in anesthesiology practice—A hospital survey. J Clin Anesth 2000;12:468-471. III

97. Ang-Lee MK, Moss J, Yuan CS: Herbal medicines and perioperative care [review]. JAMA 2001;286:208-216. V

98. Kaye AD, Kucera I, Sabar R: Perioperative anesthesia clinical considerations of alternative medicines [review]. Anesthesiol Clin North Am 2004;22:125-139. V

99. American Society of Anesthesiologists (ASA): What you should know about your patients' use of herbal medicines and other dietary supplements. Available at http://www.asahq.org/patientEducation/herbPhysician.pdf IV

Perioperative Anesthesia Management in Medical Consultation

Robert R. Gaiser and Mary K. McHugh

1. What are the risks of general anesthesia to the patient?

Search Date: March 2005

Search Strategy: *PubMed, search for "risks of general anesthesia." Limited to English language and human; 1427 citations retrieved. PubMed, search for "risk of general anesthesia" and "mortality." Limited to English language, human, and clinical studies; 72 citations retrieved. Titles and abstracts scanned; relevant bibliographies reviewed.*

Anesthesia mortality has traditionally relied on retrospective data, with death rates ranging 1 in 1000 procedures to 1 in 100,000. Two publications provide prospective information about mortality after surgery with general anesthesia.

Forrest and colleagues[1] studied 17,201 patients who received a standardized anesthetic at 15 university-affiliated hospitals. A history of cardiac failure or myocardial infarction within the past year, severe illness, and neurologic or thoracic surgery were predictors of mortality. The all-cause mortality rate in this population during the perioperative period was 1.11 deaths per 1000 patients.[1] Monk and colleagues[2] studied 1064 patients undergoing noncardiac surgical procedures. The mortality rate was 0.7% at 30 days and 5.5% at 1 year. For patients older than 65 years, the rates increased to 1.8% at 30 days and 10.3% at 1 year.[2] A limitation of these two prospective studies is that they do not distinguish anesthesia-related mortality from non–anesthesia-related mortality. In a retrospective analysis, Kawashima and coworkers[3] collected the data from all teaching Japanese hospitals over a 5-year period. A total of 2,363,038 cases were used. The average mortality rate in the perioperative period was 7.18 deaths per 10,000 cases for all causes but 0.21 per 10,000 for anesthesia-related causes.[3] Their conclusion was that although the mortality rate after surgery is high, the mortality rate attributed to anesthesia is low.

2. What is the most common risk to the patient during general anesthesia?

Search Date: March 2005

Search Strategy: PubMed, search for "risk of general anesthesia" and "dental injury." Limited to English language, human, and clinical studies; 85 citations retrieved. Titles and abstracts scanned; relevant bibliographies reviewed.

The most common risk to the patient during general anesthesia is dental injury. General anesthesia involves laryngoscopy and endotracheal intubation. During both procedures, it is possible to place stress on the teeth, resulting in dental injury. The teeth most likely to be injured are the upper incisors. Lower teeth may be injured by the endotracheal tube or by insertion of an oral airway. Risk factors for dental injury include poor dentition and a difficult intubation. Warner and colleagues[4] performed a prospective study that analyzed results for 598,904 patients undergoing general anesthesia. A total of 132 dental injuries occurred, with an incidence of 1 event per 4537 procedures. This study was important because it suggested that dental injuries are not as frequent as previously thought.

3. What is the association between general anesthesia and myocardial infarction?

Search Date: March 2005

Search Strategy: PubMed, search for "risk of general anesthesia" and "myocardial infarction." Limited to English language, human, and clinical studies; 76 citations retrieved. Titles and abstracts scanned; relevant bibliographies reviewed.

The patient with a cardiac history undergoing noncardiac surgery is of particular concern. Sprung and colleagues[5] reported the incidence of cardiac arrest among 518,294 patients undergoing noncardiac surgery. In this cohort of patients, cardiac arrest occurred in 223 patients (4.3 events per 10,000 patients). Of these cardiac arrests, only 24 were attributed to anesthesia (0.5 events per 10,000 patients). The frequency of arrest for patients receiving general anesthesia decreased over time (from 7.8 per 10,000 during 1990 to 1992 to 3.2 per 10,000 during 1998 to 2000). For survivors of perioperative cardiac arrest, the in-hospital survival rate was approximately 50%, with bleeding and profound hypotension being predictors for death.

4. What is the risk of intraoperative awareness during general anesthesia?

Search Date: March 2005

Search Strategy: PubMed, search for "risk of general anesthesia" and "intraoperative awareness." Limited to English language, human, and clinical studies; 6 citations retrieved. Titles and abstracts scanned; relevant bibliographies reviewed.

Intraoperative awareness during general anesthesia refers to the conscious recollection of operative experiences, sounds, or feelings that the patient may experience during general anesthesia. The Joint Commission on the Accreditation of Healthcare Organizations (JCAHO) issued a Sentinel Event Alert on October 6, 2004: "Preventing and Managing the Impact of Anesthesia

Awareness."[5a] This alert highlights the issue of patient awareness during general anesthesia. It also mandates hospitals to have a policy to reduce awareness and to manage it if it occurs.

Anesthesia awareness occurs in 0.1% to 0.2% of all patients undergoing general anesthesia.[6] Awareness is prevented by administering adequate anesthetic. It was previously assumed that if the patient was not hypertensive or tachycardic, the patient was also not aware of what was happening in the operating room. Numerous cases have revealed that this assumption is not valid. The bispectral index (BIS) monitor is a processed electroencephalographic derivative that assigns a numeric value to the probability of consciousness. Use of the BIS should decrease the incidence of awareness. A large, multicenter study revealed that sicker patients were at greatest risk for intraoperative awareness. Age and sex of the patient did not influence the incidence of awareness.[6]

5. What is the association between general anesthesia and perioperative blindness?

Search Date: March 2005

Search Strategy: *PubMed, search for "risk of general anesthesia" and "blindness." Limited to English language and human; 5 citations retrieved. Titles and abstracts scanned; relevant bibliographies reviewed.*

One risk of general anesthesia is catastrophic but rare: perioperative blindness. Warner and coworkers[7] studied this risk in a retrospective study of patients undergoing noncardiac surgery from 1986 to 1998. These investigators identified 410,189 patients who underwent 501,342 anesthetics. In this group, there were 405 cases of new-onset vision loss. Of these, 216 regained full vision within 30 days. If a patient does develop an alteration of vision, it will most likely return to normal within 1 month. Of the remaining patients who did not regain full vision within 30 days, 185 patients underwent surgical procedures that could account for the vision loss (i.e., ophthalmologic or neurologic procedures). Four patients developed prolonged vision loss without direct surgical trauma (incidence of 0.0008%). The proposed cause is an ischemic neuropathy, and it tends to occur in patients with anemia and hypotension that predispose to inadequate perfusion of the optic nerve.

6. What is the risk of malignant hyperthermia with general anesthesia?

Search Date: March 2005

Search Strategy: PubMed search for "general anesthesia" and "malignant hyperthermia." Limited to English language, human, and reviews; 40 citations retrieved. Titles and abstracts scanned; relevant bibliographies reviewed.

Malignant hyperthermia is a disease unique to anesthesia. It is triggered by the volatile agents (i.e., sevoflurane, halothane, isoflurane, and desflurane) and by succinylcholine. It is a hypermetabolic syndrome occurring in genetically susceptible individuals, and it is thought to result from a reduction in the reuptake of calcium into the sarcoplasmic reticulum. As the sympathetic nervous system is activated, blood pressure and heart rate increase. Through increases in metabolism, carbon dioxide accumulates, and hypercarbia ensues. These are early signs of malignant hyperthermia. An increase in temperature is a late sign in the disease process.

Malignant hyperthermia typically begins within the intraoperative period or up to 1 hour postoperatively. In one study, a total of 254 malignant hyperthermia–susceptible patients were followed in the postoperative period.[8] No malignant hyperthermia reactions occurred beyond the 1-hour period. Workup of a postoperative fever should not include malignant hyperthermia if the fever began more than 1 hour after the surgical procedure. Malignant hyperthermia is treated with dantrolene.

7. What are the risks of spinal or epidural anesthesia to the surgical patient?

Search Date: March 2005

Search Strategy: PubMed, search for "risk of spinal anesthesia" or "risk of epidural anesthesia." Limited to English language and human; 638 citations retrieved.

It is believed that spinal and epidural anesthesia have a lower-risk profile compared with general anesthesia. The major risks associated with spinal and epidural anesthesia are headache, backache, cardiac arrest, and epidural hematoma.

8. What is the association between spinal and epidural anesthesia and headache?

Search Date: March 2005

Search Strategy: PubMed, search for "spinal anesthesia" or "epidural anesthesia" and "headache." Limited to English language, human, and clinical studies; 60 citations retrieved. Titles and abstracts scanned; relevant bibliographies reviewed.

Post–dural puncture headache (PDPHA) is the most frequent adverse complication of dural puncture. PDPHA was first described by August Bier in 1898, when he was investigating spinal anesthesia by injecting cocaine into the subarachnoid space. Dr. Bier reportedly felt fine until the next morning, when he noticed a headache on arising that was relieved by lying down. He postulated the headache to be a result of cerebrospinal fluid (CSF) loss.[9] The incidence of PDPHA has been extensively studied using different gauges and designs of needles. Choi and colleagues[10] performed a meta-analysis of PDPHA in the obstetric population. They found that the size of a sharp needle affects the incidence. A 22-gauge needle was associated with an incidence of 10%, whereas use of a 27-gauge needle was associated with an incidence of 1.5% of PDPHA. Using a pencil-point needle, the incidence is approximately 1% to 2%, regardless of gauge. If conservative measures to treat the headache fail, an epidural blood patch may be used. This therapy involves the injection of autologous blood into the epidural space. The postulated mechanism for its effectiveness is compression of the thecal space and elevation of the subarachnoid pressure. Maintenance of the therapeutic effect is attributed to clot preventing further CSF leak.[11]

9. What is the association between spinal and epidural anesthesia and backache?

Search Date: March 2005

Search Strategy: PubMed, search for "spinal anesthesia" or "epidural anesthesia" and "backache." Limited to English language, human, and clinical studies; 33 citations retrieved. Titles and abstracts scanned; relevant bibliographies reviewed.

Epidural and spinal anesthesia have been associated with backache. A significant association was found between backache and epidural anesthesia (relative risk [RR] = 1.8) in a survey study sent to 30,096 women who had delivered infants between 1978 and 1985.[12] The survey response rate was 38%, leading to concerns about nonresponder bias (i.e., patients with problems after procedures may be more likely to complete a survey than patients without problems). In a prospective study, 329 women were followed for 1 year after delivery; 164 received epidural anesthesia, and 165 did not.[13] There was no difference in the incidence of backache (10% for each group).

10. What is the association between spinal anesthesia and cardiac arrest?

Search Date: March 2005

Search Strategy: PubMed, search for "spinal anesthesia" or "epidural anesthesia" and "cardiac arrest." Limited to English language and human; 86 citations retrieved. Titles and abstracts scanned; relevant bibliographies reviewed.

Cardiac arrest during spinal anesthesia was first discussed in 1988, when a series of 14 healthy patients who received spinal anesthesia were reported to have sudden cardiac arrest.[14] Of these, six suffered severe neurologic injury. The arrest was attributed to oversedation and profound sympathetic blockade from the spinal anesthetic. A prospective series was conducted in France, where 487 anesthesiologists reported on every spinal or epidural anesthetic performed during a 10-month period.[15] A total of 41,251 spinal anesthetics and 35,379 epidural anesthetics were performed. In this cohort of patients, 10 cardiac arrests occurred in the spinal group (2.7 events per 10,000 patients), and 0 cardiac arrests occurred in epidural group. Cardiac arrest due to spinal anesthesia is a real risk. It is most likely caused by the sympathectomy, mandating early intervention with intravenous epinephrine. The key to preventing cardiac arrest is limiting the upper level of anesthesia to prevent inhibition of the cardiac accelerator fibers.

11. What is the association between spinal or epidural anesthesia and nerve root injury?

Search Date: March 2005

Search Strategy: PubMed, search for "spinal anesthesia" or "epidural anesthesia" and "nerve injury." Limited to English language, human, and clinical trials; 6 citations retrieved. Titles and abstracts scanned; relevant bibliographies reviewed.

Although many believe that epidural or spinal anesthesia is associated with nerve injury, the literature does not support such a claim. A prospective study conducted in France examined nerve injury. There were 11 peripheral neuropathies in the spinal group and 0 in the epidural group. The incidence of nerve injury after spinal anesthesia appears to be low (1.4 cases per 10,000 patients) based on this study.[15]

12. Is regional anesthesia safer than general anesthesia in regard to cardiac complications?

Search Date: March 2005

Search Strategy: PubMed, search for "regional anesthesia" and "general anesthesia" and "mortality." Limited to English language, human, and randomized controlled trials; 26 citations retrieved. Titles and abstracts scanned; relevant bibliographies reviewed.

Many believe that regional anesthesia is safer than general anesthesia in regard to cardiac complications. It is thought that regional anesthesia is safer because intubation, extubation, and the hemodynamic consequences of both are avoided. This belief is based on a study published in 1987. In this study of 53 surgical patients with coronary artery disease, patients were randomized to receive epidural anesthesia or general anesthesia.[16] Compared with the general anesthesia group, there was a major reduction in the incidence of heart failure in the regional anesthesia group. Other studies have not validated these results. Bode and associates[17] randomized 423 patients with cardiac disease undergoing peripheral vascular surgery to general anesthesia ($n = 138$) or regional anesthesia ($n = 285$). Cardiovascular morbidity and mortality rates were not different between groups. In a repeat study, 1021 patients undergoing intraabdominal surgery were randomized to epidural anesthesia or general anesthesia.[18] There was no difference in overall cardiac complications. The epidural group did have better analgesia and faster recovery time. It appears that general anesthesia and regional anesthesia do not differ in terms of cardiac risk.

13. How does neuraxial anesthesia impact perioperative risk?

Search Date: February 2005

Search Strategy: PubMed, 1995-2005, search for "neuraxial" AND "anesthesia" OR "anaesthesia" OR "anesthesia" (MeSH term) OR "morbidity." Limited to English language; 32 citations retrieved. Titles and abstracts scanned; relevant bibliographies reviewed.

The use of neuraxial anesthesia provides unequivocal benefits for the perioperative patient. Pain management by central neuraxial techniques clearly reduces the incidence of postoperative pulmonary complications after thoracic and upper abdominal surgery.[19] The decreased incidence of peripheral vascular graft occlusion and improved joint mobility after major orthopedic procedures are attributed to the use of central neuraxial blockade.[20,21] Results of a literature review suggest that overall mortality after major surgery is reduced by neuraxial anesthesia.[22]

14. How does anticoagulation affect the risk profile of neuraxial anesthesia?

Search Date: February 2005

Search Strategy: PubMed, 1995 to 2005, search for "neuraxial" AND "anesthesia" OR "anaesthesia" AND "blood coagulation disorders" and "blood coagulation disorders (MeSH term) or "coagulopathy" Limit to English language; 4 citations retrieved. Titles and abstracts scanned. PubMed, search for "neuraxial" AND "anesthesia" OR "anaesthesia" AND "hematoma" OR "hematoma" (MeSH term); 35 citations retrieved. Limit to English language an human subjects. Titles and abstracts scanned; all relevant bibliographies reviewed. Bibliography accompanying ASRA Consensus Statement also reviewed.

Because of the increasing use of perioperative venous thromboprophylaxis, the American Society of Regional Anesthesia and Pain Medicine (ASRA) convened in 1998 and 2002 to assess the risk and to provide guidelines for the use of neuraxial blockade in the setting of anticoagulation.[23] Spinal hematoma represents one of the most troublesome complications of central neuraxial blockade. Defined as the symptomatic accumulation of blood in the neuraxial space, spinal hematoma has proved to be a rare event, with an estimated incidence of 1 case in 150,000 and 1 case in 220,000 anesthetics after epidural and spinal anesthesia, respectively.[23] Risk factors for the development of spinal hematoma include the following: inherent or pharmacologically induced coagulopathy, traumatic needle or catheter placement, and spinal deformity.[24] Although the development of spinal hematomas is likely the culmination of many factors, coagulopathy seems very important. In two prospective surveys performed in France, where therapeutic anticoagulation precludes the performance of neuraxial blockade, there were essentially no reported cases of spinal hematoma among more than 220,000 patients.[25,26] Extensive review of the literature supports this assertion; 68% of spinal hematomas associated with neuraxial blockade occurred in patients with compromised hemostatsis.[27]

Progressive sensory and motor deficits represent the most common and ominous symptoms of spinal hematoma; severe back and radicular pain or bowel and bladder dysfunction manifest less frequently. Unfortunately, the ongoing analgesia and anesthesia associated with neuraxial blockade often delay diagnosis. Suspicion of spinal hematoma warrants immediate diagnostic evaluation with magnetic resonance imaging (MRI) or computed tomography (CT). The ASRA advises prompt, definitive treatment with surgical decompression. Case reports suggest that clot evacuation within 8 hours of presentation ensures the most favorable outcome.[28,29]

15. What management strategies exist for the patient receiving perioperative anticoagulation and neuraxial anesthesia?

Search Date: February 2005

Search Strategy: PubMed, 1995 to 2005, search for "neuraxial" AND "anesthesia" OR "anaesthesia" AND "blood coagulation disorders" and "blood coagulation disorders (MeSH term) or "coagulopathy." Limit to English language; 4 citations retrieved. Titles and abstracts scanned. PubMed, search for "neuraxial" AND "anesthesia" OR "anaesthesia" AND "hematoma" OR "hematoma" (MeSH term); 35 citations retrieved. Limit to English language and human subjects. Titles and abstracts scanned; all relevant bibliographies reviewed. Bibliography accompanying ASRA Consensus Statement also reviewed.

Recommendations for the use of heparin during neuraxial blockade rely largely on the experience of stroke patients. In the 1980s, Ruff and Dougherty presented a series of 342 patients undergoing diagnostic lumbar puncture and subsequent therapeutic heparinization for the treatment of cerebral vascular ischemia. Among these patients, seven subsequently developed spinal hematoma. Ruff and Dougherty[23] identified several associated factors for the development of spinal hematoma in their patient population, including systemic heparinization within 60 minutes of lumbar puncture, traumatic needle placement, and concomitant use of other anticoagulants.

Given these facts and the results of several additional series supporting these assertions, the ASRA formulated the following recommendations. Full intraoperative anticoagulation with intravenous unfractionated heparin does not obviate the use of neuraxial anesthesia; needle placement should, however, should occur at least 1 hour before the administration of heparin. The presence of indwelling spinal or epidural catheters in the setting of full anticoagulation demands cooperation between surgical and medical care providers. Heparin should be discontinued for at least 2 to 4 hours, and the coagulopathy should be corrected and documented before the catheter is removed. After the catheter is removed, an interval of 1 hour should pass before resumption of anticoagulation with unfractionated heparin. Because 50% of spinal hematomas occur after removal of indwelling catheters, heightened vigilance for neurologic deterioration is recommended for at least 12 hours after catheter removal.[23]

SUBCUTANEOUS HEPARIN
Both consensus statements from the ASRA support the safety of neuraxial blockade and concurrent thromboprophylaxis with subcutaneous heparin. The experience of more than 9000 patients underscores this statement. Approximately 2% to 4% of patients receiving thromboprophylactic doses of subcutaneous heparin experience full anticoagulation, and caution and confirmation of coagulation status should be exercised when using spinal anesthesia in this population.[23]

16. What recommendations exist for the perioperative use of low-molecular-weight heparin and neuraxial blockade?

Based on its reputed safety in European trials, low-molecular-weight heparin (LMWH) gained widespread acceptance in the 1990s as a convenient modality for thromboprophylaxis. The early experience with LMWH in the Unites States, however, failed to duplicate that of its European predecessors. As the popularity of LMWH increased, the number of spinal hematomas documented through case reports or the Medwatch system (a U.S. Food and Drug Administration [FDA]–sponsored database) also increased. These dichotomous experiences likely result from different dosing regimens used in European trials.[31] The absence of a laboratory marker for therapeutic effect and the lack of an effective reversal agent also present problems with the use of LMWH.[30] Given these concerns, the ASRA has recommended caution when using LMWH in the perioperative setting; their specific guidelines follow.

TIMING OF REGIONAL ANESTHESIA WITH LMWH

Neuraxial blockade in patients receiving prophylactic doses of LMWH before surgery (30 mg of enoxaparin sodium SC every 12 hours; 75 units/kg of tinzaparin SC daily; 5000 units of dalteparin sodium SC daily; 50 units/kg of ardeparin sodium SC every 12 hours) may commence 10 to 12 hours after the last dose of LMWH. Higher doses of LMWH (1 mg/kg of enoxaparin every 12 hours; 1.5 mg/kg of enoxaparin daily; 120 units/kg of dalteparin every 12 hours; 200 units/kg of dalteparin daily; 175 units/kg of tinzaparin daily), intended for the treatment of thromboembolic events, require a 24-hour drug-free interval before neuraxial blockade. For patients receiving their initial dose of LMWH the day of surgery, neuraxial blockade is ill advised.[32]

RESTARTING LMWH POSTOPERATIVELY

The postoperative use of LMWH in patients receiving neuraxial blockade is addressed in the ASRA guidelines. For the patient who requires LMWH twice daily, ASRA recommends beginning therapy 24 hours after the surgical procedure. Removal of indwelling epidural or spinal catheters before the first dose of LMWH is advised; a

2-hour interval should separate catheter removal and drug administration.[34] Postoperative analgesia with indwelling catheters is feasible. A 10- to 12-hour interval should separate catheter removal and the previous dose of LMWH. Subsequent doses should be delayed by at least 2 hours. If there is evidence that traumatic needle or catheter placement occurred at the time of neuraxial blockade, the ASRA recommends delaying thromboprophylaxis for 24 hours after the procedure.[23]

17. What are the recommendations for the use of Warfarin during neuraxial blockade?

The use of Warfarin necessitates a drug-free interval of 4 to 5 days before neuraxial blockade and normalization of the coagulation profile. Patients may undergo neuraxial blockade with relative impunity if receiving an initial single dose of Warfarin (low dose of 5 mg or less) in the immediate perioperative setting.[32] Neuraxial blockade in the following situations requires prior documentation of normal clotting abilities: in patients receiving more than one dose preoperatively or in patients receiving their initial dose 24 hours before surgery. The use of indwelling catheters in patients receiving even low-dose Warfarin requires daily evaluation of coagulation profile. Removal of catheters in this setting demands near normalization of the coagulation profile, with an international normalized ratio (INR) less than 1.5. Frequent assessment of neurologic integrity should follow catheter removal for 24 hours.[23]

18. Does perioperative use of nonsteroidal anti-inflammatory drugs (NSAIDs) or aspirin preclude neuraxial blockade?

According to both consensus statements issued by the ASRA, the use of NSAIDs or aspirin in the perioperative setting confers no increased risk for bleeding complications during neuraxial blockade. The absence of other agents or conditions affecting hemostasis is presumed. The German Society of Anesthesiology and Intensive

Care Medicine support a drug-free interval of 2 and 3 days for NSAIDs and aspirin, respectively, before performing neuraxial blockade.[23,33,34]

19. What are the ASRA recommendations for the use of other antiplatelet drugs during neuraxial blockade?

The use of thienopyridine derivatives and glycoprotein receptor GP IIb/IIIa antagonists during neuraxial blockade has not undergone critical review. Several case reports implicate the development of spinal hematoma with the use of these medications.[35] Given these case reports, the ASRA has issued guidelines based largely on the experience of surgical and interventional radiologic communities and on package labeling. Drug-free intervals of at least 7 days for clopidogrel and 14 days for ticlopidine should allow safe performance of neuraxial blockade.[23] GP IIb/IIIa receptor antagonists should be avoided for 4 weeks after surgical or other invasive procedures; the ASRA recommends frequent assessment of neurologic status if administration of these drugs occurs during this time interval.

REFERENCES

1. Forrest JB, Cahalan MK, Rehder K, et al: Multicenter study of general anesthesia. II. Results. Anesthesiology 1990;72:262-268. **II**

2. Monk TG, Saini V, Weldon BC, Sigl JC: Anesthetic management and one-year mortality after noncardiac surgery. Anesth Analg 2005;100:4-10. **III**

3. Kawashima Y, Takahashi S, Suzuki M, et al: Anesthesia-related mortality and morbidity over a 5-year period in 2,363,038 patients in Japan. Acta Anaestheiol Scand 2003;47:809-817. **III**

4. Warner ME, Benefeld SM, Warner MA, et al: Perianesthetic dental injuries: Frequency, outcomes, and risk factors. Anesthesiology 1999;90:1302-1305. **III**

5. Sprung J, Warner ME, Contreras MG, et al: Predictors of survival following cardiac arrest in patients undergoing noncardiac surgery: A study of 518,294 patients at a tertiary referral center. Anesthesiology 2003;99: 259-269. **III**

5a. JCAHO Sentinel Event Alert. Preventing and managing the impact of anesthesia awareness. http://www.jointcommission.org/sentinelevents/sentineleventalert/sea_32.htm.

6. Sebel PS, Bowdle TA, Ghoneim MM, et al: The incidence of awareness during anesthesia: A multicenter United States study. Anesth Analg 2004;99:833-839. III

7. Warner ME, Warner MA, Garrity JA, et al: The frequency of perioperative vision loss. Anesth Analg 2001;93:1417-1421. III

8. Pollock N, Langtont E, Stowell K, et al: Safe duration of postoperative monitoring for malignant hyperthermia susceptible patients. Anaesth Intensive Care 2004;32:502-509. III

9. Turnbull DK, Shepherd DB: Post–dural puncture headache: Pathogenesis, prevention, and treatment. Br J Anaesth 2003;91:718-729. V

10. Choi PT, Galinski SE, Takeuchi L, et al: PDPH is a common complication of neuraxial blockade in parturients: A meta-analysis of obstetrical studies. Can J Anesth 2003;50:460-469. I

11. Rosenberg PH, Heavner JE: In vitro study of the effect of epidural blood patch on leakage through a dural puncture. Anesth Analg 1985;64:501-504. III

12. MacArthur C, Lewis M, Knox EG, Crawford JS: Epidural anaesthesia and long term backache after childbirth. BMJ 1990;301:9-12. III

13. MacArthur AJ, MacArthur C, Weeks SK: Is epidural anesthesia in labor associated with chronic low back pain? A prospective cohort study. Anesth Analg 1997;85:1066-7100. III

14. Caplan RA, Ward RJ, Posner K, Cheney FW: Unexpected cardiac arrest during spinal anesthesia: A closed claims analysis of predisposing factors. Anesthesiology 1988;68:5-11. VI

15. Auroy Y, Benhamou D, Bargues L, et al: Major complications of regional anesthesia in France: The SOS Regional Anesthesia Hotline Service. Anesthesiology 2002;97:1274-1280. III

16. Yeager MP, Glass DD, Neff RK, Brinck-Johnsen T: Epidural anesthesia and analgesia in high-risk surgical patients. Anesthesiology 1987;66:729-736. II

17. Bode RH, Lewis KP, Zarich SW, et al: Cardiac outcome after peripheral vascular surgery. Comparison of general and regional anesthesia. Anesthesiology 1996;84:3-13. II

18. Park WY, Thompson JS, Lee KK: Effect of epidural anesthesia and analgesia on perioperative outcome: A randomized, controlled Veterans Affairs cooperative study. Ann Surg 2001;234:560-569. II

19. Watson A, Allen PR: Influence of thoracic epidural analgesia on outcome after resection for esophageal cancer. Surgery 1994;115:429-423. III

20. Liu S, Carpenter RI, Neal JM: Epidural anesthesia and analgesia. Their role in perioperative outcome. Anesthesiology 1995;82:1474-1506. V

21. Capdevila X, Barthelet Y, Biboulet P, et al: Effects of perioperative analgesic technique on surgical outcome and duration of rehabilitation after major knee surgery. Anesthesiology 1999;91:8-15. II

22. Rogers A, Walker N, Schug S, et al: Reduction of postoperative mortality and morbidity with epidural and spinal anaesthesia: Results from overview of randomized trials. BMJ 2000;321:1493-1497. V

23. Horlocker TT, Wedel DJ, Benzon H, et al: Regional Anesthesia in the anticoagulated patient: Defining the risks (the second ASRA Consensus Conference on Neuraxial Anesthesia and Anticoagulation). Reg Anesth Pain Med 2003;28:172-197. IV

24. Wulf H: Epidural anesthesia and spinal hematoma. Can J Anesth 1996;43:1260-1271. VI

25. Auroy Y, Narchi P, Messiah A, et al: Serious complications related to regional anesthesia: Results of a prospective survey in France. Anesthesiology 1997;87:1274-1280. III

26. Vandermeulen EP, Van Aken H, Vermylen J: Anticoagulants and spinal-epidural anesthesia. Anesth Analg 1994;79:1165-1177. V

27. Liu SS, Mulroy MF: Neuraxial anesthesia and analgesia in the presence of standard heparin. Reg Anesth Pain Med 1998;23:157-163. V

28. Lawton MT, Porter RW, Heisermann JE, et al: Surgical management of spinal epidural hematoma: Relationship between surgical timing and neurological outcome. J Neurosurg 1995;83:1-7. VI

29. Tryba M, Wedel DJ: Central neuraxial block and low molecular weight heparin (enoxaparin): Lessons learned from two different dosing regimes in two continents. Acta Anaesthesiol Scand 1997;41:100-104. V

30. Herbstreit F, Kienbaum P, Merguet P, Perters J: Conservative treatment of paraplegia after removal of an

epidural catheter during low-molecular-weight heparin treatment. Anesthesiology 2002;97:733-737. VI

31. Horlocker T, Wedel DJ, Benzon H, et al: Regional anesthesia in the anticoagulated patient: Defining the risks. Reg Anesth Pain Med 2004;29:1-11. IV

32. Litz RJ, Hubler M, Koch T, Albrecht M: Spinal epidural hematoma following epidural anesthesia in the presence of antiplatelet and heparin therapy. Anesthesiology 2001;95:1031-1033. VI

33. Horlocker TT, Bajwa ZH, Ashraf Z, et al: Risk assessment of hemorrhagic complications associated with nonsteroidal anti-inflammatory medications in ambulatory pain clinic patients undergoing epidural steroid injections. Anesth Analg 2002;95:1691-1697. III

34. Benzon HT, Wong HY, Siddiqui T, Ondra S: Caution in performing epidural injections in patients on several antiplatelet drugs. Anesthesiology 1999;91:1558-1559. V

35. Litz R, Gottschlich B, Stehr S: Spinal epidural hematoma after spinal anesthesia in a patient treated with clopidogrel and enoxaparin. Anesthesiology 2004;101:1467-1470. VI

3

Perioperative Pulmonary Evaluation

Susan Krekun and Jason S. Fritz

1. How common are postoperative pulmonary complications, and do they increase length of hospital stay?

Search Date: January 2006

Search Strategy: PubMed, 1980 to 2006, search for "postoperative pulmonary complications" AND ("incidence" OR "prevalence"). Limited to human and English language; 99 citations retrieved. Titles and abstracts scanned, with relevant citations selected. Bibliographies of all relevant citations reviewed. Search of PIER section of The American College of Physicians website with bibliography review.

Postoperative pulmonary complications (PPCs) have not been uniformly defined in the literature. Early studies included PPC that may be clinically irrelevant, such as increase in temperature, productive cough, or changes in the chest physical examination findings.[1] Later studies have used definitions of PPC that contribute to morbidity or mortality or prolonged hospital stay. For instance, in a systematic review published by the American College of Physicians (ACP)[2] in 2006, 59% of the 145 trials that met inclusion criteria included respiratory insufficiency and respiratory failure in the definition of PPC. Others included pulmonary edema or pulmonary embolus. The ACP review defined the most important and morbid PPCs to be atelectasis, pneumonia, respiratory failure, and exacerbation of underlying chronic obstructive pulmonary disease (COPD).[2]

Early estimates of PPCs were derived from studies designed to assess the incidence of cardiac complications. Subsequent studies used various definitions of

PPC and different methodologies, making the true incidence difficult to define. The paucity of high-quality studies specifically designed to address PPCs suggest that they are at least as common as postoperative cardiac complications, with an incidence ranging from 2% to 19%.[3] The crude rate of PPCs in the cohort studies listed in the ACP systematic review was 3.4%.[2]

Retrospective studies have demonstrated that length of stay is longer for patients with PPCs,[3,4] with a mean of 27.9 days compared with 4.5 days ($P = .006$) for patients without PPCs,[3] and PPCs may be more likely than postoperative cardiac complications to predict long-term mortality.[2]

2. What are the risk factors for postoperative pulmonary complications?

Search Date: September 2006

Search Strategy: *PubMed, 2001 to 2006, search for "postoperative pulmonary complications" AND "risk factors." Limited to humans and English language; 30 citations retrieved. Titles and abstracts reviewed. Related articles also scanned, with relevant citations selected. Bibliographies of all relevant citations reviewed. Search of the Cochrane Database and the PIER section of The American College of Physicians website with bibliography review.*

In a systematic review that forms the basis for the current ACP Practice Guideline on risk stratification of patients for PPCs, 145 trials published from January 1980 through June 2005 met inclusion criteria. Of these, 83 were studies with univariate analysis, 27 were studies with multivariate analysis, 20 were randomized trials, and 11 were systematic reviews, for a total of 11,851 PPCs in 173,500 patients.[2] The *ACP Journal Club* has also published summary results of this data.[44] Combined results of these reviews, with odds ratios for patient- and procedure-related risk factors are listed in Table 3-1. Clinicians can use this information to estimate a patient's risk for PPCs. An in-depth discussion of this review and of the literature on individual risk factors continues here.

Table 3-1. **Risk Stratification for Postoperative Pulmonary Complications**

Risk Factors for PPCs*	Odds Ratio (CI)
Patient-Related Factors	
COPD	1.7 (1.4-2.2)
Cigarette smoking	1.2 (1.0-1.5)
Age > 60 years	2.0 (1.7-2.5)
ASA class ≥ II	4.8 (3.3-7.1)
Functionally dependent status (total)	2.5 (1.9-3.1)
Partially dependent status	1.6 (1.3-2.0)
CHF	2.9 (1.0-8.4)
Procedure-Related Factors	
Surgery > 3 hours	2.14 (1.3-3.4)
Abdominal surgery	3.0 (2.4-3.7)
Thoracic surgery	4.2 (2.9-6.2)
Neurosurgery	NR
AAA repair	6.9 (2.7-17)
Head and neck surgery	NR
Vascular surgery	NR
Emergency surgery	2.2 (1.5-3.1)
General anesthesia	1.8 (1.3-2.4)

*Patient-related and procedure-related risk factors for PPC as recommended by the American College of Physicians (ACP) clinical guidelines[19] and the ACP Journal Club.[20]

AAA, abdominal aortic aneurysm; ASA class, ASA class: classification of patient status developed by the American Society of Anesthesiologists; CHF, congestive heart failure; CI, confidence interval; COPD, chronic obstructive pulmonary disease; NR, odds ratios not reported; PPCs, postoperative pulmonary complications.

The quality of most of the univariate studies included were rated as poor or fair, with 10 of the 83 rated as good quality. For the multivariate studies included, 6 of 27 studies were rated as good quality. The three largest trials reporting multivariate analysis accounted for about 90% of the patients included and accounted for 82.3% of the PPCs.

PPC definitions varied across studies. Two of these three large studies developed risk indices with narrowly defined PPCs, including respiratory failure[5] and pneumonia.[6] These were derived from a total of 242, 524 patients, prospectively validated in 254, 656 male veterans, and are the best attempts to develop tools for identifying patients at risk for PPCs, because they report a multitude of risk factors (many of them common to both indices). The most significant limitation of these studies is that derivation and validation cohorts consisted of male veterans, making it unclear how results are applicable to broader populations (e.g., healthier patients, women).

Smaller studies have attempted to clarify the risk of individual factors rather than factors in aggregate. In one of these larger trials of 17, 638 patients who had ambulatory or low-risk operations, there was no difference in incidence of postoperative complications between patients who were younger than 65 years and those who were 65 or older, suggesting that the impact of age may depend on adjustment for the type of surgery.[7]

In studies that pooled risk factors, smoking conferred a higher risk for PPCs, with odds ratios in multivariate analysis ranging from 1.28 to 1.9; however, studies specifically addressing this risk factor are mixed. An evidence-based review of more recent literature showed that in retrospective studies with a total of 331 patients, smoking was difficult to assess in multivariate analysis as an independent risk factor. However, results of prospective studies with a total of 1374 patients suggest that smoking is an important independent risk factor for PPCs. Incidence ranged from 17.5% to 24%,[8] but differences in study methods make definitive conclusions difficult.

Examining the data for smoking cessation does not clarify the issue. Criteria for a Cochrane review included randomized, controlled trials through 2005 that recruited smokers before surgery, offered a smoking cessation intervention, measured abstinence in the preoperative and postoperative periods, and examined the effect of smoking cessation on the incidence of intraoperative and postoperative complications.[9]

Only four trials met the inclusion criteria, and of these, only two described cardiopulmonary or pulmonary complications. One of the trials had a total of 108 patients, and the primary effect of the smoking cessation intervention was a decrease in wound-related complications (5% in the intervention group versus 31% in the control group; $P = .001$). The rate for cardiopulmonary complications, described as patients needing ventilatory support or cardiac intervention, was 2%, compared with 12% in the control group ($P = .039$).[10]

In the other randomized trial of 60 patients who underwent colorectal surgery, results of the short-term smoking cessation intervention showed no differences in PPCs between groups. Eleven percent of the intervention group experienced complications, compared with 16% in the control group.[11]

Two studies examined the effect of smoking on PPCs after minor surgical procedures. In a retrospective study[12] of 811 patients undergoing hip or knee arthroplasty, the most significant postoperative complications in multivariate analysis for smokers were impaired wound healing (OR = 3.2; 95% CI: 1.8 to 6.0), transfer to the intensive care unit (ICU) (OR = 8.5; 95% CI: 1.6 to 46.7), or any complication (OR = 2.4; 95% CI: 1.4 to 3.8). The incidence of PPCs was not significantly different between groups.[12]

A prospective, cohort trial[13] enrolled 1011 patients undergoing elective minor surgery. There were no significant differences in PPCs among smokers, former smokers, and nonsmokers, but sputum production had an odds ratio of 3.8 (95% CI: 1.4 to 10.4). The clinical significance of this finding is unclear.[13]

Although COPD seems to be an established risk factor for PPCs in several higher-quality studies, asthma as a risk factor is less clear. Previous retrospective studies were limited by poorly defined diagnostic criteria for asthma, lack of assessment of severity of asthma in study participants, and various definitions of PPCs. In the largest trial published, a review of medical records from 1964 thorough 1983 (total of 706 patients with asthma), perioperative bronchospasm occurred in only 1.7% of patients (95% CI: 0.9% to 3.0%). None of the patients in this study had postoperative pneumonia, pneumothorax, or death, suggesting that asthma does not appear to be a significant risk factor for PPCs.[14]

The relationship between obstructive sleep apnea (OSA) and PPCs has not been extensively studied. In a retrospective, case-control study of 101 patients with OSA undergoing knee or hip replacement, patients with OSA required reintubation and experienced hypercapnia and episodic hypoxemia more frequently than controls, although these differences were not statistically significant. Patients with OSA had higher rates of unplanned ICU transfer (60% versus 20%, $P < .001$) and longer lengths of stay (6.8 ± 2.8 versus 5.1 ± 4.1 days; $P = .007$) than control patients. In the OSA group, one half of the unplanned ICU transfers were for reintubation, hypercapnia without reintubation, and severe hypoxemia, but the differences between OSA and control groups were not statistically significant when assessed separately as described previously.[15] In this study, the definitions of postoperative pulmonary complications did not include pneumonia, prolonged mechanical ventilation, or atelectasis. The severity of OSA was not assessed, control patients were not matched for body mass index (BMI), and the rate of complications might have been underestimated because it was a retrospective study.

Older studies of exercise capacity were retrospective and designed before modern anesthetics were being used, making that data of questionable validity today. A questionnaire study[16] of 600 patients who self-reported inability to walk four blocks or climb two flights of stairs showed a statistically insignificant increase in PPCs, with 9% of patients who were deemed to have poor exercise tolerance having pulmonary complications, compared with 6.3% in those considered to have good exercise capacity ($P = .21$). Patients in this study underwent a variety of surgical procedures, one half of which were oncology related.[16] In a prospective study, 83 patients were evaluated before undergoing high-risk surgery for the ability to climb a total of seven flights of stairs. The most significant predictor of cardiopulmonary complications was the number of flights of stairs climbed. The inability to climb two flights was associated with a positive predictive value of 80% and a sensitivity of 38%. The ability to climb five or more flights was associated with a negative predictive value of 95% and a specificity of 32%.[17]

A randomized, controlled trial comparing atracurium and vecuronium with pancuronium found that pancuronium induced a prolonged neuromuscular blockade and had a fourfold increase in PPCs.[18] A systematic review of 141 randomized trials (9559 patients) found that any neuraxial blockade, including epidural or spinal anesthesia, is associated with fewer pulmonary complications of pneumonia (OR = 0.61; 95% CI: 0.48 to 0.76) and respiratory depression (OR = 0.41; 95% CI: 0.23 to 0.73) than general anesthesia.[19] This systematic review did not exclude studies in which the participants received general anesthesia and neuraxial blockade, although all trials included were randomized. Sensitivity analysis lacked power to distinguish moderate-size differences between groups in mortality.

There is a paucity of high-quality data to confidently define the risk factors for PPCs. These risk factors are often characterized as patient- or procedure-related risk factors. The ACP has published a companion guideline with their systematic review recommending patients undergoing noncardiothoracic surgery be evaluated for the following significant risk factors for PPCs: COPD, age older than 60 years, American Society of Anesthesiologists (ASA) class II (i.e., mild systemic disease) or greater, functional dependence, and heart failure (previously designated congestive heart failure). Obesity and mild or moderate asthma are not considered significant risk factors. For patients who are clinically suspected of having hypoalbuminemia, a serum albumin measurement is recommended, because this is a strong marker of increased risk for PPCs. Clinicians should also consider the procedure to be performed when assessing risk. Procedures lasting longer than 3 hours, abdominal surgery, thoracic surgery, neurosurgery, head and neck surgery, vascular surgery, abdominal aortic aneurysm (AAA) repair, emergency surgery, and the use of general anesthesia also confer a higher risk for PPCs.[20]

Validated prediction rules derived from a large cohort of patients representative of the general population are needed to help determine which factors confer the strongest risk for PPCs and to guide clinicians in identifying risk factors that may be modified before surgery to lower risk.

3. Is incentive spirometry or chest physiotherapy effective in reducing the incidence of postoperative pulmonary complications?

Search Date: January 2006

Search Strategy: PubMed, 1980 to 2006, search for ("incentive spirometry" OR "chest physical therapy" OR "chest physiotherapy" OR "deep breathing") AND (postoperative OR post-operative) AND (complications OR pneumonia OR atelectasis OR "respiratory failure"). Limits of English and human studies; 116 citations retrieved. Titles and abstracts scanned, with relevant citations selected. Bibliographies of all relevant citations reviewed.

There is a large body of literature examining the effect of various noninvasive interventions on the reduction of PPCs. Incentive spirometry, deep-breathing or coughing exercises, and externally applied physical therapy (i.e., chest percussion) are techniques that have been studied alone or in combination. There is considerable diversity within the available evidence with respect to type of intervention used, type of control used, population studied, and the types of outcomes measured. Regarding the latter, some investigators have chosen to study the effect of the designated intervention on primarily physiologic parameters (e.g., arterial oxygen tension, pulmonary function indices), whereas others have chosen more clinically oriented end points (e.g., atelectasis, pneumonia).

SYSTEMATIC REVIEWS AND META-ANALYSES

A systematic review and meta-analysis[21] published in 1994 examined the literature through 1992 pertaining to the efficacy of incentive spirometry, intermittent positive-pressure breathing, or deep-breathing exercises in preventing PPCs after upper abdominal surgery. Criteria for inclusion in the analysis were a study population consisting of patients undergoing upper abdominal surgery; intervention consisting of any combination of incentive spirometry, intermittent positive-pressure breathing, or deep-breathing exercises; outcome defined as any type of PPC; and randomized study design. Using this method, 10 review articles and 116 primary research articles were identified. Of the primary research citations, 55 were considered potentially relevant, and 14 of these met the inclusion criteria and were included in the final analysis.

Two studies compared incentive spirometry versus no treatment, with one showing a benefit with respect to chest radiography and physical examination findings (postoperatively). The pooled common odds ratio for a pulmonary complication for these two studies combined ($N = 212$) was 0.44 (95% CI: 0.18 to 0.99; $P = .034$), suggesting a benefit of incentive spirometry over no treatment. In comparing deep-breathing exercises versus no treatment, four studies were identified. The pooled common odds ratio for a pulmonary complication for these four studies combined ($N = 564$) was 0.43 (95% CI: 0.27 to 0.63; $P = .005$), also suggesting a benefit of deep-breathing exercises over no treatment. When the studies were pooled to examine potential differences in the efficacy of incentive spirometry, intermittent positive-pressure breathing, and deep-breathing exercises (compared with each other), no significant difference could be found between any of the interventions.

The methodology of the previous studies was low as scored by the authors of the meta-analysis.[21] Compliance with the prescribed therapy was measured in only two of the studies identified by the literature search, and there was significant variability in the way in which pulmonary complications were defined. All of these factors make interpretation of the results of pooled statistical analyses difficult. In this case, incentive spirometry or deep-breathing exercises are recommended as means to reduce PPCs in patients undergoing upper abdominal surgery.

Another, more rigorous systematic review was published in 2001.[22] It examined the literature pertaining to incentive spirometry (available through June 2000). Forty-six articles were identified that examined the effect of incentive spirometry or other forms of physiotherapy on the reduction of PPCs. Of these, 35 were excluded from the review due to various methodologic flaws, including inappropriate statistical analyses, invalid outcome measures, lack of documentation of compliance with the studied treatment, bias, and study designs that were unable to isolate the effect of incentive spirometry from other interventions. After application of the exclusion criteria, five randomized trials; three randomized, controlled trials; two case studies; and one crossover study remained. Cardiac and upper abdominal surgical patients comprised the study population in most of these reports. This study did not statistically pool results in a meta-analytic fashion.

In the group of four randomized trials that studied patients after cardiac surgery, no benefit could be demonstrated for incentive spirometry or deep-breathing exercises. One study compared each of these modalities in combination with early mobilization versus early mobilization alone and found no difference among the three groups. Another study suggested that incentive spirometry was inferior to continuous positive airway pressure (CPAP) and bi-level positive airway pressure (BiPAP) with respect to changes in vital capacity and forced expiratory volume in 1 second (FEV_1) in the early postoperative course.

In the four randomized trials that studied patients after abdominal surgery, only one study (involving patients undergoing both upper and lower abdominal surgery) showed a benefit of incentive spirometry in preventing PPCs, which were defined in the study as the development of three or more of the following: cough, phlegm, dyspnea, chest pain, temperature higher than 38°C, or pulse rate greater than 100 beats/min.[22] The benefit was statistically equivalent to that observed with deep-breathing exercises or intermittent positive-pressure ventilation. The frequency of PPCs with each of these interventions was 21%, 22%, 22%, respectively, compared with 48% in the no-treatment group. Remaining studies showed no benefit for incentive spirometry as compared with CPAP or positive expiratory pressure. According to this systematic review,[22] evidence does not support the use of incentive spirometry for decreasing the incidence of PPCs.

Similar conclusions were reached in the review of the subject by Pasquina and colleagues,[23] who in 2003 reviewed the data from 18 trials published from 1978 through 2003, in which various prophylactic methods were studied in patients who underwent cardiac surgery. Methods included incentive spirometry, chest physiotherapy, CPAP, and intermittent positive-pressure breathing. Only four studies used a nonintervention control group, and each used a different intervention; none of these four studies showed a significant treatment effect with respect to the end points of atelectasis, pneumonia, oxygenation, or pulmonary function.

RECENT PRIMARY STUDIES

Few relevant primary research articles have since been published on the subject. Westerdahl and coworkers[24] studied the effect of 4 days of hourly deep-breathing exercises on pulmonary function, atelectasis, fever, and length of ICU or hospital stay in 90 patients after coronary artery bypass grafting (CABG); all study patients underwent early mobilization and instructions on coughing techniques. Statistically significant reductions in atelectasis as quantified by spiral computed tomography on the fourth postoperative day were found (basal zone: $2.6\% \pm 2.2\%$ versus $4.7\% \pm 5.7\%$ [mean $\pm$ SD], $P = .045$; apical zone: $0.1\% \pm 0.2\%$ versus $0.3\% \pm 0.5\%$, $P = .01$), as were reductions in the decrement of postoperative forced vital capacity (FVC) (to $71\% \pm 12\%$ versus $64\% \pm 13\%$ of the preoperative values, $P = .01$) and FEV_1 (to $71\% \pm 11\%$ versus $65\% \pm 13\%$ of the preoperative values, $P = .01$). However, no differences in arterial O_2 or CO_2 tension, fever, or length of stay were observed.

Similarly, Mackay and associates[25] studied 56 patients undergoing abdominal surgery and randomized them to early mobilization alone or early mobilization with deep-breathing or coughing exercises. No difference in the frequency of PPCs was found between the groups: 14% in the control group and 17% in the treatment group (95% CI: -22% to 19%).

CONCLUSION AND RECOMMENDATIONS

There are few good data to support the use of incentive spirometry or deep-breathing exercises in the reduction of PPCs in cardiac or abdominal surgery patients. Results from existing systematic reviews and a meta-analysis are conflicting. However, given the relative ease, safety, and low cost of these two techniques, it is probably reasonable to recommend incentive spirometry or deep-breathing exercises postoperatively for patients after abdominal or cardiac surgery, because the potential benefits—although certainly not clear from the available evidence—likely outweigh the risks. Specific therapeutic regimens for these methods have not been standardized, although most studies have employed deep-breathing regimens of four or five times daily or 10 maximal breaths using an incentive spirometer hourly while awake.[21]

4. What is the optimal timing of preoperative smoking cessation so that postoperative pulmonary complications are minimized?

Search Date: January 2006

Search Strategy: *PubMed search, 1980 to 2006, for smoking postoperative pulmonary complications. Limits of English and human studies; 234 citations retrieved. Titles and abstracts scanned, with relevant citations selected. Bibliographies of all relevant citations reviewed.*

Smoking is considered to be a risk factor for the development of PPCs,[8] although the extent to which this is a primary effect or results from the coexistence of other smoking-related lung disease is debatable. It should be implicit that smoking cessation would reduce the frequency of postoperative pulmonary complications. This usually is true; however, there is some debate in the literature regarding the optimal timing of smoking cessation. Specifically, the notion that smoking cessation initiated within the 8 weeks immediately before surgery *increases* the risk of PPCs is addressed.

TO QUIT OR NOT TO QUIT?
The topic of smoking cessation and timing in relation to the prevention of pulmonary complications began to be studied by Warner and colleagues with retrospective and prospective studies published in 1984[26] and 1989,[27] respectively. In the initial retrospective study of 500 patients after CABG in 1984,[26] Warner defined a PPC as purulent sputum with an oral temperature higher than 38.3°C, secretions requiring inhalation therapy and additional chest physical therapy, bronchospasm requiring bronchodilators, pleural effusion or pneumothorax requiring drainage, or segmental pulmonary collapse. Smoking status was obtained through the medical history from the patient (and subject to recall bias). Patients were divided

into groups of smokers who never stopped, those who stopped less than 2 weeks before surgery, those who stopped 2 to 4 weeks before surgery, those who stopped 4 to 8 weeks before surgery, those who stopped more than 8 weeks before surgery, and lifelong nonsmokers. The investigators observed an overall complication rate of 11.4% for the nonsmoker group, compared with a rate of 39.0% for all other smoking groups in aggregate ($P < .001$). The difference in the rates of complications between current smokers and those who quit less than 8 weeks before surgery were statistically equivalent (48.4% versus 56.4%). This led the investigators to conclude that the benefit of smoking cessation in reducing PPCs could only be realized if patients quit 8 weeks or more before surgery. Warner and colleagues[27] subsequently published a second, prospective study in which 200 consecutive patients undergoing CABG were studied; the definition of a PPC was the same described previously, and current smoking status was verified biochemically. The overall complication rate was 18.7% (95% CI: 14% to 25%). In contrast to the prior study, there apparently was a significant *increase* in the rate of PPCs in patients who quit within the 8 weeks before surgery compared with current smokers (57.1% versus 33%). For those who quit more than 8 weeks and 6 months prior before surgery, the rates were 14.5% and 11.1%, respectively; for nonsmokers, the rate was 11.9%. Detailed statistics were not provided for each calculation, but P values are presumed to be less than .05 based on the Methods section of the article. In this study, bronchospasm requiring bronchodilators, secretion retention, and segmental lobe collapse were the most common complications (accounting for about 76% of all complications).

In 1998, Bluman and colleagues[28] published a prospective cohort study of 410 veterans undergoing noncardiac elective surgery that examined the relationship between preoperative smoking habits and PPCs. Smoking status was determined with a questionnaire, and subgroups were defined at the outset as current smokers if patients smoked with 2 weeks of their interview, past smokers if patients smoked more than 2 weeks before the interview, and nonsmokers. Definition of PPC was split into two groups: *major* (i.e., pulmonary infection seen on a chest radiograph, a temperature of more than 38.5°C and/or use of antibiotics, unexpected use of intravenous aminophylline or steroids to treat wheezing, reintubation, hospital readmission due to pneumonia, or death related to pulmonary disease) and *minor* (i.e., unexpected postoperative use of aerosol treatment or new or worsening atelectasis on the chest radiograph). The investigators found complication rates of 22.0%, 12.8%, and 4.9% among current smokers, past smokers, and never smokers, respectively; however, differences were only significant with respect to minor complications. In multivariate analysis, when controlling for type of anesthesia, the presence of an abnormal chest radiograph, history of COPD, educational level, and age, current smoking remained an independent predictor for the development of a PPC, with an odds ratio of 4.2 (95% CI: 1.2 to 14.8) compared with never smokers—a finding that was consistent with the results of prior studies. The study authors performed a subgroup analysis for the current smokers group, in which about 25% of the patients were able to reduce (but not eliminate, as in the study by Warner and coworkers[27]) their cigarette consumption for various lengths of time since learning of the need for surgery. After controlling for age, educational level, type of surgery, and COPD history, those who reduced their smoking for any length of time from 1 month or more before surgery to within 1 week of surgery had a relative risk of 6.7 (95% CI: 2.6 to 17.1) for developing a PPC compared with current smokers who did not attempt to cut down. This finding appears to corroborate the results of the 1989 study by Warner and coworkers,[27] particularly considering that most complications in both studies resulting in statistically significant differences were attributed to bronchospasm or atelectasis.

COUNTERARGUMENTS TO THE 8-WEEK CUTOFF

In 2001, Nakagawa and colleagues[29] conducted a retrospective cohort study of 288 consecutive patients undergoing pulmonary surgery (i.e., tumor enucleation, wedge resection, lobectomy, or pneumonectomy). Smoking status was determined by questionnaire, and patients were categorized into the following groups: current smoker if the patient had smoked within 2 weeks before surgery, recent smoker if the patient abstained

2 to 4 weeks before surgery, ex-smoker if the patient abstained for more than 4 weeks before surgery, and never smoker. The study authors used a comprehensive definition of a PPC, which included pneumonia (based on radiography, temperature, white blood cell count, culture, or antibiotic use); atelectasis prompting bronchoscopy; a $PaCO_2$ higher than 50 mm Hg, FIO_2 higher than 60%, or alveolar-arterial (A-a) gradient greater than 300 mm Hg at 24 hours after surgery; bronchopleural fistula; various types of pleural pathology; pulmonary embolism; and mechanical ventilation for more than 72 hours for any reason. Bronchospasm or radiographic atelectasis alone was not included. The investigators found rates of PPCs of 43.2% for current smokers ($P < .05$ for comparison versus never smokers; OR = 2.4; 95% CI: 1.11 to 5.27), 53.8% for recent smokers ($P < .05$ for comparison versus never smokers; OR = 3.7; 95% CI: 1.15 to 11.95), 34.7% for ex-smokers, and 23.9% for never smokers. The current smokers had statistically equivalent rates compared with recent smokers. As indicated by the aforementioned odds ratios for the comparisons, in univariate analysis, current smoking and recent smoking as defined by the study authors remained significant predictors of PPCs, along with age, FEV_1/FVC less than 70%, duration of surgery longer than 30 minutes, and male gender. The investigators calculated "moving averages" of the incidence of PPCs based on the length of patients' smoke-free periods (i.e., 0 to 3 weeks preoperatively, 1 to 4 weeks preoperatively, 2 to 5 weeks preoperatively, and so on up to 12 to 15 weeks preoperatively). They found that the average incidence of PPCs did not begin to decrease until patients were abstinent 5 to 8 weeks before surgery or longer. However, in a multivariate analysis that controlled for the other predictors in a univariate analysis of age, gender, pulmonary function, and duration of surgery, neither current (OR = 2.09; 95% CI: 0.83 to 5.25) nor recent (OR = 2.44; 95% CI: 0.67 to 8.89) smoking status remained independent predictors of PPCs.

Barrera and associates[30] sought to further clarify the issue of optimal timing of smoking cessation given the suggestion from the previous data that there may be a paradoxical increase in the risk for PPCs when the period of smoking cessation is less than 2 months.

Like Nakagawa and colleagues,[29] Barrera and associates[30] studied a group of lung cancer patients undergoing lung resection, but they did so prospectively. The sample size was 300 patients. The definition of groups studied were current smokers (4% of the study population); recent quitters, who stopped smoking less than 2 months before surgery (13% of the study population); past quitters, who stopped smoking more than 2 months before surgery; and nonsmokers. A PPC was defined as any of the following: respiratory failure requiring ICU admission or intubation, pneumonia, atelectasis requiring bronchoscopy, pulmonary embolism, or the need for supplemental oxygen at discharge. Smoking status was obtained through the patient's history only and not chemically confirmed. The study authors found complication rates of 23% for current smokers and for recent quitters, 19% for past quitters, and 8% for nonsmokers. The overall complication rate for all smoking groups in aggregate was 19%, which was significantly different from the nonsmoking group ($P = .03$), but there were no significant differences among the subcategories of smokers, including current smokers versus recent quitters. The study authors conclude that it was safe to quit smoking within 2 months of surgery.

CONCLUSION AND RECOMMENDATIONS

In summary, two retrospective studies[26,29] of different patient populations suggest that current smokers and those who have quit within the preceding 2 months share an equivalent, elevated risk for PPCs (one study included bronchospasm and atelectasis as complications, but the other did not). Two other studies,[27,28] also of different populations, suggest an *increased* risk for patients who quit within 2 months before surgery[27] or reduce their smoking within 1 month before surgery[28] (both studies included bronchospasm and atelectasis as PPCs). A prospective study[30] of patients undergoing thoracotomy did *not* reveal an increased risk for quitters in the 2 months before surgery, although the power to detect a difference may have been hindered by the relatively small size of the current smoker group. This study did not include nonsignificant atelectasis or bronchospasm as end points.

In light of the available data, it seems reasonable to recommend that for optimal risk reduction, patients should attempt to quit smoking at least 2 months before surgery. Studies are not in agreement regarding the possible paradoxical increase in risk seen in those who quit (or cut down) within 2 months before surgery; both studies[27,28] that claim this phenomenon included more minor complications, such as radiographic atelectasis and bronchospasm. However, the study by Barrera and colleagues[30] is reassuring about this matter. Proposed mechanisms by which quitting or cutting down closer to surgery may increase the risk relative for active smokers include increased mucus production combined with a reduction in irritant-induced cough[27] and nicotine withdrawal.[30] One reviewer commented that the long-term benefits of smoking cessation—regardless of timing—are likely to outweigh the potential risks incurred if done within 2 months of surgery. More studies are needed to clarify the optimal timing of smoking cessation before surgery.

5. Is continuous positive airway pressure or bi-level positive airway pressure effective as a prophylactic intervention to reduce the incidence of postoperative pulmonary complications?

Search Date: January 2006

Search Strategy: PubMed search, 1980 to 2006, for ("positive pressure" OR "positive airway pressure" OR CPAP OR BiPAP) AND (postoperative OR post-operative OR peri-operative OR perioperative) AND (complications OR pneumonia OR atelectasis OR hypoxia OR hypoxemia OR oxygenation OR intubation OR re-intubation OR "respiratory failure" OR "pulmonary function" OR "gas exchange"). Limits of English and human studies; 477 citations retrieved. Titles and abstracts scanned, with relevant citations selected. Bibliographies of all relevant citations reviewed.

Patients undergoing surgery experience disruptions in normal pulmonary physiology that presumably underlie the development of postoperative pulmonary complications. Postoperative derangements in diaphragmatic and chest wall mechanics lead to alterations in airflow and lung volumes that can facilitate the development of atelectasis, pneumonia, ventilation-perfusion mismatch, hypoxemia or hypercarbia, and ultimately, frank respiratory failure. The location of the surgical site in relation to the diaphragm and chest wall undoubtedly influences the degree to which these derangements occur in a patient.

CPAP and BiPAP are modes of noninvasive ventilatory support that have been shown to be beneficial in treating patients with obstructive sleep apnea, those with obesity-hypoventilation syndrome, and those with acute exacerbations of heart failure and chronic obstructive pulmonary disease. The theory of using these modes of therapy as *prophylaxis* in postoperative patients is appealing; both methods use externally applied positive pressure to "splint" open the airways, theoretically promoting ventilation of alveoli and preventing their collapse at end-expiration. Given the higher risk incurred by patients undergoing thoracic or upper abdominal procedures, most of the literature studying prophylactic CPAP or BiPAP has focused on these patient populations.

CONTINUOUS POSITIVE AIRWAY PRESSURE AND UPPER ABDOMINAL SURGERY

Four studies[31-34] have examined the effect of prophylactic CPAP given in the immediate postoperative period on the incidence of PPCs among patients undergoing upper abdominal surgery. Stock and coworkers[31] randomized 65 patients to intermittent CPAP at 7.5 cm H_2O, incentive spirometry, or deep-breathing exercises; each group was treated for 15 minutes every 2 hours while awake, starting 4 hours after surgery and continuing through the third postoperative day. The study authors found CPAP increased the rate of recovery of functional residual capacity (FRC) on the second and third postoperative day, but there were no statistically significant differences in the rates of atelectasis. The overall rate of pneumonia among all cohorts was quite low, with only two patients in the entire study population developing this complication.

Ricksten and associates[32] randomized 50 patients undergoing elective upper abdominal surgery (excluding patients with clinical or radiographic signs of pulmonary vascular congestion) to CPAP at 10 to 15 cm H_2O, deep-breathing exercises with the aid of an exercising device, or positive expiratory pressure (PEP) by mask; each group was treated for 30 breaths every 1 hour while awake, starting 1 hour after surgery and continuing through the third postoperative day. In all groups the A-a O_2 difference increased postoperatively, but by the third postoperative day, the CPAP and PEP groups had improved A-a O_2 difference, arterial oxygen saturation, and FVC compared with the deep-breathing group. On postoperative day 3, the PEP and CPAP groups had a reduced incidence of atelectatic consolidation as seen on chest radiographs compared with the deep-breathing group (0%, 8%, and 40%, respectively; $P < .001$ for PEP versus deep breathing, $P < .05$ for CPAP versus deep breathing).

Denehy and colleagues[33] randomized 58 patients undergoing elective upper abdominal surgery to intermittent CPAP at 10 cm H_2O for 15 minutes four times daily with standard physiotherapy, intermittent CPAP at 10 cm H_2O for 30 minutes four times daily with standard physiotherapy, or standard physiotherapy alone. Physiotherapy included preoperative education and twice-daily sessions postoperatively lasting for 10 minutes and consisting of deep breathing, forced expiration, and coughing. Treatment was given through the third postoperative day. Patients with a preoperative FEV_1 less than 50% of predicted were excluded from the study. The outcomes in this study included FRC, vital capacity (VC), oxygen saturation, length of stay, and incidence of PPCs (defined as temperature higher than 38°C for more than 1 day with at least moderate collapse or consolidation of one lung base seen on the radiograph and at least one of the following: elevated white blood cell count, change in sputum or positive sputum culture with a potential pathogen, or escalation in antibiotic therapy). The investigators observed no significant differences among treatment groups with respect to all outcomes measured. The overall incidence of PPCs as defined previously was 22%, 11%, and 6% in the control, 15-minute CPAP, and 30-minute CPAP groups, respectively.

Böhner and coworkers[34] randomized 204 patients undergoing midline laparotomies for vascular surgery to continuous CPAP with supplemental O_2 at 10 cm H_2O for at least 12 hours after admission to the surgical ICU or to supplemental O_2 alone; oxygen was titrated to an arterial saturation of more than 95%. The population studied had an approximately 30% prevalence of pulmonary disease at baseline. The study authors found a 5% rate of "severe oxygenation disturbance" (defined as $Po_2 < 70$, despite an $Fio_2 \geq 70\%$) in the CPAP group versus a 16.2% in the control group ($P = .012$). However, there were no significant differences between groups with respect to rates of pneumonia, reintubation, cardiac arrest, death, length of ICU stay, or readmission to the ICU.

In summary, the evidence is conflicting regarding the benefit of CPAP over more conventional chest physiotherapy; no studies in this population are available comparing CPAP with no treatment. Given on an hourly[32] or continuous[34] basis, somewhat beneficial effects on arterial O_2 tension[32,34] and radiographic atelectasis may exist,[32] whereas no benefits were observed with a four-times daily regimen in a study with a more clinically oriented definition of a postoperative pulmonary complication.[33] No studies regarding the cost-effectiveness of this relatively expensive modality exist. Based on these data, routine prophylactic use of CPAP cannot be recommended in patients undergoing upper abdominal surgery.

CONTINUOUS POSITIVE AIRWAY PRESSURE AND THORACIC SURGERY

With respect to patients undergoing thoracic surgery, three randomized trials[35-37] have examined the effect of prophylactic CPAP administered in the immediate postoperative period on the incidence of PPCs. Stock and associates[35] randomized 38 patients undergoing median sternotomy to intermittent CPAP at 7.5 cm H_2O, incentive spirometry, or cough or deep-breathing exercises. All treatments were given for 15 minutes every 2 hours for 72 hours after extubation. No differences were observed among treatments groups with respect to changes in pulmonary function tests, chest radiograph evidence of atelectasis, physical examination findings, or body temperature. Only 1 of the 38 patients developed pneumonia according to the study authors' criteria.

Pinilla and colleagues[36] randomized 58 patients with normal FEV_1/FVC ratios undergoing coronary artery bypass surgery to continuous mask CPAP for 12 hours at 7.5 cm H_2O or higher pressure or to oxygen therapy;

both groups received routine chest physiotherapy (not defined). The PaO_2/FIO_2 ratio was modestly improved in the CPAP group compared with the control group from 30 minutes after extubation through 24 hours after extubation (234 ± 57 versus 212 ± 56; $P < .01$ for the latter time point), but the difference disappeared after 24 hours. No significant differences between groups were observed with respect to incidence of radiographic atelectasis, consolidation, pulmonary edema, or frequency of positive sputum cultures.

Jousela and coworkers[37] randomized 30 patients (excluding those with pulmonary function test results less than 80% of predicted values) undergoing CABG to continuous CPAP at 10 cm H_2O with an FIO_2 of 30% or oxygen alone. Treatment was given for 12 hours after extubation. Both groups received conservative pulmonary therapy (not defined). In those treated with CPAP, the PaO_2 value decreased less after extubation at the end of the intervention period. The PaO_2/FIO_2 ratio increased during CPAP treatment but decreased in the control group during the same period. However, these differences were not observed by the second postoperative morning. Radiographic evidence of atelectasis was seen with equal frequency on the second postoperative day in both groups.

Olsén and associates[38] studied a "hybrid" population presumably at an even higher risk for PPCs: patients undergoing thoracoabdominal resection of the esophagus. In this approach, midline abdominal and right thoracotomy incisions were performed in each patient. Seventy patients were randomized to intermittent CPAP at 5 to 10 cm H_2O for 30 minutes at a time or inspiratory resistance–positive expiratory pressure (IR-PEP) for 30 breaths; treatments were given every 2 hours for at least 3 days while in the ICU. After being transferred to the surgical ward, all patients were converted to IR-PEP. All patients underwent early mobilization and chest physiotherapy (not defined). Roughly 15% of patients in both groups were classified as having pulmonary disease at baseline. The study authors observed a significant difference in the study's primary end point of need for reintubation and prolonged mechanical ventilation: 2.9% in the CPAP group versus 19.4% in the IR-PEP group ($P < .05$). There were no differences in mortality or length of ICU or hospital stay between groups.

Similarly, Kindgen-Milles and colleagues[39] examined the effect of prophylactic continuous nasal CPAP compared with intermittent mask CPAP on pulmonary complications in patients undergoing thoracoabdominal aortic surgery. Each group contained 25 patients. The treatment group received continuous nasal CPAP at 10 cm H_2O for 12 to 24 hours, beginning immediately after extubation. The control group received intermittent mask CPAP at 10 cm H_2O every 4 hours for 10 minutes for 12 to 24 hours. Both groups received supplemental oxygenation, chest physical therapy, intravenous mucolytics, and antibiotic prophylaxis with ampicillin or sulbactam. The overall rate of PPCs (defined as pneumonia, atelectasis, Pa_{O_2}/F_{IO_2} ratio < 100, or reintubation) was 28% for the treatment group and 96% for the control group ($P = .019$). Total hospital length of stay was significantly reduced in the treatment group (22 ± 2 versus 34 ± 5 days; $P = .048$).

In summary, for patients undergoing abdominal surgery, the weight of evidence does not support the routine use of prophylactic CPAP for the prevention of postoperative pulmonary complications. Some studies[37,37] suggest a transient benefit with respect to oxygenation in the immediate postoperative period, but no sustained benefits have been demonstrated after CPAP therapy has been terminated. Limited data suggest CPAP may reduce the incidence of reintubation[38,39] and overall pulmonary complications and reduce the length of stay[39] after combined thoracoabdominal procedures. However, the interventions and controls used in these two studies were not equivalent, the patient populations were different, and neither study employed a no-treatment arm. These data are intriguing, but additional confirmatory studies are needed before this approach can be recommended for widespread use.

BI-LEVEL POSITIVE AIRWAY PRESSURE

Three randomized controlled trials are identified that examine the use of prophylactic BiPAP.[40-43] The first two[40,41] are based on otherwise healthy, obese patients submitted for bariatric surgery, whereas the third[42] is based on a population of patients undergoing CABG.

Joris and coworkers[40] randomized 33 obese but otherwise healthy patients undergoing open gastroplasty to oxygen by face mask, BiPAP at a pressure setting of 8/4 cm H_2O, or BiPAP at 12/4 cm H_2O administered for 24 hours postoperatively; all groups received identical regimens of incentive spirometry and chest physiotherapy. Consistent with the findings of other studies documenting decline in pulmonary function parameters postoperatively, these studies found a decrease in FVC, FEV_1, peak expiratory flow rate (PEFR), and oxygenation saturation in all three groups in the immediate postoperative period. However, BiPAP at a setting of 12/4 cm H_2O (but not 8/4 cm H_2O) resulted in an attenuation of the drop in FVC, FEV_1, and arterial oxygen saturation, an effect that persisted 2 days after cessation of therapy. BiPAP at a setting of 8/4 cm H_2O improved oxygen saturation but had no effect on pulmonary function. This study did not investigate whether these physiologic effects were translated into a reduced rate of more clinically defined pulmonary complications.

Ebeo and associates[41] randomized 27 obese patients undergoing Roux-en-Y gastric bypass surgery to BiPAP at 12/4 cm H_2O in combination with incentive spirometry for 12 to 24 hours or to incentive spirometry alone. As in the previously described study, these investigators also observed a drop in pulmonary function indices and oxygen saturation postoperatively that was attenuated by the use of BiPAP. No differences in length of stay or rates of cardiopulmonary complications (zero in both groups) were observed. In the BiPAP treatment group, there was a 29% dropout rate due to an inability to tolerate the intervention for at least 12 hours.

In a series of CABG patients, Matte and colleagues[42] randomized 96 patients to CPAP at 5 cm H_2O, BiPAP at 12/5 cm H_2O, or incentive spirometry; all groups received the same chest physiotherapy. Treatments in the CPAP and BiPAP groups were given for 1 of every 3 hours on the first postoperative day. Both CPAP and BiPAP attenuated the drop seen in VC and FEV_1 postoperatively. Both CPAP and BiPAP reduced venous admixture, presumably by improvements in intrapulmonary shunting. The study authors observed a 15% rate of atelectasis in the CPAP and BiPAP groups compared with 30% in the incentive spirometry group; however, no statistics were provided in the article, suggesting this was not a statistically significant result.

In summary, the total body of literature examining prophylactic BiPAP is quite limited, and studies are generally small. In the types of populations studied, a physiologic benefit from a pulmonary function perspective may be gained, along with marginal increases in arterial saturation. However, no studies have convincingly showed that any of these potential benefits translate into reduction of mortality, length of hospital stay, pneumonia, atelectasis, or other relevant effects. Until more data are available, especially considering the cost of the intervention, routine use of prophylactic BiPAP cannot be recommended.

REFERENCES

1. Smetana GW: Preoperative pulmonary evaluation. N Engl J Med 1999;340:937-943. Ⓥ

2. Smetana GW, Lawrence VA, Cornell JE:. Preoperative pulmonary risk stratification for noncardiothoracic surgery: Systematic review for the American College of Physicians. Ann Intern Med 2006;144:581-595. Ⓘ

3. McAlister FA, Bertsch K, Man J, Jacka M: Incidence of and risk factors for pulmonary complications after nonthoracic surgery. Am J Respir Crit Care Med 2005; 171:514-517. Ⓘ

4. Fleishmann KE, Goldman L, Young B, Lee TH: Association between cardiac and noncardiac complications in patients undergoing noncardiac surgery: Outcomes and effects on length of stay. Am J Med; 2003 115: 515-520. Ⓘ

5. Arolzullah AM, Daley J, Henderson WG, Khuri SF: Multifactorial risk index for predicting postoperative respiratory failure in men after major noncardiac surgery. Ann Surg 2000;2:242-253. Ⓘ

6. Arozullah AM, Shukri SF, Henderson WG, Delay J: Development and validation of a multifactorial risk index for predicting postoperative pneumonia after major noncardiac surgery. Ann Intern Med 2001; 135:847-857. Ⓘ

7. Chung F, Mezei G, Tong D: Adverse events in ambulatory surgery. A comparison between elderly and younger patients. Can J Anesth 1999;46:309-321. Ⓘ

8. Morres L: Smoking and pulmonary and cardiovascular complications: An evidence-based review of the recent literature. Clin Chest Med 2000;21:139-146. Ⓥ

9. Moller A, Villebro N, Pedersen T: Interventions for preoperative smoking cessation. Cochrane Database Syst Rev 2005;(3):CD002294. (II)

10. Moller A, Villebro N, Pederson T, Tonnesen H: Effect of preoperative smoking intervention on postoperative complications: A randomized controlled trial. Lancet 2002;359:114-117. (II)

11. Sorensen LT, Jorgensen T: Short-term pre-operative smoking cessation intervention does not affect postoperative complications in colorectal surgery: A randomized trial. Colorectal Dis 2003;5:347-352. (II)

12. Moller A, Pederen T, Villebro N, Munksgard A: Effect of smoking on early complications after elective orthopedic surgery. J Bone Joint Surg Br 2003;85:178-181. (III)

13. Yamashita S, Yamaguchi H, Sakaguchi M, et al: Effect of smoking on intraoperative sputum and postoperative pulmonary complication in minor surgical patients. Respir Med 2004;98:760-766. (III)

14. Warner DO, Warner MA, Barnes RD, et al: Perioperative respiratory complications in patients with asthma. Anesthesiology 1996;85:460-467. (III)

15. Gupta RM, Parvizi J, Hanssen AD, Gay PC: Postoperative complications in patients with obstructive sleep apnea syndrome undergoing hip or knee replacement: A case-control study. Mayo Clin Proc 2001;76:897-905. (III)

16. Reilly DF, McNeely MJ, Doerner D, et al: Self-reported exercise tolerance and the risk of serious perioperative complications Arch Intern Med 1999;159:2185-2192. (III)

17. Girish M, Trayner E, Dammann O, et al: Symptom-limited stair climbing as a predictor of postoperative cardiopulmonary complications after high-risk surgery. Chest 2001;120:1147-1151. (III)

18. Berg H, Roed J, Viby-Mogensen J, et al: Residual neuromuscular block is a risk factor for postoperative pulmonary complications. A prospective randomized, and blinded study of postoperative pulmonary complications after atracurium, vecuronium, and pancuronium. Acta Anaesthesiol Scand 1997;41:1095-1103. (II)

19. Rodgers A, Walker N, Schug S, et al: Reduction of postoperative mortality and morbidity with epidural or spinal anaesthesia: Results from overview of randomized trials. BMJ 2000;321:1-12. (I)

20. Qaseem A, Snow V, Fitterman N, et al, for the Clinical Efficacy Subcommittee of the American College of Physicians: Risk Assessment for and strategies to reduce perioperative pulmonary complications for patients undergoing noncardiothoracic surgery: A guideline from the American College of Physicians. Ann Intern Med 2006;144:575-580. **I**

21. Thomas JA, McIntosh JM: Are incentive spirometry, intermittent positive pressure breathing, and deep breathing exercises effective in the prevention of postoperative pulmonary complications after upper abdominal surgery? A systematic overview and meta-analysis. Phys Ther 1994;74:8-15. **I**

22. Overend TJ, Anderson CM, Lucy SD, et al: The effect of incentive spirometry on postoperative pulmonary complications: A systematic review. Chest 2001; 120:971-978. **I**

23. Pasquina P, Tramer MR, Walder B: Prophylactic respiratory physiotherapy after cardiac surgery: Systematic review. BMJ 2003;327:1379-1384. **I**

24. Westerdahl E, Lindmark B, Eriksson T, et al: Deep-breathing exercises reduce atelectasis and improve pulmonary function after coronary artery bypass surgery. Chest 2005;128:3482-3488. **II**

25. Mackay MR, Ellis E, Johnston C: Randomised clinical trial of physiotherapy after open abdominal surgery in high risk patients. Aust J Physiother 2005;51: 151-159. **II**

26. Warner MA, Divertie MB, Tinker JH: Preoperative cessation of smoking and pulmonary complications in coronary artery bypass patients. Anesthesiology 1984;60:380-383. **III**

27. Warner MA, Offord KP, Warner ME, et al: Role of preoperative cessation of smoking and other factors in postoperative pulmonary complications: A blinded prospective study of coronary artery bypass patients. Mayo Clinic Proc 1989;64:609-711. **III**

28. Bluman LG, Mosca L, Newman N, Simon DG: Preoperative smoking habits and postoperative pulmonary complications. Chest 1998;113:883-889. **III**

29. Nakagawa M, Tanaka H, Tsukuma H, Kishi Y: Relationship between the duration of the preoperative smoke-free period and the incidence of postoperative pulmonary complications after pulmonary surgery. Chest 2001;120:705-710. **III**

30. Barrera R, Shi W, Amar D, et al: Smoking and timing of cessation: Impact on pulmonary complications after thoracotomy. Chest 2005;127:1977-1983. **III**

31. Stock MC, Downs JB, Gauer PK, et al: Prevention of postoperative pulmonary complications with CPAP, incentive spirometry, and conservative therapy. Chest 1985;87:151-157. **II**

32. Ricksten SE, Bengtsson A, Soderberg C, et al: Effects of periodic positive airway pressure by mask on postoperative pulmonary function. Chest 1986;89:774-781. **II**

33. Denehy L, Carroll S, Ntoumenopoulos G, Jenkins S: A randomized controlled trial comparing periodic mask CPAP with physiotherapy after abdominal surgery. Physiother Res Int 2001;6:236-250. **II**

34. Böhner H, Kindgen-Milles D, Grust A, et al: Prophylactic nasal continuous positive airway pressure after major vascular surgery: Results of a prospective randomized trial. Langenbecks Arch Surg 2002;387:21-26. **II**

35. Stock MC, Down JB, Cooper RB, et al: Comparison of continuous positive airway pressure, incentive spirometry, and conservative therapy after cardiac operations. Crit Care Med 1984;12:969-972. **II**

36. Pinilla JC, Oleniuk FH, Tan L, et al: Use of a nasal continuous positive airway pressure mask in the treatment of postoperative atelectasis in aortocoronary bypass surgery. Crit Care Med 1990;18:836-840. **II**

37. Jousela I, Rasanen J, Verkkala K, et al: Continuous positive airway pressure by mask in patients after coronary surgery. Acta Anaesthesiol Scand 1994;38:311-316. **II**

38. Fagevik Olsen MF, Wennberg E, Johnsson E, et al: Randomized clinical study of the prevention of pulmonary complications after thoracoabdominal resection by two different breathing techniques. Br J Surg 2002;89: 1228-1234. **II**

39. Kindgen-Milles D, Muller E, Buhl R, et al: Nasal-continuous positive airway pressure reduces pulmonary morbidity and length of hospital stay following thoracoabdominal aortic surgery. Chest 2005;128:821-828. **II**

40. Joris JL, Sottiaux TM, Chiche JD, et al: Effect of bi-level positive airway pressure (BiPAP) nasal ventilation on the postoperative pulmonary restrictive syndrome in obese patients undergoing gastroplasty. Chest 1997;111:665-670. **II**

41. Ebeo CT, Benotti PN, Byrd RP Jr, et al: The effect of bi-level positive airway pressure on postoperative

pulmonary function following gastric surgery for obesity. Respir Med 2002;96:672-676. **II**

42. Matte P, Jacquet L, Van Dyck M, Goenen M: Effects of conventional physiotherapy, continuous positive airway pressure and non-invasive ventilatory support with bilevel positive airway pressure after coronary artery bypass grafting. Acta Anaesthesiol Scand 2000;44:75-81. **II**

43. Steinberg DI: Review: Surgical site, advanced age, and comorbid conditions increase risk for postoperative pulmonary complications. ACP J Club 2006;145:37. **II**

Preoperative Cardiovascular Risk Assessment

Atif Qasim and David Horowitz

1. Does perioperative beta blockade reduce morbidity or mortality rates for patients undergoing noncardiac surgery?

Search Date: March 2006

Search Strategy: *PubMed, search for "beta blocker AND noncardiac surgery" (86 items, 41 when the term "mortality" was included), "preoperative beta blockers" (567 items), and "beta blocker, surgery AND mortality OR morbidity" (701 items). Titles and abstracts were reviewed; relevant bibliographies were scanned and related article searches were performed when applicable. ACC/AHA guidelines were also scanned for references.*

Whether to administer perioperative beta blockers to patients undergoing noncardiac surgery is one of the most common decisions the medical consultant has to make. Perioperative beta blockers have been considered an effective strategy to reduce perioperative cardiac events, and clinical criteria and guidelines for their use have enjoyed wide acceptance by clinicians. However, several recent meta-analyses indicate that perioperative beta blockers may not be beneficial and may be harmful in certain patient groups. Because of this, the American College of Cardiology/American Heart Association (ACC/AHA) has put forth new guidelines to better delineate the use of perioperative beta blockers.[1] Ultimately, the use of beta blockers depends on clinicians being familiar with the literature and making patient-specific risk-benefit assessments.

RANDOMIZED CONTROLLED TRIALS

A randomized, controlled trial by Stone and colleagues[2] of 128 patients was one of the first to recognize an increased risk of myocardial ischemia in patients with uncontrolled hypertension undergoing surgery. This risk was significantly reduced by giving atenolol compared with no treatment for blood pressure. Eleven of 39 untreated hypertensive patients had electrocardiographic evidence of ischemia compared with none of the 44 given atenolol, 30 of whom were given the drug acutely on the morning of surgery. In 1995, a larger, prospective, case-control study was published by Yeager and coworkers[3], and it suggested a 50% reduction ($P = .03$) of perioperative myocardial infarction (MI) with preoperative or intraoperative beta blocker use.

The first blinded, randomized study was performed by Mangano and colleagues[4] in 1996; in it, 200 San Francisco Veterans Administration (VA) patients who had known coronary artery disease (CAD) or were at high risk for CAD were given placebo or intravenous atenolol 30 minutes before surgery and then orally postoperatively for up to 7 days.[4] Twenty-three percent of patients were on beta blockers before surgery, and approximately 15.5% continued on atenolol after surgery during a follow-up of 2 years. Only six patients died before discharge, and there was no difference found between groups in 30-day mortality or morbidity rates. Overall mortality, however, was less in the atenolol group at follow-up starting at 6 months (1% versus 10% in the placebo arm; $P < .001$). Although there was no difference in the rate of death between both groups after 8 months, this initial difference over the first 6 to 8 months persisted until the 2-year end point of the study, ultimately translating into a mortality difference of 9% versus 21% in favor of the atenolol arm (number needed to treat [NNT] = 8.3; $P = .019$). Cardiac events in the first 6 months were also greater in the placebo group and persisted 2 years after surgery. Limitations of the study included the fact that more patients in the placebo group were on calcium channel blockers postoperatively and that more in the atenolol group were taking beta blockers and angiotensin-converting enzyme (ACE) inhibitors after discharge.

Devereaux and associates[11] point out that the Mangano trial was not an intention-to-treat analysis because six deaths in the study arm were excluded, and they conclude that the reduction in mortality due to atenolol is no longer significant when these deaths are included. Nevertheless, a follow-up study by Wallace and colleagues[5] looked at postoperative ischemia in this same population (diagnosed by electrocardiographic [ECG] changes and cardiac enzymes) and found the incidence of MI was reduced with atenolol, with an effect seen as early as 2 days postoperatively (17% atenolol-arm patients versus 34% placebo-arm patients; $P = .008$).

Poldermans and colleagues[6] subsequently published a randomized (although not blinded) multicenter study of 112 high-risk patients who had positive dobutamine stress test results and were scheduled to undergo elective abdominal aortic aneurysm (AAA) or vascular surgery. Patients were assigned to standard care or bisoprolol given orally at least 1 week (but an average of 37 days) before surgery, with a target heart rate of less than 60 beats/min. Patients continued this regimen postoperatively for 1 month. Intravenous metoprolol could be used in the bisoprolol group as needed to keep the heart rate less than 80 beats/min in the postoperative setting. The study authors found a reduced incidence of perioperative cardiac death (17% versus 2%; $P < .02$) and nonfatal MI (17% versus 0%; $P < .001$), and they found no significant adverse events from beta blocker use. They excluded those already taking beta blockers long term and those with severe wall motion abnormalities seen on echocardiography. Because there were no noncardiac causes of deaths in this period, all-cause mortality was not evaluated. A follow-up study over a mean of 22 months using the same population did, however, find a difference between cardiac events of 12% versus 32% ($P = .025$), with an odds ratio for cardiac death and MI of 0.30 (95% CI: 0.11 to 0.83) favoring the bisoprolol arm.[7] Overall mortality was not discussed.

No other randomized, controlled studies have data specifically on mortality for preoperative beta blocker use. A review by Auerbach and Goldman[8] highlights an additional two randomized, controlled studies that gave beta blockers immediately postoperatively. Raby and coworkers[9] looked at 26 vascular surgery patients with preoperative ischemia given esmolol for 48 hours postoperatively and found a suggestion of reduction in postoperative ischemia (33% versus 73% in the control arm; $P < .05$). Similarly, Urban and associates[10] looked at 120 patients undergoing elective knee arthroplasty, who were given esmolol within 1 hour after surgery, followed by oral metoprolol titrated to a heart rate of less than 80 beats/min for 48 hours and continued until discharge. In contrast to previous studies, they were unable to demonstrate a difference between the control and beta blocker groups of postoperative MI ($P = .35$) or cardiac morbidity ($P = .51$) as evidence by ECG changes, elevated cardiac enzymes, chest pain, or heart failure. However, about one third of the control patients were treated with other beta blockers postoperatively to maintain heart rate and blood pressure. Immediate postoperative ischemia, as evidenced by ECG findings, appeared to be significantly decreased initially postoperatively ($P = .04$), but this was not the case after 2 days ($P = .135$). Both studies were likely underpowered to detect significant differences between groups.

META-ANALYSES

Several meta-analyses have been published within the past year to help answer this question. Although they differ in the trials that they include, all are unable to demonstrate a reduction on mortality. Devereaux and associates[11] looked at 22 trials of perioperative beta blocker use and could not determine the effect of perioperative beta blocker use on all-cause mortality. Wide confidence intervals include the possibility that perioperative beta blockers could increase all-cause mortality. There was, however, a clear and statistically significant risk of hypotension and bradycardia requiring treatment[11] (Table 4-1). This meta-analysis included data for patients at all levels of cardiac risk, and it leaves open the question of whether beta blockers may benefit only high-risk patients. Consistent with this possibility is the finding from a retrospective cohort study of more than 100,000 patients that beta blockers reduced risk of in-hospital death among high-risk patients, but not those at low risk.[12]

Another meta-analysis by McGory and associates[13] took a stricter approach, looking at only eight trials, of which six were randomized, controlled trials. They found no reduction in overall mortality (relative risk [RR] = 0.52; 95% CI: 0.20 to 1.35) but did find a reduction in cardiac

Table 4-1. Composite Data on Perioperative Cardiovascular Events and Symptomatic Bradycardia: Perioperative Beta Blockers versus Placebo or Usual Care (Control) for Noncardiac Surgery at 30 Days

Outcomes	No. of Trials (N)	Weighted Event Rates		RRR (95% CI)	NNT (95% CI)
		Beta Blockers	Control		
All-cause death	4 (907)	2.4%	4.2%	44% (−131 to 86)	NS
CV death	4 (907)	1.2%	2.9%	60% (−15 to 86)	NS
Nonfatal MI	6 (853)	3.4%	9.0%	62% (−29 to 89)	NS
Nonfatal cardiac arrest	2 (299)	1.6%	3.3%	50% (−129 to 89)	NS
				RRI (95% CI)	NNH (95% CI)
CHF	5 (861)	5.4%	3.4%	54% (−17 to 187)	NS
Nonfatal stroke	1 (200)	4.0%	1.0%	308% (−54 to 3487)	NS
Hypotension needing treatment	10 (1712)	26%	20%	27% (4 to 56)	19 (9 to 24)
Bradycardia needing treatment	9 (1196)	12%	5.4%	127% (53 to 236)	15 (8 to 35)

CHF, congestive heart failure; CI, confidence interval; CV, cardiovascular; MI, myocardial infarction; NNH, number needed to harm; NNT, number needed to treat; NS, not significant; RRI, relative risk increase; RRR, relative risk reduction.
Adapted from Kalra S, Kitchens J. Review: evidence of benefit for perioperative beta-blockers in noncardiac surgery is unreliable. ACP J Club 2006;144:17.

mortality (RR = 0.25; 95% CI: 0.07 to 0.87), as well as MI and ischemia. Stevens and colleagues[14] looked at 11 trials, including nonblinded studies, in which beta blockers were used perioperatively and found a benefit for high-risk patients (NNT = 8 for perioperative ischemia prevention; NNT = 23 for MI prevention), but their results were not significant with elimination of the two most positive trials. Schouten and colleagues[15] looked at 15 studies that included 1077 patients. They complement the findings by McGory but do not remark on reduction in overall mortality.

AHA GUIDELINES

Until this past year, ACC/AHA recommendations[1] were primarily still based on the observations by Mangano and Poldermans. The additional information from several meta-analyses mentioned previously is reflected in the latest ACC/AHA guidelines,[16] which cite lack of power in past randomized, controlled trials and the lack of evidence in low- and intermediate-risk populations. The language used in their newer recommendation is weaker and leaves more room for clinicians' interpretations. Beta blockers are considered class I (see Chapter 1, Table 1-3) in the latest guidelines for those with symptomatic angina, arrhythmia, or hypertension undergoing surgery or those demonstrated to have ischemia on preoperative testing while undergoing vascular surgery. Class IIa recommendations suggest beta blockers are probably indicated for those shown to have coronary disease or high cardiac risk because of multiple clinical risk factors, and class IIb recommendations suggest beta blockers can be considered for those with intermediate or low cardiac risk.

With beta blocker use more prevalent than at the time these studies were performed, an additional question is whether individuals on chronic beta-blocker therapy receive the same benefits. A review of 18 case-control and observational studies analysis has suggested that continuing beta blocker therapy in the perioperative period may not provide the same cardioprotective effects seen with acute preoperative therapy.[17] This issue remains to be rigorously studied, because current guidelines do not distinguish between acute and chronic beta-blocker therapy.

> Box 4-1. **Summary Points**
> - Patients who are clearly high risk for intraoperative and postoperative cardiac ischemia should receive perioperative beta-blocker therapy.
> - For patients at moderate risk, clinicians should weigh the benefits and risks (e.g., hypotension, bradycardia, bronchospasm) of beta-blocker therapy for each case.
> - For low-risk patients, no data support the use of perioperative beta-blocker therapy.

RECOMMENDATIONS

In summary, the new clinical guidelines reflect the lack of data and suggest clinicians must carefully weigh the risks and benefits of perioperative beta blockade in patients undergoing noncardiac surgery. Although gaps in the data still exist, a reasonable strategy is to administer beta blockers to patients that are clearly at high risk for postoperative cardiac events and to withhold them from patients who are clearly at low risk. For intermediate-risk patients, the risk and benefits must be weighed, and when possible, patients should be informed about the questionable benefit and potential harms of beta blockers in the perioperative setting. Beta-blocker therapy should be withheld or used with caution in patients at risk for bradycardia or hypotension or in patients for whom these side effects would be catastrophic (e.g., recent ischemic stroke, preexisting cardiac conduction defects, history of very severe asthma) (Box 4-1).

2. Does an asymptomatic 65-year-old woman incidentally found to AS on a preoperative echocardiography (AVA 0.9 cm^2, gradient of 60 mm Hg) require further additional medical or surgical intervention before her hip replacement surgery?

Search Date: March 2006

Search Strategy: *PubMed, search for "aortic stenosis AND noncardiac surgery" (55 items); also "aortic balloon valvuloplasty" and "noncardiac surgery" (23 items). Titles and abstracts were reviewed, relevant bibliographies* *scanned, and searches for related articles were done when appropriate. The most current ACC/AHA guidelines were also scanned for references.*

Aortic stenosis, which has a prevalence of 2% to 9% in adults older than 65 years,[18,19] is considered an important risk factor for postoperative cardiac complications. Early studies estimated the risk of perioperative death at 13%.[20] A case-control series by Kertai and colleagues[21] suggests a similar risk. In this study, 108 mostly symptomatic patients with moderate to severe aortic stenosis had a higher perioperative mortality rate and rate of nonfatal MI than age-matched controls (14% versus. 2%; $P < .001$).

Although it is agreed that surgical aortic valve replacement (AVR) is the optimal treatment in symptomatic, critical aortic stenosis (i.e., those presenting with chest pain, congestive heart failure [CHF], or syncope), there are no randomized, controlled trials to help guide management in patients with moderate to severe aortic stenosis who are asymptomatic or who have mild symptoms and require noncardiac surgery. Results of three small case studies have questioned the need for preoperative AVR or valvuloplasty in such patients. Raymer and colleagues[22] looked at a case-control series of 55 patients with aortic stenosis (mean aortic valve area [AVA] of 0.9 cm²) and found no difference in risk of cardiac complications with age-matched controls. O'Keefe and coworkers[23] looked at 48 consecutive aortic stenosis patients (mean gradient of 76 mm Hg, 22 patients with general anesthesia), 75% of whom had symptomatic aortic stenosis and were undergoing noncardiac operations. Although there were no intraoperative deaths, five had perioperative hypotension that was transient and easily treated intraoperatively. Torsher and associates[24] looked at a case series of 19 patients (AVA < 0.5 cm² or gradient > 50 mm Hg, with 84% of patients being symptomatic) in which there were no perioperative events, but 2 patients died after long, complicated postoperative courses. The authors of these studies suggest that careful hemodynamic monitoring was key to managing perioperative complications such as hypotension and that selected patients can undergo surgery with acceptable risk. A later case-control study was published by Zahid and colleagues,[25] in which

5149 patients with aortic stenosis undergoing noncardiac surgery were taken from a national registry and compared with twice as many controls. Those with aortic stenosis had a higher incidence of acute MI after surgery compared with controls (3.86% versus 2.03%; $P < .001$), but overall mortality was no different. This result was determined after statistically correcting for age, heart failure, diabetes, hypertension, and known CAD. Unfortunately, because the definition of aortic stenosis was based on ICD codes in this study, it is unclear how severe the aortic stenosis was or whether patients were symptomatic at the time of surgery or optimally medically managed. It is possible that there were additional comorbidities that were not accounted for or a greater degree of subclinical atherosclerosis present in those with aortic stenosis compared with controls.

AORTIC BALLOON VALVULOPLASTY

There is also little consensus on the role of aortic balloon valvuloplasty and whether it should be used as a temporizing measure or in addition to medical management in those who are not candidates for AVR. Limited data come from two small, retrospective, non–case-control series that examined patients who refused AVR, who were poor surgical candidates before necessary noncardiac surgery, or who required emergency noncardiac surgery. The results are mixed. Hayes and coworkers[26] looked at 15 patients with severe aortic stenosis and a contraindication to AVR who had valvuloplasty resulting in improved AVA and gradient before surgery. Three patients had left ventricular (LV) perforation (resulting in one death); one developed CHF, and another developed a femoral aneurysm. Only nine patients ultimately underwent surgery successfully. Roth and associates[27] reported a series of seven patients for whom valvuloplasty also reduced AVA and mean gradient. All patients had uncomplicated noncardiac surgery thereafter, and only one patient required redo valvuloplasty. It is unclear whether medical management alone would have had similar outcomes, because there were no case controls.

Current ACC/AHA guidelines suggest that in symptomatic critical aortic stenosis, AVR is ideally done first if the surgery can wait,[1] but for those who are not candidates or refuse, the mortality rate for noncardiac surgery is approximately 10%, a number based on the studies cited previously. In asymptomatic patients, noncardiac surgery may be performed safely with appropriate intraoperative monitoring and medical management. There are insufficient data to recommend use of valvuloplasty as a preoperative measure, and it should be performed only on a selected basis. A review article describes a convenient algorithm for clinical use (Fig. 4-1).[28]

3. Are preoperative arrhythmias predictive of perioperative morbidity and mortality?

Search Date: March 2006

***Search Strategy:** PubMed, search for "atrial" (46 items) or "ventricular" (73 items) with the terms "arrhythmia" and "noncardiac surgery"; also "preoperative atrial" (574 items) or "ventricular" (659 items) and "arrhythmia." Titles and abstracts reviewed, and relevant bibliographies scanned. The most current ACC/AHA guidelines were scanned for references.*

Early case series found that patients with preoperative arrhythmias had higher morbidity and mortality rates and that supraventricular and ventricular arrhythmias were independent risk factors for coronary events. Goldman and coworkers[20] found that five or more premature ventricular contractions (PVCs), the presence of any nonsinus rhythm, or the presence of premature atrial contractions (PACs) on a preoperative ECG was associated with increased morbidity and mortality. In their studies, 7 of 44 patients with PVCs and 11 of 112 patients with PACs were at risk of life-threatening cardiac complications.[20] However, two later studies suggested otherwise.

One prospective, cohort trial of VA patients examined 230 men—one half with known CAD and one half at high risk for CAD—and recorded their rhythms before, during, and after surgery.[29] Forty-four percent of patients had frequent ventricular ectopy, defined as more than 30 extra beats per hour. Ectopy was more common in smokers, those with CHF, and those with evidence of ischemia. There were only nine events of nonfatal MI or

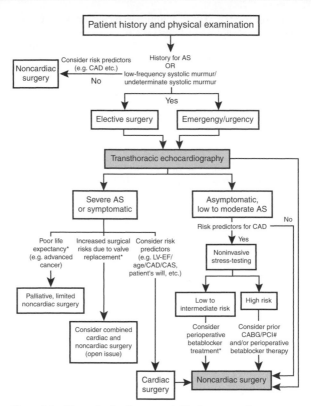

Figure 4-1. Diagnostic algorithm suggested for the preoperative evaluation of patients with suspected or established aortic stenosis who have been scheduled for noncardiac surgery. Antimicrobial prophylaxis is mandatory in the recommended surgical procedures. Palliative noncardiac surgery (e.g., partial cancer resection for relief of symptoms) may be performed in patients with severe aortic stenosis whose short-term to mid-term life expectancy is poor. In selected patients who are at very high risk, a nonsurgical palliative approach may be chosen. Because the strategies have not been evaluated in prospective studies, decisions should be made in an interdisciplinary manner, including the opinions or wishes of the patient and the patient's family. AS, aortic stenosis; CABG, coronary artery bypass grafting; CAD, coronary artery disease; CAS, carotid artery stenosis; LVEF, left ventricular ejection fraction; PCI, percutaneous coronary intervention; *, risks of anticoagulation during neurosurgery and concerns

Continued

posed by prosthetic valves (e.g., infection from abdominal surgery) may represent an indication for a combined procedure in selected patients, with the noncardiac operation performed immediately after the valve surgery; #, the decision about medical or interventional therapy should be made according to the American College of Cardiology/American Heart Association recommendations. (Adapted from Christ M, Sharkova Y, Geldner G, Maisch B: Preoperative and perioperative care for patients with suspected or established aortic stenosis facing noncardiac surgery. Chest 2005; 128:2944-2953.)

death and no significant differences among those with or without preoperative arrhythmias (OR = 1.6; 95% CI: 0.4 to 6.2). Given the few number of events for this combined outcome, they likely did not have enough power to detect a difference between groups with or without arrhythmias. However, the study showed that preoperative arrhythmias were also associated with intraoperative (OR = 7.3; 95% CI: 3.3 to 16) and postoperative (OR = 6.4; 95% CI: 2.7 to 15) arrhythmias.

Subsequently, Mahla and colleagues[30] performed a prospective study enrolling 60 patients with structural heart disease and ventricular ectopy. Using a Holter monitor, they also assessed arrhythmias before, during, and after surgery. Preoperative and intraoperative arrhythmias occurred in 35% of patients, and arrhythmias occurred in 87% postoperatively. Five patients had adverse events (i.e., one with unstable angina and four with heart failure). There were no differences in the frequency of perioperative ventricular dysrhythmias in patients with or without adverse cardiac outcomes. Patients with an ejection fraction (EF) of less than 40% had more ventricular dysrhythmias preoperatively than those with an EF of more than 40% ($P = .05$).

Both studies had too few events to demonstrate differences in morbidity and mortality between those with or without preoperative arrhythmias. They do show, however, that most postoperative cardiac complications in these patients were not directly related to arrhythmias, but rather to ischemia or heart failure. The importance of preoperative atrial or ventricular ectopy or arrhythmias may therefore be as markers of underlying structural heart disease, and they should provide a

> **Box 4-2. Summary Points for Frequent Preoperative Atrial or Ventricular Ectopy**
>
> - Frequent preoperative atrial or ventricular ectopy is associated with perioperative arrhythmias.
> - It should prompt an evaluation (i.e., history, physical examination, and echocardiography) for underlying structural heart disease in otherwise low- to moderate-risk patients.
> - It does not add to risk stratification models for already high-risk patients undergoing elective surgery.

source for investigation in otherwise low- to moderate-risk patients. It is not clear whether their presence adds to risk stratification models for already high-risk patients. Because preoperative arrhythmias and ectopy seem to be associated with the appearance of postoperative arrhythmias, their presence provides good reason for the medical consultant to follow these patients postoperatively and, in certain cases, to obtain postoperative ECGs (Box 4-2).

4. Is preoperative systolic dysfunction a risk factor for morbidity and mortality in patients undergoing noncardiac surgery?

Search Date: March 2006

Search Strategy: PubMed, search for "ejection fraction" and "noncardiac surgery" (89 items) in addition to "multiple gated acquisition scan" (89 items), "gated heart blood pool scan" (100 items), and the terms "radionuclide ventriculography" (5 items), "angiocardiography" (5 items), and "echocardiography" (189 items), combined with the term "noncardiac surgery." Titles and abstracts were reviewed; relevant bibliographies were scanned. The most current ACC/AHA guidelines were also scanned for references.

Although active heart failure has been associated with postoperative morbidity and mortality, less is known about the prognostic significance of a low resting EF alone in the preoperative setting. Early data from Goldman and colleagues[20] showed that patients with an S_3 or elevated jugular venous pressure preoperatively had a 20% incidence of cardiac death and 14% incidence of cardiac morbidity.[20] Detsky and associates[31] furthered this notion using a multifactorial cardiac index prospectively on 455 patients and found that pulmonary edema within 1 week of surgery was also an independent risk factor for cardiac events.

A low EF in an otherwise euvolemic patient is not a consistent predictor of surgical mortality or morbidity. Most data are derived from a large number of small, retrospective and prospective studies but no randomized, controlled trials. Early studies used radionuclide scanning for assessment of EF and suggested increased mortality with lower EF values. Pasternack and colleagues[32] retrospectively assessed 100 patients who underwent lower extremity revascularization and found a high incidence of perioperative MI (6 of 8 patients) in those with EF values of less than 35% compared with those with normal EF values (0 of 50 patients) ($P < .02$). Additional small series by Mosely and colleagues[33] ($n = 41$ $P < .001$), Kazmers and coworkers[34] ($n = 35$, $P = .029$), and Fletscher and associates[35] ($n = 72$, $P < .001$) of patients undergoing AAA repair suggested increased mortality for those with an EF value less than 30%, 29%, and 35%, respectively. Lazor and colleagues[36] used multiple gates acquisition scan (MUGA) for 196 patients undergoing surgery up to 60 days after EF determination and found mortality rates of 19.5% for those with an EF less than 35%, 5.4% for those with an EF of 36% to 54%, and 2.2% for those with a normal EF value ($P < .005$). There was no difference in mortality rates for patients undergoing cardiac surgical procedures. A later study by Pederson and associates[37] suggested that in addition to a low EF, those with high EF values (>70%)—and presumably diastolic dysfunction—also had a greater risk of cardiovascular complications, such as CHF and pulmonary edema.

Countering data come from a prospective study by Halm and colleagues[38] of a cohort of 330 men with suspected CAD undergoing noncardiac surgery. The investigators found that EF, as determined by echocardiography, had limited prognostic value, and that although an EF of 40% or less was associated with poorer outcomes, measurement of EF did not alter risk assessment beyond currently used models.[38] For example, EF was not a significant predictor of CHF (OR = 2.1; 95% CI: 0.7 to 6.0) or ventricular arrhythmias (OR = 1.8; 95% CI: 0.7 to 4.7), but it was a predictor of all cardiac outcomes combined (OR = 2.5; 95% CI: 1.2 to 5.0). Another study by Franco and colleagues[39] looked at 85 patients undergoing vascular surgery and found no difference in groups based on EF. In their study population, 9 of 50 patients with normal EF values had cardiac events but no deaths. There were two deaths in the low-EF group of 15 patients, which was not statistically significant.

Differences between these studies may reflect that they were underpowered and that advances in preoperative and perioperative medical management occurred from the mid-1980s to the 1990s, when these studies were published. There may also have been differences in patient volume status at the time of surgery.

META-ANALYSES

Meta-analyses have been performed to work around these limitations. One such analysis by Karkos and associates[40] assessed the ability of MUGA to predict cardiac risk before elective surgery. They evaluated 22 trials, which included 3096 patients. Although there were individual study limitations such as selection bias and differences in imaging type and cut-off points, the study authors found overall that resting EF was not a significant predictor of perioperative ischemic events.[40] Similarly, Kertai and colleagues[41] looked at six different testing modalities of preoperative cardiac risk assessment, including ambulatory ECG and stress echocardiography. They found that one of these modalities, radionuclide ventriculography, had a low sensitivity but high specificity for perioperative cardiac complications, and that it did not add anything above and beyond other risk-stratification methodologies or stress-testing techniques. Both groups postulate this is because resting EF may provide minimal information about how the heart performs under stress.

RECOMMENDATIONS

In summary, early studies suggested that the greatest risk of adverse postoperative events occurs in patients with an EF of less than 35%. Later meta-analyses questioned this notion. Although patients with signs and symptoms of heart failure before surgery warrant evaluation and treatment with the goal of euvolemia, for the asymptomatic, otherwise euvolemic patient, there are no data to suggest that measurement of the resting EF adds to current risk-stratification methodology for morbidity and mortality. In patients with suspected or newly diagnosed systolic dysfunction, it is perhaps more important for the medical consultant to recognize whether the cause is ischemic in nature or not.

5. Does percutaneous coronary angioplasty or intervention before elective noncardiac surgery reduce perioperative morbidity or mortality?

Search Date: March 2006

Search Strategy: PubMed, search for "percutaneous coronary intervention AND noncardiac surgery" (10 items) "percutaneous coronary angioplasty OR angioplasty AND noncardiac surgery" (113 and 147 items, respectively). Titles and abstracts reviewed, as were related articles to those of interest. Relevant bibliographies were also scanned. The most current ACC/AHA guidelines were also scanned for references.

PREOPERATIVE PTCA

Preoperative percutaneous transluminal coronary angioplasty (PTCA) or percutaneous coronary intervention (PCI) (i.e., stenting) before noncardiac surgery is a controversial topic. Until recently, most data were derived from a series of small retrospective and case-control studies (Table 4-2), which were inconclusive overall. Some suggested only limited morbidity or mortality before surgery, whereas others did not. One reason for significant differences was related to the time between revascularization and noncardiac surgery. With the advent of PCI, the increased the risk of bleeding from antiplatelet agents had to be balanced with the risk for subacute thrombosis and MI. Since drug-eluting stents have become the standard of care in many instances, this question has become even more complicated.

Table 4-2. Morbidity and Mortality of Surgery after Angioplasty (PTCA) or Stenting (PCI)

Study, Year	No. with PTCA	No. with PCI	Mortality	Morbidity (Events)	Time to surgery
Allen et al, 1991[42]	148	—	0.7%	10.1% (arrhythmia, ischemia)	72 were < 90 days; range, 4 to 1867 days
Huber et al, 1992[43]	50	—	2%	4% (MI)	9 days (median)
Elmore et al, 1993[44]	14	—	0%	0	10 days (median)
Jones et al, 1993[43]	108	—	0.9%	2.7% (MI)	14.5 days (mean); range, 0 to 41 days
Gottlieb et al, 1998[46]	194	—	0.5%	13.4% (MI,CHF)	11 days (median)
Posner et al, 1999[47]	686	—	2.9%	31.5% (angina, CHF, MI)	1 year (median); range, 2 days to 6.6 years; 451 within 90 days
Hassan et al (BARI), 2001[48]	251	—	0.8%	0.8% (MI)	29 months (median)
Birlakis et al, 2005[49]	350	—	0.3%	0.6%	All were with in 60 days of angioplasty

Kaluza et al, 2000[50]	—	40	15%	2.5% (bleeding, MI)	13 days (mean); range, 1 to 39 days
Sharma et al, 2003[51]	—	47	13%	4.2% (bleeding, MI)	27 were < 3 weeks; 20 were > 3 weeks
Wilson et al, 2003[54]	—	207	3%	1% (MI)	Range of 1 to 60 days; 168 within 6 weeks
McFalls et al, 2004[55]	—	141	22% (at 2.7 years)	12% (MI at 30 days)	41 days (median)
Godet et al, 2005[53]	—	78	5.1%	9% (MI)	5 weeks (mean)
Reddy et al, 2005[52]	—	56	7%	14.3% (MI, major bleeding)	Up to 42 days

CHF, congestive heart failure; MI, myocardial infarction; PCI, percutaneous coronary intervention; PTCA, percutaneous transluminal coronary angioplasty.

Allen and associates[42] first looked retrospectively at a cohort of preoperative PTCA cases and found no significant increase in cardiac mortality or morbidity in those performed less than 90 days before noncardiac surgery compared with those performed later. Several small cohort studies followed, in which PTCA was done within a mean of 2 weeks of noncardiac surgery, and all showed limited cardiovascular morbidity (0% to 13.4%) and mortality (0% to 2%).[43-46] A larger, retrospective, case-control study by Posner and colleagues[47] countered these findings. The study authors looked at 686 patients, many of whom had PTCA within 90 days of noncardiac surgery (overall mean time to noncardiac surgery after PTCA was 1 year) and found no difference in death or MI compared with those with CAD and no intervention. They did see, however, a decreased risk of angina (OR = 0.51; 95% CI: 0.34 to 0.76) and heart failure (OR = 0.40; 95% CI: 0.27 to 0.58) in PTCA patients. More importantly, the morbidity seen with PCI overall was higher than previously reported at 31.5%. Significant limitations of this study were the lack of control for CAD severity, comorbidities, and medical management in control versus PTCA groups. Moreover, the median time to noncardiac surgery from PTCA was about 1 year, much longer than in previous studies.

The first randomized, controlled trial that indirectly included an assessment of morbidity and mortality with PTCA before noncardiac surgery was the Bypass Angioplasty Revascularization Investigation (BARI) study.[48] Designed to compare PTCA with CABG before noncardiac surgery, the study looked at 501 patients who had revascularization by PTCA ($n = 251$) or CABG ($n = 250$) a median of 29 months before their noncardiac surgery. The investigators found no difference in 30-day cardiac mortality rates or cardiac events after the first noncardiac surgery between CABG (4 of 250 patients) and PTCA groups (4 of 251 patients) in a multivariate model that adjusted for major cardiac risk factors (OR for CABG versus PTCA = 1.4; 95% CI: 0.3 to 6.1; $P = .64$). Overall mortality was also comparatively low in both groups (0.8%) compared with the findings in Posner's study, and the median time to surgery was similar.

PREOPERATIVE PCI

When PCI overtook PTCA as the standard of care, similar questions arose about its use before noncardiac surgery. Later studies of PCI done before noncardiac surgery found various incidences of adverse outcomes, depending on when the PCI was performed. For example, two small, nonrandomized studies found a higher incidence of mortality when surgery was done within 2 to 3 weeks of stenting,[50,51] usually resulting in major bleeding and fatal and nonfatal MI—thought to be from thrombosis when antiplatelet therapy was stopped. Outcomes appeared to be equivocal or better than for those who waited several weeks after PCI, as suggested in later retrospective studies.[52,53] For instance, Wilson and colleagues[54] studied in 207 PCI patients and found all events occurred in patients undergoing PCI less than 6 weeks before noncardiac surgery, whereas no events occurred in those who waited 7 to 9 weeks after PCI.

The only randomized, controlled trial was published by McFalls and colleagues,[55] and it addressed questions similar to those of the BARI study, but with PCI instead of PTCA. In the trial, 510 VA patients with stable CAD (at least > 70% stenosis and suitable for revascularization) awaiting elective major vascular surgery were assigned to no revascularization ($n = 252$) or revascularization ($n = 258$, 59% by PCI and 41% by CABG) before surgery. The median time to noncardiac surgery was 54 days for the revascularized group, compared with 18 days for the nonrevascularized group. At follow-up of 2.7 years, mortality was not different between groups. There was also no difference in 30-day postoperative MI. Overall rates of mortality, however, were approximately 22% in both groups (RR = 0.98; 95% CI: 0.70 to 1.37). All patients in this study had stable coronary disease and an overall normal EF. Higher-risk patients with low EF or those with acute coronary syndrome were not included, and it was underpowered to detect differences in event rates in high-risk subgroups.

RECOMMENDATIONS

Overall, for high-risk patients, data are lacking for whether preoperative angioplasty or PCI makes a difference in morbidity and mortality for noncardiac surgery.

Given the known complications with acute coronary syndrome, several of the current ACC/AHA recommendations for coronary angiography and potential intervention are similar, whether the patient is to go for elective surgery or not.[1] For example, class I recommendations include the following situations: a significantly positive noninvasive test result, angina not responsive to medical therapy, unstable angina in moderate- to high-risk surgery, and equivocal noninvasive test results in those considered to be at high risk for a coronary event undergoing high-risk surgery.[1] Studies comparing PCI with medical management before noncardiac surgery in high-risk populations are difficult to perform given the current standard to care. When revascularization is thought to be necessary, the ideal time to wait before surgery is debatable, especially in the era of drug-eluting stents that delay endothelialization and require longer periods of antiplatelet therapy compared with bare metal stents. Most cardiologists recommend waiting 4 to 6 weeks.[56] When elective surgery is required sooner, some may opt to use a bare metal stent, for which the duration for antiplatelet therapy is less, to balance the risk of ischemia with that of bleeding during surgery.[57]

6. How long should a patient wait after a myocardial infarction before having elective noncardiac surgery?

Search Date: March 2006

Search Strategy: *PubMed, search for "myocardial reinfarction" and "surgery" (606 items) or with "noncardiac and surgery" (9 items). Titles and abstracts reviewed, and relevant bibliographies scanned; as were related articles. The most current ACC/AHA guidelines were scanned for references.*

No randomized, controlled trials have been performed to answer the question of how long to delay elective surgery after an MI. Guidelines are heavily based on data from observational or retrospective series from the late 1970s and 1980s in which the risk of reinfarction or mortality after an MI during subsequent noncardiac surgery was assessed.

Initial reports by Goldman and colleagues[58] and Rao and coworkers[59] suggested a reinfarction rate of 30% and 36% when surgery was performed within 3 months of an MI, respectively. These rates decreased to 15% and 26% when surgery was done within 3 to 6 months. After 6 months, the rate was lower (approximately 5%). Steen and associates[60] published similar rates of morbidity in their series of 587 patients. Those operated on within 3 months of an MI had a reinfarction rate of 27%, which decreased to 4% to 5% after waiting 6 months until surgery.[60]

Subsequent data suggest this high mortality may actually be lower. In the same publication, Rao and colleagues[59] looked at a second series patients operated on later (between 1977 and 1982) and found a reinfarction rate of 5.7% for operations done within 3 months and 2.3% when done within 3 to 6 months of an MI ($P < .05$). However, there was variation in the type of operations patients underwent, and many procedures were minor, making interpretation and application of the findings difficult.

Other studies had similar findings. Wells and colleagues[61] found no reinfarctions in their group of 48 patients who had surgery within 3 months of an MI. Schoeppel and coworkers[62] found an overall reinfarction rate of 3.8% in the 53 post-MI patients in their study. In another study, Shah and associates[63] took 275 patients with MIs and found overall that 4.7% had reinfarctions with surgery. The rates were 4.3% within 3 months, 0% from 3 to 6 months, and 5.7% after 6 months. Procedures included major vascular operations. The urgency of the procedure was not a variable that showed statistical significance in their study with respect to overall mortality.

Apparent decreases in perioperative morbidity seen in later studies may reflect the nature of changes in surgery and anesthetic techniques and better medical management, including use of beta blockers, statins, and ACE inhibitors. Many of these studies do not rigorously quantify the size and extent of infarction or associated complications, such as arrhythmias, to use as comparisons between studies. Taken together, these data have impelled some to suggest that elective surgery be delayed, if possible, up to 6 months after MI. If surgery is necessary sooner, stress testing or revascularization, or both, as needed should be performed first in such patients.

7. Does smoking cessation before noncardiac surgery have any effect on perioperative cardiovascular morbidity or mortality?

Search Date: March 2006

Search Strategy: PubMed, search for "smoking AND cessation AND surgery" (479 items); "tobacco and cessation and surgery" (327 items). Additional search terms were "perioperative," "preoperative," "noncardiac," and "cardiac risk," which yielded fewer results. Searches were performed on related articles of interest. Titles and abstracts reviewed; relevant bibliographies scanned.

Tobacco use has been associated with cardiovascular disease in general, and the benefits of smoking cessation on overall morbidity and mortality compel physicians to recommend smoking cessation to all patients. Whether smokers gain any specific benefit from preoperative smoking cessation in the short term, however, is a matter of interest. There is only one small, randomized, controlled trial and one prospective, case-control series that include cardiovascular morbidity among other factors assessed in preoperative smoking cessation.

Moller and colleagues[64] randomized 120 patients undergoing hip or knee alloplasty to a smoking intervention arm or a control arm. The intervention arm involved counseling and nicotine replacement therapy, and patients had to quit or reduce tobacco intake by 50% at approximately 6 to 8 weeks before their elective surgery and for at least 10 days after the surgery. In the intervention group, 36 of 60 patients stopped smoking, and 14 reduced their intake; 4 of 60 patients in the control arm stopped smoking. Five patients in the control group had complications of MI or heart failure, compared with none in the intervention group; however, this was not statistically significant ($P = .08$). There was also no difference found with respect to respiratory complications ($P = .97$). Instead, the major difference found was with respect to would healing and related complications: 3% in the intervention arm versus 16% in the control arm ($P = .001$; relative risk reduction [RRR] = 83%; NNT = 4; 95% CI: 2 to 8). Overall event rates were low because this was a small study with relatively healthy patients. Only 15 had heart disease of any kind, only 12 had underlying COPD, and only 4 had diabetes, suggesting the study might have been underpowered to detect such differences. Several other studies,[65-67] including a retrospective study of 188 patients, confirmed the finding of fewer wound complications in patients who stopped smoking 3 weeks before head and neck surgery but did not address overall mortality or cardiovascular complications

Moore and colleauges[68] prospectively studied 233 smokers who underwent a cessation program of their choice before pelvic reconstruction surgery. Smoking cessation started 1 month before surgery and continued for 1 month after surgery. Postoperative complications were compared with those of 654 nonsmokers in the postoperative setting. The investigators found no difference in any type of smoking-related cardiovascular complications, including CHF, atrial fibrillation, syncope, or other arrhythmia (OR = 0.47; 95%CI: 0.07 to 2.78). Moreover, they found no difference with respect to wound complications (OR = 0.98; 95% CI: 0.5 to 1.9).

RECOMMENDATIONS

Data are limited on the effect of preoperative smoking cessation on the cardiovascular complications of surgery, and there is no firm evidence that preoperative smoking is an independent risk factor for major cardiac events during surgery. Current major indices of preoperative cardiac risk therefore have not used smoking status before surgery as one of the main predictors of cardiovascular outcome.[69] Further study using larger cohorts or randomized, controlled trials is needed. There does appear to be some benefit with respect to wound healing, and several trials have looked at postoperative pulmonary complications with conflicting results,[70-73] but the appropriate timing of smoking cessation before surgery is not clear. Several of the studies mentioned have arbitrarily used 3 weeks to several months before surgery. In either case, smoking cessation is a necessary recommendation for all patients, regardless of whether they are undergoing surgery. The prospect of elective surgery may be a good opportunity to motivate the patient to quit tobacco use.

8. Does preoperative use of statins reduce postoperative cardiac events or mortality?

Search Date: March 2006

Search Strategy: PubMed, search for "statin AND "preoperative cardiac risk" (11 items), "statin AND preoperative" (25 items), "statin AND cardiac risk" (182 items), "statin AND noncardiac" (14 items), and "statin AND surgery" (288 items). Titles and abstracts reviewed; searches performed on related articles of interest. Relevant bibliographies were scanned.

The diverse therapeutic benefits of HMG-CoA reductase inhibitors (statins) have become evident and continue to evolve. Beyond their favorable effect on lipid profiles, statins appear to affect several pathways involved in myocardial injury. Reduced platelet aggregation, diminished inflammatory response, improved endothelial function, and overall stabilization of atherosclerotic plaques are likely results of statin therapy. Several studies support the multiarmed effects of statins, with reduction in cardiac events and symptoms preceding quantifiable changes in angiographically demonstrated atherosclerotic plaques.[74,75]

Although the use of statins on perioperative events is still in its inception, early clinical trials offer compelling results and are summarized in Table 4-3. In 2002, Poldermans and colleagues[76] performed a case-control, retrospective analysis, evaluating the impact of statin therapy on perioperative mortality after major vascular surgery. A fourfold reduction in mortality was observed among statin users. A subsequent study by Ward and associates[77] looked retrospectively at 446 patients undergoing infrainguinal vascular bypass surgery and found that statin therapy was independently associated with fewer overall cardiovascular complications (OR = 0.36; 95% CI: 0.14 to 0.93; $P = .035$) and shorter length of stay. The study authors were unable to detect a difference in perioperative cardiovascular or all-cause mortality, likely because overall mortality was small (2.5%). In the Poldermans study, however, it was 5.8%. Several other retrospective analyses, including one performed by Lindanauer and coworkers,[79] have found improved event-free survival rates and reduced overall mortality

Table 4-3. Studies of Preoperative Statin Use

Study	Design	Population	Results
Poldermans et al, 2003[76]	Retrospective	2816 patients undergoing major vascular surgery, 160 cases matched with controls	Statin therapy less common in case than control: 8% vs. 25%, $P < .001$. Odds ratio for perioperative mortality was 0.22 (95% CI: 0.10 to 0.47).
Lindanauer et al, 2004[77]	Retrospective	Of 780,591 patients undergoing surgery, 77,082 were identified by pharmacy records as receiving statin therapy the first 2 hospital days.	Mortality rates were less among statin users. OR = 0.62 (95% CI: 0.58 to 0.67), with NNT = 85 (77 to 98).
Durrazzo et al, 2004[82]	Randomized	Of 100 patients, 50 patients received placebo and 50 received 20 mg of atorvastatin, regardless of serum cholesterol level. Surgery was performed on average of 30 days after randomization. Patients were followed for 6 months.	There was no difference in cardiac death ($P = 1.0$), unstable angina ($P = 1.0$), or nonfatal MI ($P = .2$). Statin use reduced a composite end point of cardiac death, nonfatal MI, unstable angina, and stroke ($P = .031$).
Kertai et al, 2004[78]	Retrospective	570 patients undergoing abdominal aortic aneurysm surgery; outcome end points were perioperative mortality and MI	Statin users had decreased composite end points of mortality and MI: 3.7% vs. 11.0%, with an odds ratio after covariate correction of correction 0.24 (95% CI: 0.10 to 0.70).
Ward et al, 2005[77]	Retrospective	446 patients undergoing infrainguinal vascular bypass surgery	Overall mortality rate was 2.5%. Statin therapy was associated with fewer combined cardiovascular complications (6.9% vs. 20.1%, $P = .008$) and shorter length of stay (6.4 vs. 9.7 days, $P = .007$), but not with cardiovascular or overall mortality rates.

MI, myocardial infarction; NNT, number needed to treat.

rates among patients using statins who undergo major vascular surgery.

A retrospective study by McGirt and associates[80] looked at preoperative statin therapy (within at least 1 week of surgery) in 1566 patients undergoing carotid endarterectomy. They found that statin use was associated with a decreased incidence of perioperative stroke and transient ischemic attacks and with all-cause mortality (0.3% versus 2.1%; $P < .01$).[80] A similar study by Kennedy and colleagues[81] showed statin use at the time of admission was associated with reduced in-hospital mortality after carotid endarterectomy, but it was not clear at what point patients were started on statins.

In 2004, Durazzo and colleagues[82] published the results of a randomized, controlled trial examining statin use before vascular surgery. Approximately 100 patients were randomly assigned to receive statins or placebo for at least 30 days before major vascular surgery. Randomization occurred regardless of baseline cholesterol levels. The four primary end points were death from cardiac cause, nonfatal MI, ischemic cerebral vascular accident, and unstable angina. The follow-up period was 6 months. Statin users demonstrated reductions in the occurrence of all four end points combined but not each individually, likely because the number of events was too small for a difference to be detected (see Table 4-3).[82]

Before the use of statins in the perioperative setting becomes customary, further investigation is necessary. The evidence suggests that the cardioprotective effects of statins may extend to the perioperative setting.

REFERENCES

1. Eagle KA, Berger PB, Calkins H, et al: ACC/AHA guideline update for perioperative cardiovascular evaluation for noncardiac surgery—Executive summary a report of the American College of Cardiology/American Heart Association Task Force on Practice Guidelines (Committee to Update the 1996 Guidelines on Perioperative Cardiovascular Evaluation for Noncardiac Surgery). Circulation 2002;105:1257-1267. IV

2. Stone JG, Foex P, Sear JW, et al: Risk of myocardial ischaemia during anaesthesia in treated and untreated hypertensive patients. Br J Anaesth 1988; 61:675-679. III

3. Yeager RA, Moneta GL, Edwards JM, et al: Reducing perioperative myocardial infarction following vascular surgery. The potential role of beta-blockade. Arch Surg 1995;130:869-872; discussion 872-873. III

4. Mangano DT, Layug EL, Wallace A, Tateo I: Effect of atenolol on mortality and cardiovascular morbidity after noncardiac surgery. Multicenter Study of Perioperative Ischemia Research Group. N Engl J Med 1996;335:1713-1720. II

5. Wallace A, Layug B, Tateo I, et al: Prophylactic atenolol reduces postoperative myocardial ischemia. Anesthesiology 1998;88:7-17. II

6. Poldermans D, Boersma E, Bax JJ, et al: The effect of bisoprolol on perioperative mortality and myocardial infarction in high-risk patients undergoing vascular surgery. Dutch Echocardiographic Cardiac Risk Evaluation Applying Stress Echocardiography Study Group. N Engl J Med 1999;341:1789-1794. II

7. Poldermans D, Boersma E, Bax JJ, et al, for the Dutch Echocardiographic Cardiac Risk Evaluation Applying Stress Echocardiography Study Group. Bisoprolol reduces cardiac death and myocardial infarction in high-risk patients as long as 2 years after successful major vascular surgery. Eur Heart J 2001;22:1353-1358. II

8. Auerbach AD, Goldman L: Beta-blockers and reduction of cardiac events in noncardiac surgery: Scientific review. JAMA 2002;287:1435-1444. I

9. Raby KE, Brull SJ, Timimi F, et al: The effect of heart rate control on myocardial ischemia among high-risk patients after vascular surgery. Anesth Analg 1999;88:477-482. III

10. Urban MK, Markowitz SM, Gordon MA, et al: Postoperative prophylactic administration of beta-adrenergic blockers in patients at risk for myocardial ischemia. Anesth Analg 2000;90:1257-1261. II

11. Devereaux PJ, Beattie WS, Choi PT, et al: How strong is the evidence for the use of perioperative beta blockers in non-cardiac surgery? Systematic review and meta-analysis of randomised controlled trials. BMJ 2005; 331:313-321. I

12. Giles JW, Sear JW, Foex P: Effect of chronic beta-blockade on peri-operative outcome in patients undergoing non-cardiac surgery: An analysis of observational and case control studies. Anaesthesia 2004;59:574-583. III

13. McGory ML, Maggard MA, Ko CY: A meta-analysis of perioperative beta blockade: What is the actual risk reduction? Surgery 2005;138:171-179. I

14. Stevens RD, Burri H, Tramer MR: Pharmacologic myocardial protection in patients undergoing noncardiac surgery: A quantitative systematic review. Anesth Analg 2003;7:623-633. I

15. Schouten O, Shaw LJ, Boersma E, et al: A meta-analysis of safety and effectiveness of perioperative beta-blocker use for the prevention of cardiac events in different types of noncardiac surgery. Coron Artery Dis 2006; 17:173-179. I

16. Fleisher LA, Beckman JA Brown KA, et al: ACC/AHA 2006 guideline update on perioperative cardiovascular evaluation for noncardiac surgery: focused update on perioperative beta-blocker therapy: A report of the American College of Cardiology/American Heart Association Task Force on Practice Guidelines (Writing Committee to Update the 2002 Guidelines on Perioperative Cardiovascular Evaluation for Noncardiac Surgery) developed in collaboration with the American Society of Echocardiography, American Society of Nuclear Cardiology, Heart Rhythm Society, Society of Cardiovascular Anesthesiologists, Society for Cardiovascular Angiography and Interventions, and Society for Vascular Medicine and Biology. J Am Coll Cardiol 2006;47:2343-2355. IV

17. Lindenauer PK, Pekow P, Wang K, et al: Perioperative beta-blocker therapy and mortality after major noncardiac surgery. N Engl J Med 2005;353:349-361. III

18. Stewart BF, Siscovick D, Lind BK, et al: Clinical factors associated with calcific aortic valve disease. Cardiovascular Health Study. J Am Coll Cardiol 1997;29:630-634. III

19. Lindroos M, Kupari M, Heikkila J, Tilvis R: Prevalence of aortic valve abnormalities in the elderly: An echocardiographic study of a random population sample. J Am Coll Cardiol 1993;21:1220-1225. III

20. Goldman L, Caldera DL, Nussbaum SR, et al: Multifactorial index of cardiac risk in noncardiac surgical procedures. N Engl J Med 1977;297: 845-850. III

21. Kertai MD, Bountioukos M, Boersma E, et al: Aortic stenosis: An underestimated risk factor for perioperative complications in patients undergoing noncardiac surgery. Am J Med 2004;116:8-13. III

22. Raymer K, Yang H: Patients with aortic stenosis: Cardiac complications in non-cardiac surgery. Can J Anaesth 1998;45:855-859. III

23. O'Keefe JH Jr, Shub C, Rettke SR: Risk of noncardiac surgical procedures in patients with aortic stenosis. Mayo Clin Proc 1989;64:400-405. III

24. Torsher LC, Shub C, Rettke SR, Brown DL: Risk of patients with severe aortic stenosis undergoing noncardiac surgery. Am J Cardiol 1998;81:448-452. III

25. Zahid M, Sonel AF, Saba S, Good CB: Perioperative risk of noncardiac surgery associated with aortic stenosis. Am J Cardiol 2005;96:436-438. III

26. Hayes SN, Holmes DR Jr, Nishimura RA, Reeder GS: Palliative percutaneous aortic balloon valvuloplasty before noncardiac operations and invasive diagnostic procedures. Mayo Clin Proc 1989;64:753-775. III

27. Roth RB, Palacios IF, Block PC. Percutaneous aortic balloon valvuloplasty: Its role in the management of patients with aortic stenosis requiring major noncardiac surgery. J Am Coll Cardiol 1989;13:1039-1041. III

28. Christ M, Sharkova Y, Geldner G, Maisch B: Preoperative and perioperative care for patients with suspected or established aortic stenosis facing noncardiac surgery. Chest 2005;128:2944-2953. V

29. O'Kelly B, Browner WS, Massie B, et al: Ventricular arrhythmias in patients undergoing noncardiac surgery. The Study of Perioperative Ischemia Research Group. JAMA 1992;268:217-221. III

30. Mahla E, Rotman B, Rehak P, et al: Perioperative ventricular dysrhythmias in patients with structural heart disease undergoing noncardiac surgery. Anesth Analg 1998;86:16-21. III

31. Detsky AS, Abrams HB, Forbath N, et al: Cardiac assessment for patients undergoing noncardiac surgery. A multifactorial clinical risk index. Arch Intern Med 1986;146:2131-2134. III

32. Pasternack PF, Imparato AM, Riles TS, et al: The value of the radionuclide angiogram in the prediction of perioperative myocardial infarction in patients undergoing lower extremity revascularization procedures. Circulation 1985;72(Pt 2):II13- II17. III

33. Mosley JG, Clarke JM, Ell PJ, Marston A: Assessment of myocardial function before aortic surgery by radionuclide angiocardiography. Br J Surg 1985;72: 886-887. III

34. Kazmers A, Cerqueira MD, Zierler RE: Perioperative and late outcome in patients with left ventricular ejection fraction of 35% or less who require major vascular surgery. J Vasc Surg 1988;8:307-315. III

35. Fletcher JP, Antico VF, Gruenewald S, Kershaw LZ: Risk of aortic aneurysm surgery as assessed by preoperative gated heart pool scan. Br J Surg 1989;76:26-28. III

36. Lazor L, Russell JC, DaSilva J, Radford M: Use of the multiple uptake gated acquisition scan for the preoperative assessment of cardiac risk. Surg Gynecol Obstet 1988;167:234-238. III

37. Pedersen T, Kelbaek H, Munck O: Cardiopulmonary complications in high-risk surgical patients: The value of preoperative radionuclide cardiography. Acta Anaesthesiol Scand 1990;34:183-189. III

38. Halm EA, Browner WS, Tubau JF, et al: Echocardiography for assessing cardiac risk in patients having noncardiac surgery. Study of Perioperative Ischemia Research Group. Ann Intern Med 1996;125:433-441. III

39. Franco CD, Goldsmith J, Veith FJ, et al: Resting gated pool ejection fraction: A poor predictor of perioperative myocardial infarction in patients undergoing vascular surgery for infrainguinal bypass grafting. J Vasc Surg 1989;10:656-661. III

40. Karkos CD, Baguneid MS, Triposkiadis F, et al: Routine measurement of radioisotope left ventricular ejection fraction prior to vascular surgery: Is it worthwhile? Eur J Vasc Endovasc Surg 2004;27:227-238. I

41. Kertai MD, Boersma E, Bax JJ, et al: A meta-analysis comparing the prognostic accuracy of six diagnostic tests for predicting perioperative cardiac risk in patients undergoing major vascular surgery. Heart 2003; 89:1327-1334. I

42. Allen JR, Helling TS, Hartzler GO: Operative procedures not involving the heart after percutaneous transluminal coronary angioplasty. Surg Gynecol Obstet 1991; 173:285-288. III

43. Huber KC, Evans MA, Bresnahan JF, et al: Outcome of noncardiac operations in patients with severe coronary artery disease successfully treated preoperatively with coronary angioplasty. Mayo Clin Proc 1992;67:15-21. III

44. Elmore JR, Hallett JW Jr, Gibbons RJ, et al: Myocardial revascularization before abdominal aortic aneurysmorrhaphy: Effect of coronary angioplasty. Mayo Clin Proc 1993;68:637-641. III

45. Jones SE, Raymond RE, Simpfendorfer CC, Whitlow PL: Cardiac outcome of major noncardiac surgery in patients undergoing preoperative coronary angioplasty. J Invasive Cardiol 1993;5:212-218. III

46. Gottlieb A, Banoub M, Sprung J, et al: Perioperative cardiovascular morbidity in patients with coronary artery disease undergoing vascular surgery after percutaneous transluminal coronary angioplasty. J Cardiothorac Vasc Anesth 1998;12:501-506. III

47. Posner KL, Van Norman GA, Chan V: Adverse cardiac outcomes after noncardiac surgery in patients with prior percutaneous transluminal coronary angioplasty. Anesth Analg 1999;89:553-560. III

48. Hassan SA, Hlatky MA, Boothroyd DB, et al: Outcomes of noncardiac surgery after coronary bypass surgery or coronary angioplasty in the Bypass Angioplasty Revascularization Investigation (BARI). Am J Med 2001;110:260-266. II

49. Brilakis ES, Orford JL, Fasseas P, et al: Outcome of patients undergoing balloon angioplasty in the two months prior to noncardiac surgery. Am J Cardiol 2005;96:512-514. III

50. Kaluza GL, Joseph J, Lee JR, et al: Catastrophic outcomes of noncardiac surgery soon after coronary stenting. J Am Coll Cardiol 2000;35:1288-1294. III

51. Sharma AK, Ajani AE, Hamwi SM, et al: Major noncardiac surgery following coronary stenting: When is it safe to operate? Catheter Cardiovasc Interv 2004;63:141-145. III

52. Reddy PR, Vaitkus PT: Risks of noncardiac surgery after coronary stenting. Am J Cardiol 2005;95:755-757. III

53. Godet G, Riou B, Bertrand M, et al: Does preoperative coronary angioplasty improve perioperative cardiac outcome? Anesthesiology 2005;102:739-746. III

54. Wilson SH, Fasseas P, Orford JL, et al: Clinical outcome of patients undergoing non-cardiac surgery in the two months following coronary stenting. J Am Coll Cardiol 2003;42:234-240. III

55. McFalls EO, Ward HB, Moritz TE, et al: Coronary-artery revascularization before elective major vascular surgery. N Engl J Med 2004;351:2795-2804. II

56. Mendoza CE, Virani SS, Shah N, et al: Noncardiac surgery following percutaneous coronary intervention. Catheter Cardiovasc Interv 2004;63:267-273. V

57. Satler LF: Recommendations regarding stent selection in relation to the timing of noncardiac surgery postpercutaneous coronary intervention. Catheter Cardiovasc Interv 2004;63:146-147. V

58. Goldman L: Cardiac risks and complications of noncardiac surgery. Ann Intern Med 1983;98:504-513. III

59. Rao TL, Jacobs KH, El-Etr AA: Reinfarction following anesthesia in patients with myocardial infarction. Anesthesiology 1983;59:499-505. III

60. Steen PA, Tinker JH, Tarhan S: Myocardial reinfarction after anesthesia and surgery. JAMA 1978;239: 2566-2570. III

61. Wells PH, Kaplan JA: Optimal management of patients with ischemic heart disease for noncardiac surgery by complementary anesthesiologist and cardiologist interaction. Am Heart J 1981;102(Pt 1):1029-1037. III

62. Schoeppel SL, Wilkinson C, Waters J, Meyers SN: Effects of myocardial infarction on perioperative cardiac complications. Anesth Analg 1983;62:493-498. III

63. Shah KB, Kleinman BS, Sami H, et al: Reevaluation of perioperative myocardial infarction in patients with prior myocardial infarction undergoing noncardiac operations. Anesth Analg 1990;71:231-235. III

64. Moller AM, Villebro N, Pedersen T, Tonnesen H: Effect of preoperative smoking intervention on postoperative complications: A randomised clinical trial. Lancet 2002;359:114-117. II

65. Sorensen LT, Horby J, Friis E, et al: Smoking as a risk factor for wound healing and infection in breast cancer surgery. Eur J Surg Oncol 2002;28:815-820. III

66. de Cassia Braga Ribeiro K, Kowalski LP, Latorre Mdo R: Perioperative complications, comorbidities, and survival in oral or oropharyngeal cancer. Arch Otolaryngol Head Neck Surg 2003;129:219-228. III

67. Padubidri AN, Yetman R, Browne E, et al: Complications of postmastectomy breast reconstructions in smokers, ex-smokers, and nonsmokers. Plast Reconstr Surg 2001;107:342-349. III

68. Moore S, Mills BB, Moore RD, et al: Perisurgical smoking cessation and reduction of postoperative complications. Am J Obstet Gynecol 2005;192:1718-1721. III

69. Warner DO: Perioperative abstinence from cigarettes: Physiologic and clinical consequences. Anesthesiology 2006;104:356-3567. V

70. Kuri M, Nakagawa M, Tanaka H, et al: Determination of the duration of preoperative smoking cessation to improve wound healing after head and neck surgery. Anesthesiology 2005;102:892-896. III

71. Barrera R, Shi W, Amar D, et al: Smoking and timing of cessation: Impact on pulmonary complications after thoracotomy. Chest 2005;127:1977-1983. III

72. Bluman LG, Mosca L, Newman N, Simon DG: Preoperative smoking habits and postoperative pulmonary complications. Chest 1998;113:883-889. III

73. Warner MA, Offord KP, Warner ME, et al: Role of preoperative cessation of smoking and other factors in post operative pulmonary complications: A blinded prospective study of coronary artery bypass patients. Mayo Clin Proc 1989;64:609-616. III

74. O'Neil-Callahan K, Katsimaglis G, Tepper MR, et al: Statins decrease perioperative cardiac complications in patients undergoing noncardiac vascular surgery. J Am Coll Cardiol 2005;45:336-342. V

75. Furberg CD, Adams HP, Applegate WB, et al: and Asymptomatic Carotid Artery Progression Study (ACAPS) Research Group. Effect of lovastatin on early carotid atherosclerosis and cardiovascular events. Circulation 1994;90:1679-1687. II

76. Poldermans D, Bax JJ, Kertai MD, et al: Statins are associated with a reduced incidence ofperioperative mortality in patients undergoing major noncardiac vascular surgery. Circulation 2003;107:1848-1854. III

77. Ward RP, Leeper NJ, Kirkpatrick JN, et al: The effect of preoperative statin therapy on cardiovascular outcomes in patients undergoing infrainguinal vascular surgery. Int J Cardiol 2005;104:264-268. III

78. Kertai MD, Boersma E, Westerhout CM, et al: A combination of statins and beta-blockers is independently associated with a reduction in the incidence of perioperative mortality and nonfatal myocardial infarction in patients undergoing abdominal aortic aneurysm surgery. Eur J Vasc Endocasc Surg 2004;28:343-352. III

79. Lindenauer PK, Pekow P, Wang K, et al: Lipid-lowering therapy and in-hospital mortality following major noncardiac surgery. JAMA 2004;291:2092-2099. III

80. McGirt MJ, Perler BA, Brooke BS, et al: 3-Hydroxy-3-methylglutaryl coenzyme A reductase inhibitors reduce the risk of perioperative stroke and mortality after carotid endarterectomy. J Vasc Surg 2005;42:829-36; discussion 836-837. III

81. Kennedy J, Quan H, Buchan AM, et al: Statins are associated with better outcomes after carotid endarterectomy in symptomatic patients. Stroke 2005;36:2072-2076. III

82. Durazzo AE, Machado FS, Ikeoka DT, et al: Reduction in cardiovasscular eventsafter vascular surgery with atorvastin: A randomized trial. J Vasc Surg 2004;39:967-975. II

5

Other Topics in Cardiology Consultation

Deborah H. Kwon and Lee Goldberg

1. How does perioperative myocardial ischemia affect short-term and long-term mortality?

Search Date: February 2006

Search Strategy: PubMed, search for "perioperative myocardial ischemia" AND "mortality." Titles and abstracts were reviewed; relevant bibliographies were scanned. ACC/AHA guidelines were scanned for references.

Each year, approximately 50,000 patients undergoing elective noncardiac surgery have postoperative myocardial infarctions (MIs). The estimated perioperative mortality rate is 30% to 50% for these patients.[1]

Mangano and associates[2] prospectively studied 474 patients with coronary artery disease (CAD) or at high risk for CAD who underwent noncardiac surgery. Data were collected during hospitalization and for 6 to 24 months after the surgery. Eighty-three patients (18%) experienced postoperative cardiac events. Fifteen patients experienced cardiac death, MI, or unstable angina; 30 patients had congestive heart failure; and 38 patients experienced ventricular tachycardia. Postoperative ischemia was demonstrated in 41% and was associated with a 2.8-fold increase in all cardiac adverse events (95% CI: 1.6 to 4.9; $P < .0002$) and 9.2-fold increase in the odds of an ischemic event (95% CI: 2.0 to 42.0; $P < .004$).[2]

In a prospective cohort study, Mangano and colleagues[3] evaluated the 2-year cardiac prognosis for high-risk patients undergoing noncardiac operations. Cardiac death, MI, unstable angina, progressive angina requiring coronary artery bypass grafting (CABG) or angioplasty, and new unstable angina requiring hospitalization were the outcomes. Eleven percent of patients experienced cardiac complications. Twenty-four patients suffered cardiac death, 11 had nonfatal MIs, 6 developed progressive angina requiring CABG or percutaneous transluminal coronary angioplasty (PTCA), and 6 had new unstable angina requiring hospitalization. Patients who survived a postoperative MI had a 29-fold increase in the rate of subsequent cardiac complications within 6 months after surgery, a 15-fold increase within 1 year, and a 14-fold increase within 2 years (95% CI: 5.8-32; $P < .00001$).[3]

McFalls and coworkers[4] examined the effect of a perioperative MI on long-term mortality in patients who have undergone elective vascular surgery. For 4 years, the study followed 115 consecutive patients who underwent elective vascular procedures at a Veterans Affairs Medical Center. The 30-day postoperative mortality rate was 3%, the 1-year mortality rate was 19%, the 2-year mortality rate was 26%, the 3-year mortality rate was 35%, and the mortality rate at 4 years was 39%. Perioperative MI was only a marginally significant independent predictor of 1-year mortality ($P = .06$). Patients who demonstrated clinical indicators of symptomatic CAD and nonfatal perioperative MI (e.g., abnormal electrocardiogram [ECG], moderate to large size defect on exercise thallium perfusion, and left ventricular ejection fraction < 40%) were at risk for increased mortality in the first postoperative year. Forty-five patients died within 4 years after surgery. The causes of death were cardiac events (40%), cancer (18%), cerebrovascular events (13%), and peripheral vascular disease (11%). In this patient population, the need for non–abdominal aortic aneurysm (AAA) surgery was a stronger independent predictor at 4 years.[4] This study examined a very specific patient population undergoing vascular surgery, and these findings therefore may not be generalized to patients without vascular disease undergoing noncardiac, nonvascular operations.

In summary (Box 5-1), the current data demonstrate that postoperative myocardial ischemia is associated with decreased short- and long-term survival.

BOX 5-1. Summary Points

- Patients with coronary artery disease (CAD) or at high risk for CAD are at increased risk for postoperative cardiac events.

- Patients who have postoperative myocardial infarction (MI) have a substantially increased risk for another MI in the future.

- Postoperative myocardial ischemia is associated with decreased short- and long-term survival.

2. In a postoperative patient with myocardial infarction, what are the effects of aspirin, beta blockers, statins, ACE inhibitors, and clopidogrel on death and recurrent myocardial infarction?

Search Date: February 2006

Search Strategy: PubMed, search for "perioperative myocardial ischemia" AND "mortality." Titles and abstracts were reviewed; relevant bibliographies were scanned. ACC/AHA guidelines were scanned for references.

No studies have evaluated the use of aspirin, beta blockers, statins, angiotensin-converting enzyme (ACE) inhibitors, and clopidogrel specifically in noncardiac postoperative patients who have had an MI. We only found one study evaluating the safety of aspirin in this particular patient population. However, the data for the use of aspirin, beta blockers, statins, and ACE inhibitors are well established in patients after MI, and it is therefore reasonable to extrapolate a beneficial effect to patients with postoperative MIs.

One study examined the safety of using aspirin or other antiplatelet medications perioperatively in patients who underwent noncardiac surgery. Neilipovitz and colleagues[5] studied patients undergoing infrainguinal revascularization surgery. These patients are at risk for perioperative thrombotic complications. Although aspirin is known to decrease thrombotic events, it is often discontinued to avoid perioperative bleeding. These investigators used a decision analysis to determine whether aspirin should be discontinued before infrainguinal revascularization surgery. Two strategies were compared: aspirin cessation 2 weeks before surgery and aspirin continuation throughout the perioperative period. Clinical events examined included MI, thrombotic cerebrovascular accident, hemorrhagic cerebrovascular accident, gastrointestinal hemorrhage, and incisional hemorrhagic complications. The study evaluated perioperative mortality, life expectancy, and quality-adjusted life expectancy. According to the model, continued aspirin use decreased perioperative mortality rates from 2.78% to 2.05%. Because the study authors did not cite a *P* value or confidence intervals, it is difficult to evaluate the significance of this decrease in perioperative mortality rate.

Aspirin increased the number of hemorrhagic complications by 2.46%, but none was life threatening. This study was conducted in a very specific patient population undergoing vascular surgery, and the results therefore may not be generalized to other patient populations. It is recommended that only patients who are at high risk for developing postoperative ischemia and whose risk of perioperative bleeding is manageable should have aspirin therapy continued.

A meta-analysis questioned the beneficial effects of perioperative beta blockers in patients who have undergone noncardiac surgery.[6] However, it appeared that patients who were at high risk for perioperative MI benefited the most from perioperative beta blockade. Based on these findings and on the known effect of beta blockers in patients with acute coronary syndromes,[7-10] the early administration of beta blockers in patients with evidence of postoperative ischemia is indicated to improve short- and long-term outcomes (Box 5-2).

Box 5-2. **Summary Points**

- Patients who are at high risk for developing postoperative ischemia and whose risk of perioperative bleeding is manageable should have aspirin therapy continued.

- The early administration of beta blockers in patients with evidence of postoperative ischemia is indicated to improve short- and long-term outcomes.

3. How sensitive and specific are the cardiac enzymes troponin and creatinine kinase for the diagnosis of cardiac ischemia in the postoperative setting?

Search Date: February 2006

Search Strategy: PubMed, search for "perioperative myocardial ischemia" AND "creatinine kinase" OR "troponin." Titles and abstracts were reviewed; relevant bibliographies were scanned. ACC/AHA guidelines were scanned for references.

Lucreiziotti and colleagues[11] reviewed the main studies that have evaluated the sensitivity and specificity of cardiac troponins (i.e., troponin I and troponin T). One study compared the diagnostic role of troponins with other traditional modalities in 96 patients who underwent vascular surgery and 12 patients who underwent spinal surgery.[12] The diagnostic gold standard was segmental wall motion abnormality on echocardiography. The positive likelihood ratio for troponin I was 99, and that of the creatine kinase myocardial band isoenzyme (CK-MB) was 3.95. The negative likelihood ratios for troponin I and CK-MB were 0.01 and 0.31, respectively. These results suggest that an elevated troponin I level is much more likely to identify myocardial ischemia than an elevated CK-MB level. A normal troponin I level is more likely to rule out myocardial ischemia than a normal CK-MB level. In a patient with a high pretest probability, myocardial ischemia may still be present even if the patient has a normal CK-MB level.

The main limitation of this study is that a segmental wall motion abnormality on echocardiography is not an accepted gold standard for the diagnosis of an acute coronary syndrome. Although suggestive of ischemia, segmental wall motion abnormalities can be caused by other conditions, or they may be absent in small MIs.

In another study, CK, CK-MB, and cardiac troponin T were measured prospectively in 1175 patients undergoing elective or urgent major noncardiac surgery. Acute MI was diagnosed in 17 patients (1.4%) by a reviewer who was blinded to the troponin T data and who used CK-MB and electrocardiographic criteria to diagnose acute MI. However, because this article did not cite *P* values or confidence intervals, it is difficult to conclude from these data that an elevated cardiac troponin T level can predict major in-hospital cardiac complications.[13] The positive likelihood ratio and negative likelihood ratio of troponin T in this study were 4.6 and 0.15, respectively. This study suggests that, as seen for troponin I, troponin T has a high negative predictive value, suggesting that either troponin assay is reasonable to rule out a perioperative MI. However, the small number of MIs in this study makes it difficult to generalize the findings to a larger population.

We evaluated a study that looked at troponins I and T as biochemical markers of myocardial damage in 80 patients undergoing vascular or major orthopedic surgery. There were no associations between postoperative ischemia and cardiac protein concentrations. There were no significant associations between postoperative ischemia and cardiac protein concentrations. In this study, troponin T was the only prospective marker for both major and minor cardiovascular complications.

The previously mentioned studies have some contradictory results, and it is therefore uncertain whether the absence of postoperative elevations of troponin I or T correlates with fewer cardiovascular events. An elevation of these markers, although not always specific, warrants additional postoperative monitoring and investigation. Larger prospective studies that examine patients of differing preoperative risk, who are clinically suspected of having cardiac ischemia, are needed to definitively determine the usefulness of cardiac enzymes for the detection of myocardial ischemia in patients undergoing noncardiac operations (Table 5-1).

4. Does recent percutaneous coronary intervention reduce postoperative cardiac complications (PCI)?

Search Date: February 2006

Search Strategy: *PubMed, search for "perioperative complications" AND "revascularization" AND "noncardiac surgery." Titles and abstracts were reviewed; relevant bibliographies were scanned. ACC/AHA guidelines were scanned for references.*

Table 5-1. Diagnostic Power of Cardiac Enzymes for the Diagnosis of Myocardial Infarction in the Postoperative Setting

Study	No. of Patients	Prevalence of Enzyme Elevation	Gold Standard	Cardiac Enzyme	+LR	−LR	OR
Adams et al, 1994[12]	108	8%	Wall motion abnormality on postoperative echocardiogram	Trop I	4.6	0.15	17
Lee et al, 1996[13]	1175	6% (initial measurement) 17% (≥ 2 measurements)	CK-MB + ECG changes	Trop T	99	0.01	13.2
Neil et al, 2000[39]	80	21%	Holter ECG monitoring	CK-MB	3.95	0.31	5.64 CI: 1.07 to 31.00
		5%		Trop I	19	0.81	17 CI: 2.20 to 116.54
		7.5%		Trop T	28.5	0.71	13 CI: 1.26 to 252.88

CK-MB, isoenzyme of creatine kinase with muscle and brain subunits; ECG, electrocardiographic; +LR, positive likelihood ratio; −LR, negative likelihood ratio; OR, relative odds ratio for postoperative ischemia; Trop, troponin.

Although many clinicians believe that preoperative revascularization can reduce the risk of postoperative cardiovascular complications, a randomized, controlled trial cast doubt on this assumption. Patients who had an increased risk for perioperative cardiac complications or clinically significant CAD were randomized to undergo revascularization or no revascularization before elective major vascular surgery. The primary end point was long-term mortality. A total of 5859 patients scheduled for vascular operations at 18 Veterans Affairs Medical Centers were screened, and 510 (9%) met the criteria for the study and were randomly assigned to coronary artery revascularization before surgery or no revascularization before vascular surgery. Percutaneous coronary intervention (PCI) was performed in 59%, and bypass surgery was performed in 41%. At 2.7 years, the mortality rate for the revascularization group was 22%, and it was 23% in the no-revascularization group (relative risk [RR] = 0.98; 95% CI: 0.70 to 1.37; P = .92). The outer ends of the confidence interval suggest that revascularization in this population could reduce mortality by up to 30%, in which case we would consider it for everyone, or increase mortality by as much as 37%, in which case we would avoid it. Postoperative MI within 30 days of vascular surgery, defined by elevated troponin levels, occurred in 12% of the revascularization group and 14% of the no-revascularization group (P = .37). Unfortunately, this large trial was unable to determine the effect of preoperative PCI on mortality or postoperative MI.[14]

In a retrospective cohort study, Posner and associates[15] investigated the differences in the prevalence of adverse cardiac outcomes (i.e., death, MI, angina, congestive heart failure, malignant dysrhythmia, cardiogenic shock, coronary artery bypass graft, or PTCA) within 30 days after noncardiac surgery among patients with prior percutaneous transluminal coronary angioplasty (PTCA), patients with non-revascularized CAD, and normal controls. Patients with prior PTCA had a twofold increase in adverse cardiac outcomes compared with healthy patients after noncardiac surgery. However, patients with prior PTCA had one half of the risk of adverse cardiac outcomes compared with patients with untreated CAD. Patients with PTCA had a twofold increase in the risk of adverse cardiac outcome compared with normal controls (odds ratio [OR] = 1.98; $P < .001$), as well as an increase in risk of angina (OR = 7.84), congestive heart failure (OR = 2.06), and MI (OR = 3.86). However, these patients had a lower risk of death (OR = 0.46; $P < 0.001$). Patients with PTCA had 50% risk of adverse cardiac outcomes compared with patients with CAD (OR = 0.50; $P < .001$), decreased risk of angina (OR = 0.51), and congestive heart failure (OR = 0.40; $P < .001$), but there was no difference in MI ($P = .304$) or death ($P = .436$). No difference was found between 142 patients with recent PTCA ($\leq$ 90 days before noncardiac surgery) matched to patients with CAD (OR = 0.90; $P = .396$). Patients revascularized by PTCA more than 90 days before noncardiac surgery seem to have a lower risk of poor outcome than non-revascularized patients, although not as low as normal controls.[15] Results of this study suggest that patients who have had a PTCA more than 90 days preoperatively are at lower risk than those who have had recent PTCA and that both groups were at lower risk than those who had CAD but no PTCA. This study is limited by the fact it was retrospective and used case-matched controls, potentially introducing selection bias. This study also did not control for CAD severity, medical management, or comorbidities that may have affected the results.

TIMING OF NONCARDIAC SURGERY AFTER PCI

Two studies demonstrated that the timing of noncardiac surgery after coronary artery intervention could affect morbidity and mortality. The first study analyzed the clinical course of 40 patients who had undergone coronary stent placement less than 6 weeks before noncardiac surgery (range, 1 to 39 days; average, 13 days). In this case series, there were 7 MIs, 11 major bleeding episodes, and 8 deaths. All deaths and MIs, as well as 8 of 11 bleeding episodes, occurred in patients subjected to surgery fewer than 14 days from stenting. Four patients died after undergoing surgery 1 day after stenting. Stent thrombosis was thought to have accounted for most of the fatal events, based on electrocardiographic, enzymatic, and angiographic evidence.[16] Another observational study of 207 patients suggested that surgery should be delayed for 6 weeks after stent placement. Eight patients (4.0%) died or suffered a MI or stent thrombosis. All eight patients (4.8%; 95% CI: 2.1 to 9.2) underwent surgery within 6 weeks after stent placement. The frequency of these events ranged from 3.8% to 7.1% per week during each of the 6 weeks. No events occurred in the 39 patients who had surgery 7 to 9 weeks after stent placement.[17] These studies are retrospective and observational, but they suggest that postponing elective noncardiac surgery for at least 6 weeks after coronary stenting is recommended to permit completion of the mandatory antiplatelet regimen, allow for vessel and endothelial healing, and therefore reduce the risk of stent thrombosis and bleeding complications.

Gottlieb and colleagues[18] reviewed a vascular surgery database for patients who underwent vascular surgery preceded by PTCA without stenting between 1984 and 1995. PTCA was performed before surgery in 94 patients who underwent aortic abdominal surgery, carotid endarterectomy (CEA), or peripheral vascular surgery. A total of 104 (54%) had previous MIs. Twenty-six patients (13.4%) had perioperative cardiac morbidity. One patient had an MI (0.5%; 95% CI: 0.0 to 2.8). One patient (0.5%) died of congestive heart failure followed by multisystem organ failure. The median interval between PTCA and surgery was 11 days (interquartile range, 3 to 49 days). Patients who developed perioperative cardiac morbidity were older than those who did not ($P = .02$). Patients who had a history of CABG (before PTCA) had a higher incidence of postoperative angina ($P = .04$). The degree of preoperative left ventricular dysfunction was linearly related to the incidence of new postoperative congestive heart failure ($P = .01$). High-risk cardiac patients undergoing vascular surgery who have had PTCA performed up to 18 months preoperatively have a low incidence of perioperative cardiac morbidity. This study suggests that prophylactic PTCA without stenting may be beneficial in patients with CAD who are at high risk for perioperative cardiac complications.[18] This raises the question of whether patients who cannot wait for the minimum of 6 weeks after coronary intervention to have their vascular surgery should have PTCA without stenting to allow them to have vascular surgery. This study was retrospective and used case-matched controls. As in the previous studies, CAD severity, medical management, or comorbidities were not controlled for, which might have affected the results (Box 5-3).

Box 5-3. **Summary Points**

- A large, randomized, controlled trial could not determine the effect of coronary artery revascularization before elective vascular surgery on mortality.

- Two retrospective studies demonstrated that patients who have had percutaneous transluminal coronary angioplasty are at lower risk for postoperative adverse cardiac events than those with untreated coronary artery disease.

- Postponing elective noncardiac surgery for at least 6 weeks after coronary stenting is recommended to reduce the risk of stent thrombosis and bleeding complications.

5. How sensitive and specific are electrocardiographic changes for diagnosing postoperative cardiac ischemia?

Search Date: February 2006

Search Strategy: *PubMed, search for "perioperative myocardial ischemia" AND "electrocardiogram." Titles and abstracts were reviewed; relevant bibliographies were scanned. ACC/AHA guidelines were scanned for references.*

Only one study[19] has examined the accuracy of ECG alone in the diagnosis of myocardial ischemia in the postoperative patient. The investigators examined the ability of intermittent 12-lead ECG recordings to identify perioperative myocardial ischemia and subsequent myocardial cell damage in 55 vascular surgery patients at risk for or with a history of CAD. Twelve-lead ECG recordings were taken preoperatively and at 15 minutes, 20 hours, 48 hours, 72 hours, and 84 hours postoperatively. The sensitivity of the 12-lead ECG to detect myocardial ischemia was compared with continuous 3-channel Holter monitoring and serial creatine kinase myocardial band isoenzyme (CK-MB) and cardiac troponins T and I. Elevations of cardiac enzyme levels presumably were used to define the presence of myocardial ischemia. The incidence of perioperative myocardial ischemia detected by 12-lead ECG was 44% and was identifiable in most patients (88%) 15 minutes after surgery. The incidence of perioperative myocardial ischemia detected by continuous monitoring was 53%. The concordance of the 12-lead method with continuous monitoring was 72%. The concordance of CK-MB with 12-lead ECG recordings was 75%, and the corresponding value for Holter monitoring was 68%. The concordance of cardiac troponin T and I levels with the 12-lead method was 85% and 87%, respectively, and concordance with Holter monitoring was 72% and 66%, respectively.[19] It was unclear how these percentages were obtained, and it was therefore difficult to assess the sensitivity and specificity of ECG changes. Results of this study suggest that postoperative 12-lead ECG can identify perioperative myocardial ischemia in most patients undergoing vascular surgery but that combining this modality with cardiac enzymes can improve the sensitivity and specificity of either approach alone (Box 5-4).

Box 5-4. **Summary Point**
- A postoperative 12-lead electrocardiogram can identify perioperative myocardial ischemia in most patients, but cardiac enzyme determinations should also be obtained.

---

6. Does cardiac catheterization after a postoperative ischemic event improve mortality and reduce recurrent myocardial infarction?

Search Date: February 2006

Search Strategy: *PubMed, search for "perioperative myocardial ischemia" AND "cardiac catheterization." Titles and abstracts were reviewed; relevant bibliographies were scanned. ACC/AHA guidelines were scanned for references.*

No clinical trials have specifically examined the efficacy of coronary angiography for postoperative acute coronary syndromes, probably because of the need for antithrombotic agents during and after the procedure. Clinical practice has evolved such that patients with an obvious perioperative MI that leads to hemodynamic or electrical instability are likely to be evaluated for emergent PTCA. In this very-high-risk population, the risks of mandatory anticoagulants and antiplatelet agents to perform the PTCA need to be balanced against the risks of major postoperative bleeding and other complications. For these reasons, it may be difficult to conduct a clinical trial to evaluate the role of postoperative acute ischemic events. Most clinicians consider a perioperative ischemic event as equivalent to a positive stress test, and once the postoperative issues have resolved, these patients should be evaluated and managed like any others with a positive stress test result.

7. Does postoperative heart failure increase mortality?

Search Date: February 2006

Search Strategy: *PubMed, search for "postoperative heart failure" AND "mortality." Titles and abstracts were reviewed; relevant bibliographies were scanned. ACC/AHA guidelines were scanned for references.*

Postoperative heart failure identifies patients with limited cardiac reserve in the setting of physiologic stress. Mangano and coworkers[3] prospectively studied 474 patients with CAD or at high risk for CAD who underwent noncardiac surgery. This group gathered data during hospitalization and for 6 to 24 months after the surgery. Eighty-three patients (18%) experienced postoperative cardiac events: 15 patients experienced cardiac death, MI, or unstable angina; 30 patients had congestive heart failure; and 38 patients had ventricular tachycardia. In a multivariate analysis evaluating postoperative heart failure, there was no association with long-term adverse outcomes when controlling for other risk factors.[3]

Many clinicians consider the presence of perioperative heart failure as an indication that the patient will require future evaluation and management after recovery from surgery.

8. Is it safe to use perioperative beta blockers in a patient who has heart failure and has never used beta blockers before?

Search Date: February 2006

Search Strategy: PubMed, search for "perioperative myocardial ischemia" AND "beta blockers" AND "heart failure." Titles and abstracts were reviewed; relevant bibliographies were scanned. ACC/AHA guidelines were scanned for references.

Several randomized, controlled trials have shown that beta-blocker therapy in the perioperative setting decreases perioperative mortality and the incidence of MI in patients at high risk for cardiac events. However, there were only 30 patients with heart failure in these trials.[20-24] We did not find any studies addressing the safety of using beta blockers perioperatively in patients with heart failure who had not been on beta-blocker therapy previously. However, we found one study addressing the use of beta blockers perioperatively in patients diagnosed with chronic heart failure. This group of investigators studied the data of the CIBIS II study. They analyzed the effect of bisoprolol on perioperative outcome in patients with moderate to severe heart failure. A total of 2647 patients with New York Heart Association (NYHA) class III or IV heart failure (see Chapter 1, Table 1-2) and left ventricular ejection fraction equal to or greater than 35% were randomized to bisoprolol or placebo. Of these patients, 165 underwent surgery (bisoprolol, $n = 87$; placebo, $n = 78$). Bisoprolol did not significantly decrease mortality in patients undergoing surgery, placebo-treated group compared with the bisoprolol-treated group (7.7% versus 5.8%; $P = .76$). Bisoprolol also did not significantly affect postoperative hospital readmission (placebo, 24.4%; bisoprolol, 34.5%; $P = .17$) or time to postoperative hospital admission (placebo, ≥ 30 days, $n = 2$; 31 to 180 days,

$n = 11$; > 180 days, $n = 6$; bisoprolol, $n = 9/10/11$; $P = .14$).[4] This study was a subgroup analysis, and the results therefore may not hold true in a randomized, controlled study powered to look specifically at patients with heart failure receiving beta-blocker therapy. The small sample size and low incidence of deaths also make these results hard to interpret. A randomized, controlled trial of perioperative beta-blocker treatment in heart failure patients is necessary to validate this observation.

Despite the lack of direct data for the use of perioperative beta blockade in heart failure, the current ACC/AHA heart failure guidelines recommend the use of beta blockade in all patients who have systolic dysfunction.[24] In heart failure, beta blockers have been shown to decrease morbidity and mortality. As for all cases of systolic heart failure, beta blockers should be administered initially at a low dose to a patient who is hemodynamically stable and not exhibiting signs or symptoms of volume overload. If possible, preoperative initiation to assess tolerability is preferred. After beta blockers are initiated, abrupt withdrawal should be avoided because this has been associated with adverse events, including MI, arrhythmia, and death (Box 5-5).

Box 5-5. **Summary Points**

- There are few direct data to support the administration of perioperative beta blockers to patients with systolic dysfunction.

- Patients with known ischemic cardiomyopathy are at high risk for postoperative cardiac events and should be considered for perioperative beta-blocker therapy.*

See Chapter 4 for further information about the use of perioperative beta blockers.

---

9. Do intraoperative pulmonary artery catheters reduce mortality and improve outcomes for surgical patients with coronary artery disease or heart failure?

Search Date: February 2006

Search Strategy: PubMed, search for "noncardiac surgery" AND "pulmonary catheter." Titles and abstracts were reviewed; relevant bibliographies were scanned. ACC/AHA guidelines were scanned for references.

Several randomized, controlled studies have evaluated the role of pulmonary catheters in patients undergoing noncardiac surgery.[25-28] All of these trials show no significant reduction of adverse events in patients with pulmonary catheters.

A group of investigators examined 4059 patients who underwent noncardiac surgery. Of these patients, 221 had right heart catheterizations (RHCs). Major cardiac events (i.e., MI, unstable angina, cardiogenic pulmonary edema, ventricular fibrillation or tachycardia, cardiac arrest, and sustained complete heart block) occurred in 171 patients. RHC seemed to be associated with a threefold increase in major cardiac events (34 [15.4%] versus 137 [3.6%]; $P < .001$). The adjusted odds ratios for cardiac and noncardiac events in patients with RHCs were 2.0 (95% CI: 1.3 to 3.2) and 2.1 (95% CI: 1.2 to 3.5), respectively. The investigators also matched the patients who underwent RHC with patients in this study with similar propensity for RHC and type of procedure. This study demonstrates that patients with RHC had an increased risk of postoperative congestive heart failure (OR = 2.9; 95% CI: 1.4 to 6.2) and major noncardiac events (OR = 2.2; 95% CI: 1.4 to 4.9).[29] Because this was an observational study, selection bias cannot be ruled out.

The ACC/AHA guidelines suggest that although very few studies have analyzed patient outcomes after treatment with or without pulmonary artery catheters, the benefit-risk profile of pulmonary artery catheter use should be determined by the severity of cardiac disease, the extent of anticipated surgery, and the setting in which the patient is being monitored.[30] Patients most likely to benefit from perioperative use of a pulmonary artery catheter are those with a recent MI resulting in heart failure, patients with significant CAD undergoing surgical interventions associated with significant hemodynamic stress, and patients with systolic or diastolic left ventricular dysfunction, cardiomyopathy, or valvular disease undergoing high-risk operations (Box 5-6).[10]

Box 5-6. **Summary Points**

- There have been no randomized, controlled trials to determine the safety of using pulmonary catheters for hemodynamic monitoring in patients undergoing non-cardiac surgery.

- One observational study suggests that pulmonary catheters are associated with an increased risk for adverse events, but selection bias cannot be ruled out.

10. Does cardioversion of postoperative atrial fibrillation decrease the risk of recurrent atrial fibrillation, stroke, morbidity, or mortality?

Search Date: February 2006

Search Strategy: *PubMed, search for "postoperative" AND "atrial fibrillation" AND "mortality" AND "cardioversion." Titles and abstracts were reviewed; relevant bibliographies were scanned. ACC/AHA guidelines were scanned for references.*

For those in whom the atrial fibrillation is well tolerated, there is a paucity of randomized, controlled studies evaluating the effect of rate control versus rhythm control in this group of patients. A few retrospective studies have suggested that rate control may be equivalent to restoring sinus rhythm. We did not come across any studies specifically evaluating patients undergoing noncardiac surgery. We also did not find any studies that analyzed the effect of restoring sinus rhythm on stroke risk in this patient population.

Lee and coworkers[31] randomized patients with atrial fibrillation after cardiac surgery to rate control or to rhythm control. Fifty patients with atrial fibrillation after heart surgery were randomized to antiarrhythmic therapy with or without electrical cardioversion or to ventricular rate control. Both groups received anticoagulation. The primary end point was time to conversion to sinus rhythm. Recurrence of atrial fibrillation was followed over a 2-month period. In this study, there was no significant difference between an antiarrhythmic-conversion strategy ($n = 27$) and a rate-control strategy ($n = 23$) or time to conversion to sinus rhythm (11.2 ± 3.2 versus

11.8 ± 3.9 hours; P = .8). The investigators used a Cox multivariate analysis to control for the effects of age, sex, beta-blocker usage, and type of surgery. The antiarrhythmic strategy showed a trend toward reducing the time from treatment to restoration of sinus rhythm (P = .08). The length of hospital stay was reduced in the antiarrhythmic arm compared with the rate-control strategy (9.0 ± 0.7 versus 13.2 ± 2.0 days; P = .05). In-hospital relapse rates in the antiarrhythmic arm were 30% compared with 57% in the rate-control arm (P = .24). There were no significant differences in relapse rates at 1 week (24% versus 28%), 4 weeks (6% versus 12%), and 6 to 8 weeks (4% versus 9%). At the end of the study, 91% of the patients in the rate-control arm were in sinus rhythm, compared with 96% in the antiarrhythmic arm (P = .6). This was a small pilot study that demonstrated no difference between a rate-control strategy and a strategy to restore sinus rhythm. In both treatment arms, most patients remained in sinus rhythm after 2 months. A larger randomized, controlled study is needed to assess the impact of restoration of sinus rhythm on length of stay.

SUGGESTED MANAGEMENT OF POST-OPERATIVE ATRIAL FIBRILLATION

Atrial fibrillation is a common postoperative complication in patients with a history of cardiovascular disease. Risk factors for the development of postoperative atrial fibrillation include prior history of atrial fibrillation, CAD, valvular heart disease, hypertension, and pulmonary disease. Thoracic surgery also increases the risk. New atrial fibrillation in a postoperative patient should trigger an evaluation to rule out coronary ischemia or a new pulmonary process, including pneumonia or pulmonary embolus.

Atrial fibrillation after cardiac surgery is associated with an increased risk for stroke, morbidity, and mortality.[32] We believe that this increased risk also applies to patients following noncardiac surgery. There are two clinical challenges: rate control and anticoagulation. The risk-benefit ratio for anticoagulation in this postoperative group of patients needs to be carefully evaluated based on the specific surgery, postoperative time, and other comorbidities. In patients who are hemodynamically unstable, have ischemia, or cannot be safely anticoagulated, urgent cardioversion should be considered.

The current practice in treating postoperative cardiac surgery patients with atrial fibrillation is to attempt restoration of sinus rhythm within 48 hours by means of electric direct cardioversion or antiarrhythmic therapy. Although there are no definitive data regarding the duration of antiarrhythmic drug and anticoagulation therapy, most centers continue antiarrhythmic therapy for 4 to 6 weeks after surgery.[33] There are no studies looking specifically at atrial fibrillation after noncardiac surgery, and physicians can only extrapolate the data gathered from cardiac patients to apply to noncardiac postoperative patients (Box 5-7).

Box 5-7. **Summary Points**

- There are no studies evaluating atrial fibrillation in patients who have undergone noncardiac surgery.

- Patients who are hemodynamically unstable, experience coronary ischemia, cannot be adequately rate controlled, or cannot be anticoagulated should be urgently cardioverted.

- In stable patients, current practice guidelines recommend restoring sinus rhythm within 48 hours by direct cardioversion or antiarrhythmic therapy to avoid the need for long-term anticoagulation.

- Current practice guidelines recommend the use of antiarrhythmic therapy for 4 to 6 weeks after surgery.

---

11. Should patients with postoperative atrial fibrillation be anticoagulated?

Search Date: February 2006

Search Strategy: *PubMed, search for "postoperative atrial fibrillation" AND "stroke" AND "anticoagulation." Titles and abstracts were reviewed; relevant bibliographies were scanned. ACC/AHA guidelines were scanned for references.*

No clinical trials have specifically studied the risk of stroke in patients with postoperative atrial fibrillation.

However, the large body of data for anticoagulating patients with new-onset atrial fibrillation can be reasonably extrapolated to postoperative patients.

The risk of stroke in patients with atrial fibrillation is increased if the patient has cardiovascular disease.[34] The use of oral anticoagulation therapy with warfarin or aspirin, or both, for patients with sustained atrial fibrillation and one of these comorbidities has been well studied.[34-37] The type of anticoagulation therapy should be based on the patients risk for developing a left atrial thrombus, which is outlined in Table 5-2.[34] Patients at low risk for thromboembolism can be treated with aspirin alone. For high-risk patients, warfarin is recommended. The treatment strategy for intermediate-risk patients is controversial and depends on the risks and benefits of therapy. In patients with chronic atrial fibrillation, anticoagulation therapy with warfarin recommended if no contraindications exist. This recommendation also can be applied to patients with postoperative atrial fibrillation and those in whom atrial fibrillation is thought likely to persist postoperatively.

The current guidelines recommend that if atrial fibrillation persists for 48 hours, patients should receive heparin and warfarin to achieve an international normalized ratio of 2.0 to 3.0 as recommended for nonoperative patients.[34] If the patient is at risk for bleeding with heparin, warfarin therapy can be started alone. No studies have been performed to determine the duration of anticoagulation therapy. If the patient has a risk for bleeding, anticoagulation therapy can be stopped if normal sinus rhythm returns. Anticoagulation should be continued for 1 month after sinus rhythm has been restored, because studies have demonstrated that impaired atrial contraction can persist for several weeks after the restoration of sinus rhythm (Box 5-8).

12. What is the prognostic significance of postoperative, nonsustained ventricular tachycardia? Is it a predictor of cardiac ischemia or mortality?

Search Date: February 2006

Search Strategy: *PubMed, search for "noncardiac surgery" AND "ventricular tachycardia." Titles and*

Table 5-2. Risk Stratification Schemes for Primary Prevention of Thromboembolism in Patients with Nonvalvular Atrial Fibrillation

Source	High Risk	Intermediate Risk	Low Risk
Atrial Fibrillation Investigators (1994)	Age ≥ 65 yr, history of hypertension, coronary artery disease, and diabetes	Age ≥ 65 yr, history of hypertension, coronary artery disease, and diabetes	Age < 65 yr and no high-risk features
American College of Chest Physicians (1998)	Age > 75 yr, history of hypertension, left ventricular dysfunction, > 1 intermediate risk factor	Age 65-75 yr, diabetes, coronary artery disease, or thyrotoxicosis	Age < 65 yr and no risk factors
Stroke Prevention in Atrial Fibrillation (1995)	Women > 75 yr, systolic blood pressure > 160 mm Hg, left ventricular dysfunction	History of hypertension and no high-risk features	No high-risk factors and no history of hypertension

Adapted from Fuster V, Ryden LE, Asinger RW, et al: ACC/AHA/ESC guidelines for the management of patients with atrial fibrillation: executive summary: A report of the American College of Cardiology/American Heart Association Task Force on Practice Guidelines and the European Society of Cardiology Committee for Practice Guidelines and Policy Conferences (Committee to Develop Guidelines for the Management of Patients with Atrial Fibrillation), developed in collaboration with the North American Society of Pacing and Electrophysiology. J Am Coll Cardiol 2001;38:1231-1266.

> **Box 5-8. Summary Points**
>
> - There are no studies evaluating anticoagulating patients with atrial fibrillation after noncardiac surgery.
> - Current guidelines suggest anticoagulating patients who have remained in atrial fibrillation for more than 48 hours.
> - Anticoagulation should be continued for 1 month after the restoration of sinus rhythm if possible.

abstracts were reviewed; relevant bibliographies were scanned. ACC/AHA guidelines were scanned for references.

Mangano and colleagues[3] prospectively studied 474 patients with CAD or at high risk for CAD who underwent noncardiac surgery. This group gathered data during hospitalization and for 6 to 24 months after surgery. Eighty-three patients (18%) experienced postoperative cardiac events: 15 patients experienced cardiac death, MI, or unstable angina, 30 patients had congestive heart failure, and 38 patients experienced ventricular tachycardia. Multivariate analysis did not demonstrate an association with long-term adverse outcomes in patients who experienced ventricular tachycardia that was determined to be nonischemic in origin.[3]

Amar and colleagues[38] examined 412 patients undergoing noncardiac thoracic surgery. These patients underwent lobectomy or pneumonectomy and were monitored with Holter recorders for 72 to 96 hours. Sixty-one patients (15%) experienced ventricular tachycardia (defined as three or more wide complexes); all episodes lasted less than 30 seconds. It was not clear how long these patients were followed. Ventricular tachycardia was not associated with adverse outcomes in the postoperative period.[38]

Nonsustained ventricular tachycardia (NSVT) may be a marker of coronary ischemia, electrolyte abnormalities, drug effects, or hypoxia. Clinicians should rapidly evaluate postoperative patients who develop NSVT for these conditions (Box 5-9).

Box 5-9. Summary Points

- Episodes of ventricular tachycardia that are not sustained and are not of ischemic origin are not associated with poor outcomes for patients who have undergone noncardiac surgery.

- Reversible causes of ventricular ectopy should be urgently evaluated, including coronary ischemia, electrolyte abnormalities, drug effects, and hypoxia.

REFERENCES

1. Mangano DT: Perioperative cardiac morbidity. Anesthesiology 1990;72:153-184. III

2. Mangano DT, Browner WS, Hollenberg M, et al: Association of perioperative myocardial ischemia with cardiac morbidity and mortality in men undergoing noncardiac surgery. The Study of Perioperative Ischemia Research Group. N Engl J Med 1990;323:1781-1788. III

3. Mangano DT, Browner WS, Hollenberg M, et al: Long-term cardiac prognosis following noncardiac surgery. The Study of Perioperative Ischemia Research Group. JAMA 1992;268:233-239. III

4. McFalls EO, Ward HB, Santilli S, et al: The influence of perioperative myocardial infarction on long-term prognosis following elective vascular surgery. Chest 1998;113: 681-686. III

5. Neilipovitz DT, Bryson GL, Nichol G: The effect of perioperative aspirin therapy in peripheral vascular surgery: A decision analysis. Anesth Analg 2001;93:573-580. III

6. Devereaux PJ, Beattie WS, Choi PT, et al: How strong is the evidence for the use of perioperative beta blockers in non-cardiac surgery? Systematic review and meta-analysis of randomised controlled trials. BMJ 2005;331: 313-321. I

7. Bertrand ME, Simoons ML, Fox KA, et al: Management of acute coronary syndromes in patients presenting without persistent ST-segment elevation. Eur Heart J 2002;23:1809-1840. IV

8. Ryan TJ, Anderson JL, Antman EM, et al: ACC/AHA guidelines for the management of patients with acute myocardial infarction: Executive summary. A report of the American College of Cardiology/American Heart Association Task Force on Practice Guidelines (Committee on Management

of Acute Myocardial Infarction). Circulation 1996;94: 2341-2350. IV

9. Ryan TJ, Antman EM, Brooks NH, et al: 1999 update: ACC/AHA Guidelines for the Management of Patients with Acute Myocardial Infarction: Executive Summary and Recommendations: A report of the American College of Cardiology/American Heart Association Task Force on Practice Guidelines (Committee on Management of Acute Myocardial Infarction). Circulation 1999;100: 1016-1030. IV

10. Eagle KA, Berger PB, Calkins H, et al: ACC/AHA guideline update for perioperative cardiovascular evaluation for noncardiac surgery—Executive summary: A report of the American College of Cardiology/American Heart Association Task Force on Practice Guidelines (Committee to Update the 1996 Guidelines on Perioperative Cardiovascular Evaluation for Noncardiac Surgery). J Am Coll Cardiol 2002;39:542-553. IV

11. Lucreziotti S, Foroni C, Fiorentini C. Perioperative myocardial infarction in noncardiac surgery: The diagnostic and prognostic role of cardiac troponins. J Intern Med 2002;252:11-20. I

12. Adams JE 3rd, Sicard GA, Allen BT, et al: Diagnosis of perioperative myocardial infarction with measurement of cardiac troponin I. N Engl J Med 1994;330:670-674. III

13. Lee TH, Thomas EJ, Ludwig LE, et al: Troponin T as a marker for myocardial ischemia in patients undergoing major noncardiac surgery. Am J Cardiol 1996;77: 1031-1036. III

14. McFalls EO, Ward HB, Moritz TE, et al: Coronary-artery revascularization before elective major vascular surgery. N Engl J Med 2004;351:2795-2804. II

15. Posner KL, Van Norman GA, Chan V: Adverse cardiac outcomes after noncardiac surgery in patients with prior percutaneous transluminal coronary angioplasty. Anesth Analg 1999;89:553-560. III

16. Kaluza GL, Joseph J, Lee JR, et al: Catastrophic outcomes of noncardiac surgery soon after coronary stenting. J Am Coll Cardiol 2000;35:1288-1294. IV

17. Wilson SH, Fasseas P, Orford JL, et al: Clinical outcome of patients undergoing non-cardiac surgery in the two months following coronary stenting. J Am Coll Cardiol 2003;42:234-240. IV

18. Gottlieb A, Banoub M, Sprung J, et al: Perioperative cardiovascular morbidity in patients with coronary artery disease undergoing vascular surgery after percutaneous

transluminal coronary angioplasty. J Cardiothorac Vasc Anesth 1998;12:501-506. **III**

19. Bottiger BW, Motsch J, Teschendorf P, et al: Postoperative 12-lead ECG predicts peri-operative myocardial ischaemia associated with myocardial cell damage. Anaesthesia 2004;59:1083-1090. **III**

20. Raby KE, Brull SJ, Timimi F, et al: The effect of heart rate control on myocardial ischemia among high-risk patients after vascular surgery. Anesth Analg 1999;88: 477-482. **II**

21. Mangano DT, Layug EL, Wallace A, Tateo I: Effect of atenolol on mortality and cardiovascular morbidity after noncardiac surgery. Multicenter Study of Perioperative Ischemia Research Group. N Engl J Med 1996;335: 1713-1720. **II**

22. Poldermans D, Boersma E, Bax JJ, et al: The effect of biso-prolol on perioperative mortality and myocardial infarc-tion in high-risk patients undergoing vascular surgery. Dutch Echocardiographic Cardiac Risk Evaluation Applying Stress Echocardiography Study Group. N Engl J Med 1999;341:1789-1794. **II**

23. Bohm M, Maack C, Wehrlen-Grandjean M, Erdmann E: Effect of bisoprolol on perioperative complications in chronic heart failure after surgery (Cardiac Insufficiency Bisoprolol Study II [CIBIS II]). Z Kardiol 2003;92:668-676. **II**

24. Hunt SA, Abraham WT, Chin MH, et al: ACC/AHA 2005 guideline update for the diagnosis and management of chronic heart failure in the adult: A report of the American College of Cardiology/American Heart Association Task Force on Practice Guidelines (Writing Committee to Update the 2001 Guidelines for the Evaluation and Management of Heart Failure): Developed in collaboration with the American College of Chest Physicians and the International Society for Heart and Lung Transplantation: Endorsed by the Heart Rhythm Society. Circulation 2005;112:e154-e253. **IV**

25. Joyce WP, Provan JL, Ameli FM, et al: The role of central haemodynamic monitoring in abdominal aortic surgery. A prospective randomised study. Eur J Vasc Surg 1990;4: 633-636. **II**

26. Ziegler DW, Wright JG, Choban PS, Flancbaum L: A prospective randomized trial of preoperative "optimization" of cardiac function in patients undergoing elective peripheral vascular surgery. Surgery 1997;122:584-592. **II**

27. Bender JS, Smith-Meek MA, Jones CE: Routine pulmonary artery catheterization does not reduce morbidity and mortality of elective vascular surgery: Results of a prospective, randomized trial. Ann Surg 1997;226: 229-236; discussion 236-237. II

28. Valentine RJ, Duke ML, Inman MH, et al: Effectiveness of pulmonary artery catheters in aortic surgery: a randomized trial. J Vasc Surg 1998;27:203-211; discussion 211-212. II

29. Polanczyk CA, Rohde LE, Goldman L, et al: Right heart catheterization and cardiac complications in patients undergoing noncardiac surgery: an observational study. JAMA 2001;286:309-314. III

30. Practice guidelines for pulmonary artery catheterization. A report by the American Society of Anesthesiologists Task Force on Pulmonary Artery Catheterization. Anesthesiology 1993;78:380-394. IV

31. Lee JK, Klein GJ, Krahn AD, et al: Rate-control versus conversion strategy in postoperative atrial fibrillation: A prospective, randomized pilot study. Am Heart J 2000;140:871-877. III

32. Hogue CW Jr, Hyder ML: Atrial fibrillation after cardiac operation: Risks, mechanisms, and treatment. Ann Thorac Surg 2000;69:300-306. III

33. Martinez EA, Bass EB, Zimetbaum P: Pharmacologic control of rhythm: American College of Chest Physicians guidelines for the prevention and management of postoperative atrial fibrillation after cardiac surgery. Chest 2005;128:48S-55S. IV

34. Fuster V, Ryden LE, Asinger RW, et al: ACC/AHA/ESC guidelines for the management of patients with atrial fibrillation: Executive summary. A Report of the American College of Cardiology/American Heart Association Task Force on Practice Guidelines and the European Society of Cardiology Committee for Practice Guidelines and Policy Conferences (Committee to Develop Guidelines for the Management of Patients with Atrial Fibrillation), developed in collaboration with the North American Society of Pacing and Electrophysiology. J Am Coll Cardiol 2001;38:1231-1266. IV

35. Hirsh J, Dalen J, Guyatt G: The sixth (2000) ACCP guidelines for antithrombotic therapy for prevention and treatment of thrombosis. American College of Chest Physicians. Chest 2001;119:1S-2S. IV

36. Hart RG, Benavente O, McBride R, Pearce LA: Antithrombotic therapy to prevent stroke in patients with

atrial fibrillation: A meta-analysis. Ann Intern Med 1999;131:492-501. **I**

37. Pearce LA, Hart RG, Halperin JL: Assessment of three schemes for stratifying stroke risk in patients with nonvalvular atrial fibrillation. Am J Med 2000;109:45-51. **III**

38. Amar D, Zhang H, Roistacher N: The incidence and outcome of ventricular arrhythmias after noncardiac thoracic surgery. Anesth Analg 2002;95:537-543. **III**

39. Neill F, Sear JW, French G, et al. Increases in serum concentrations of cardiac proteins and the prediction of early postoperative cardiovascular complications in noncardiac surgery patients. Anaesthesia 2000;55:641-647.

6

Prevention of Venous Thromboembolism in the Surgical Patient

Matthew L. Ortman
and Todd E. H. Hecht

1. What is the background of thromboprophylaxis in the surgical patient?

Thromboprophylaxis in the surgical patient has long been recognized as an effective intervention to reduce the incidence of deep venous thrombosis (DVT) and pulmonary embolism (PE), collectively referred to as venous thromboembolism (VTE). Existing guidelines are somewhat contradictory,[1-3] and physician compliance has traditionally been poor.[4]

Many factors contribute to the lack of uniformity in VTE thromboprophylaxis, but primary among them has been the lack of consensus regarding which clinically relevant end points should be used as a surrogate marker for efficacy. Effective thromboprophylaxis is ultimately a balance between efficacy and safety, and many surgeons question the necessity of preventing a potentially asymptomatic and clinically irrelevant event at the cost of increased risk of bleeding. The low incidence of PE makes it difficult to identify a statistically significant risk reduction short of performing a prospective trial involving thousand of patients, which for logistical and technical reasons is often implausible. Prospective studies commonly use as their end point venographically identified DVT or a composite end point of symptomatic DVT, asymptomatic proximal DVT, and PE. This has often been a point of contention among surgeons, who argue that asymptomatic, distal DVT would remain clinically silent regardless of thromboprophylaxis.

There are fundamental problems with the consistency of study design. With improvements in surgical and anesthetic techniques, the rate of VTE has declined steadily and significantly over the past several decades,[5,6] placing the relevance of older studies into question. Multiple options exist for thromboprophylaxis, and for each drug or device, there are more options for dosing, timing, and duration, resulting in hundreds of possible permutations for study design. There are also variations in the timing and use of diagnostic modalities. Trials that use screening venography generally report higher incidences of DVT than those that use less-sensitive modalities, such as fibrinogen uptake scanning (FUS), impedance plethysmography, and ultrasonography, likely due to the nonocclusive nature of the postoperative DVT.[7-9] Such noninvasive modalities systematically underestimate the treatment effect of a particular intervention.[10] Studies that rely exclusively on unilateral rather than bilateral venography may suffer from similar bias.[11] Because of the low incidence of PE, meta-analysis is a potentially powerful means of achieving the necessary power to establish a statistically meaningful reduction of risk, but this, too, is not without limitations. A meta-analysis of orthopedic meta-analyses found that less than one half rely exclusively on randomized, controlled studies and that meta-analyses with lower scores of quality more often report positive findings.[12]

This chapter attempts to elucidate the overwhelming volume of research that exists, using existing consensus statement guidelines, randomized trials, meta-analyses, review articles, and editorials from medical and surgical journals. Whereas other chapters in this handbook are structured around a reproducible literature search, we have, for reasons of practicality and necessity, relied on the exhaustive bibliography of the Seventh American College of Chest Physicians (ACCP) Conference on Antithrombotic and Thrombolytic Therapy. We also have performed independent literature searches to identify articles that may have followed the release of the September 2004 ACCP guidelines. For each major category of surgery, we review the existing recommendations of the major consensus guidelines and supplement them with a review of the major studies, meta-analyses, and review articles that exist for each subject. Commentary about the grades of recommendation for the ACCP guidelines can be found elsewhere.[13] We specifically address the optimal timing, duration, and choice of prophylaxis based on existing evidence and recommendations. At the conclusion of each section, we provide our own recommendations. As is always the case, no guideline can account for every conceivable clinical situation, and the choice of thromboprophylaxis must be tailored to the objectives of physician and patient.

2. What is the significance of thromboembolism in the surgical patient?

The clinical and economic significance of VTE encompasses issues of morbidity and mortality. The association of asymptomatic DVT with PE is clear,[14] and fatal PE can be the initial sign of VTE in surgical patients.[15] Although small distal thrombi in the calves incur less risk, studies have suggested that these thrombi, if left untreated, propagate to the proximal thigh in as many as 20% of cases[16] and are associated with a 30% rate of recurrent DVT or PE in 3 months.[17]

The post-thrombotic syndrome is a syndrome involving pain, swelling, claudication, and ulceration of the affected leg, the mechanism of which may involve valvular destruction, venous hypertension, and venous reflux.[18] These symptoms most commonly manifest within 1 year after development of VTE. The true prevalence of the disorder is unknown, but a meta-analysis by Wille-Jorgensen and colleagues comprising seven studies of more than 1500 patients calculated a statistically significant, relative risk increase of post-thrombotic syndrome of 158% (95% CI: 124 to 202) in patients with untreated, asymptomatic, postoperative DVT followed over 2 to 10 years.[19] One consensus guideline suggests an incidence of 34% to 69% at 3 years and 49% to 100% at 5 to 10 years, depending on the size and distribution of the thrombus.[3]

3. What is the frequency of deep venous thrombosis and pulmonary embolism in surgical populations?

The frequency of DVT varies considerably among surgical populations, ranging from 15% to 40% among general surgical, gynecologic, urologic, and neurosurgical patients to as high as 40% to 80% among trauma patients and patients undergoing hip or knee arthroplasty, repair of hip fracture, or spinal cord surgery.[1] These estimates are based on objective tests of asymptomatic and untreated patients and do not likely represent the clinical experience of most surgeons.

Trials that measure symptomatic DVT consistently and predictably register lower estimates than those that rely on venography. The Scottish Intercollegiate Guidelines Network (SIGN) report a 5.9% incidence of symptomatic DVT among all surgery patients receiving no prophylaxis.[2] The Pulmonary Embolism Prophylaxis (PEP) trial, which is discussed in more detail later in this chapter, documented an incidence of symptomatic DVT of 1.5% in hip fracture and 0.97% in hip and knee arthroplasty patients receiving placebo over 35 days, though a significant number of patients assigned received alternative prophylactic measures.[20] The incidence of VTE in laparoscopy seems to be *at least* one order of magnitude less than other surgical populations.[1]

The incidence of fatal PE is predictably even lower. Without prophylaxis, the incidence of fatal PE is less than 0.01% among low-risk patients and 0.2% to 5% among high-risk patients, a group that usually includes patients who have sustained trauma or spinal cord injury or patients undergoing hip fracture repair or joint arthroplasty.[1] Similar figures have been obtained in large, retrospective studies.[21,22]

4. What are the various pharmacologic and nonpharmacologic options to prevent venous thromboembolism?

Several pharmacologic options are available for prophylaxis, each with a unique mechanism of action, bioavailability, half-life, means of administration, side-effect profile, and efficacy. The most commonly employed agents in North America include low-dose unfractionated heparin (LDUH), low-molecular-weight heparin (LMWH), and vitamin K antagonists (VKAs). Direct thrombin inhibitors (DTIs) and factor Xa inhibitors have already been approved or are on the horizon.[23] For reasons of practicality, we discuss only agents that have been approved for use or are commonly used in the clinical setting, because some drugs have fallen out of favor or are largely used in the research setting.

Unfractioned Heparin

LDUH acts through multiple mechanisms, including binding and activating antithrombin (AT) and directly inactivating Xa. It is metabolized by the liver, excreted in the urine, and has a half-life of approximately 90 minutes. Dosing is adjusted according to overall VTE risk and body habitus of the patient. Heparin-induced thrombocytopenia (HIT) can develop in 1% to 15% of patients receiving LDUH, with subsequent development of arterial or venous thrombosis in approximately 0.4% of those who develop HIT.[24]

Low Molecular Weight Heparin

LMWHs exert their effect predominantly through the inhibition of factor Xa and, to a lesser degree, through the inhibition of factor IIa by means of AT. Many agents are available in this class, but enoxaparin (Lovenox) and dalteparin (Fragmin) are the two agents most commonly used in North America. Little is known about whether differences in efficacy and safety exist within the class,[25] but some authorities suggest that differences in their preparation, structure, and pharmacologic properties likely translate into real clinical difference.[26] LMWHs are parenterally administered, metabolized by the liver, excreted by the kidney, and have a half-life approximately twice that of LDUH. They must be dosed at lower doses in dialysis patients or patients with a creatinine clearance rate less than 30 mL/min and are associated with a lower incidence of HIT than occurs with LDUH.[27]

Vitamin K Antagonists

VKAs are orally administered agents that prevent the gamma-carboxylation of the vitamin K–dependent coagulation factors II, VII, IX and X, resulting in functionally inactive proteins. Warfarin (Coumadin) is the most commonly used agent in the United States. It is rapidly absorbed, is protein bound, is metabolized by the liver, and has an extended half-life of 36 to 42 hours.

However, its multiple drug interactions and relatively narrow therapeutic index detract from its safety and convenience. The use of a dosing nomogram may increase safety and efficacy and simplify administration of the drug postoperatively.[28]

Aspirin

Aspirin (acetylsalicylic acid) is an antiplatelet agent traditionally used for primary and secondary prevention of coronary and cerebral vascular disease. Its use is controversial in the prophylaxis of VTE, a matter which we will discuss at greater length later in the chapter.[1,2]

Factor Xa Inhibitors

Factor Xa inhibitors are synthetic pentasaccharides that mediate the interaction of heparin with AT, thereby preventing the generation of thrombin.[23,29] Fondaparinux (Arixtra) has been studied in patients undergoing elective hip and knee arthroplasty and hip fracture. It has a half-life of 17 hours, allowing for daily parenteral administration.

Direct Thrombin Inhibitors

The past several years have seen the emergence of DTIs, which bind free and bound thrombin. Ximelagatran (Exanta) was the first orally active DTI. Melagatran is its parenterally administered, biologically active equivalent. Both drugs have a dose-dependent response and predictable bioavailability and have been studied as VTE prophylaxis in knee and hip arthroplasty, as stroke prevention in atrial fibrillation, and as treatment of VTE. The U.S. Food and Drug Administration (FDA) withheld approval for ximelagatran in October 2004, and AstraZeneca withdrew application in February 2006 due to concerns about hepatic toxicity; 6% to 9.6% of patients had asymptomatic elevations in alanine aminotransferase levels between 6 weeks and 6 months after initiation of the drug, the significance of which is unclear.[23,30]

Mechanical Prophylaxis

Intermittent pneumatic compression (IPC) devices prevent venous stasis and activate local and systemic fibrinolysis.[31] The system promotes venous return through the sequential inflation and deflation of bladders that can partially or completely surround the foot, calf, and thigh at low or high pressures or combinations thereof. Their efficacy in reducing DVT has been demonstrated in high-risk surgical populations.[32] Issues of cost and compliance detract from their use, especially foot systems such as the A-V Impulse System Foot Pump (AVFP) that employ high-pressure rapid inflation.[33,34] IPCs are used more commonly in North America than in Europe.

Graded elastic compression stockings (GCS) prevent venous stasis and thrombus formation by providing uniform or graded pressure profiles below or above the knee. They are inexpensive, convenient, and easy to use, though they can be technically difficult to fit. GCS are used more commonly in Europe than in North America.

5. What are the options for preventing VTE in general surgery patients based on the available evidence?

BACKGROUND

The rate of VTE in general surgery has been documented in numerous studies and is summarized in a meta-analysis by Clagett and Reisch: 25% for asymptomatic DVT, 6.9% for asymptomatic proximal DVT, 1.6% for all PE, and 0.87% for fatal PE.[35] Although many of these data come from the 1970s and 1980s, competing trends since then in factors that would diminish risk of VTE (e.g., shorter hospital stays leading to earlier ambulation) and those that would increase risk (e.g., older and sicker patients) do not seem likely to alter the need for prophylaxis in many surgical patients.

EVIDENCE

The prophylactic strategies with the strongest evidence of benefit are LDUH dosed at 5000 units every 8 to 12 hours and LMWH. We first will explore the data on these methods, followed by the data on other pharmacologic therapies and then the data on nonpharmacologic therapies such as IPC and GCS.

Unfractionated Heparin

Of all the therapies studied, LDUH has the most literature to support its use. A meta-analysis of almost

50 studies involving general surgery patients compared LDUH, combining all dosing frequencies, with placebo or no treatment.[36] Although there was much heterogeneity, it demonstrated a 59% ± 8% reduction in the odds of developing an asymptomatic DVT. This meta-analysis then combined the outcomes for the general surgery, orthopedic surgery, and urology patients to demonstrate a 40% ± 11% reduction in the odds of nonfatal PE and a 64% ± 15% reduction in the odds of fatal PE. The study authors were also able to demonstrate a statistically significant 21% reduction in total mortality with the use of LDUH ($P < .02$). This was accompanied, however, by a 62% ± 11% increase in the odds of major bleeding in general surgery patients. The meta-analysis by Clagett and Reisch[35] showed a statistically significant decrease in the rate of DVT, but this meta-analysis also combined studies employing different LDUH dosing regimens. When factoring in only double-blinded trials, the odds ratio (OR) of developing a DVT on LDUH compared with control was 0.40 (95% CI: 0.30 to 0.54). Because this meta-analysis did not weight the studies beyond the number of patients enrolled, we are able to calculate a relative risk reduction (RRR), an absolute risk reduction (ARR), and a number needed to treat or harm (NNT or NNH). An odds ratio of 0.40 corresponds to a RRR of 53%, an ARR of 13.0%, and a NNT of 8. For all PE, the odds ratio was 0.42 (95% CI: 0.26-0.68), with an RRR of 58%, an ARR of 0.7%, and an NNT of 141. For fatal PE, the odds ratio was 0.30 (95% CI: 0.15 to 0.58), with an RRR of 70%, an ARR of 0.5%, and an NNT of 200. There was no statistically significant increase in the risk of major bleeding, although wound hematomas were significantly more likely, with an odds ratio of 1.56 (95% CI: 1.27 to 1.97), a relative risk increase of 54%, and an absolute risk increase of 2.2%. To put the rates from the second meta-analysis in perspective, the NNT to prevent one DVT is 8, to prevent one proximal DVT is 20 (data not shown), to prevent one PE is 141, and to prevent one fatal PE is 200, whereas the NNT to cause one wound hematoma is 45. A pooled analysis incorporating later data was published in the Sixth ACCP Conference guidelines and demonstrated an approximately two-thirds (68% per the guidelines) reduction in the rate of DVT with LDUH in patients undergoing general surgery.[37]

A Cochrane systematic review demonstrated an odds ratio of 0.35 (95% CI: 0.20 to 0.62) with the use of heparin compared with placebo or no treatment.[38] However, all of these analyses used pooled data from all studies employing LDUH, regardless of dosing frequency and often regardless of study design or quality.

The dosing frequency of LDUH in studies has varied between every-8-hour dosing (i.e., three times daily) and every-12-hour dosing (i.e., two times daily). The two major meta-analyses on the subject attempted to compare these two dosing regimens, although they have never been directly compared in a study.[35,36] Clagett and Reisch[35] pooled 34 studies employing every-12-hour dosing and compared this with a pool of 15 studies of every-8-hour dosing. They found a DVT rate of 11.8% (95% CI: 10.6 to 13.1%) with every-12-hour dosing, whereas patients receiving every-8-hour dosing had a rate of 7.5% (95% CI: 6.4% to 8.6%). Bleeding rates were comparable with identical wound hematoma rates and slightly higher major bleeding rates with every-8-hour dosing, although the 95% confidence intervals for the latter crossed each other. Collins and associates[36] found the odds reduction in DVT to be 72% ± 5% with every-8-hour dosing compared with 63% ± 5% for every-12-hour dosing; bleeding rates were comparable. As a consequence of the possible superiority of LDUH three times daily inferred from these studies, the ACCP recommends every-8-hour dosing for higher-risk patients (discussed later).[1] The Cochrane review compiled trials of LDUH compared with placebo or no treatment.[38] Of all the trials included, only those employing three times daily dosing had statistically significant reduction in the risk of DVT with LDUH. There is also compelling evidence in medical patients that LDUH two times daily is no different from 20 mg of enoxaparin.[39] Because the 20-mg dose of enoxaparin was shown to be equivalent to placebo in another medical cohort,[40] we think there is limited evidence supporting the use of LDUH two times daily. We therefore feel that LDUH should be employed only as a regimen using dosing three times daily.

Low Molecular Weight Heparin
Several meta-analyses and systematic reviews have explored the benefit of LMWH in general surgery patients,

although most of these comparisons were against other therapies (usually LDUH) rather than placebo.[38,41-48] LMWH is typically dosed based on anti-Xa units, with 2000 anti-Xa units corresponding to 20 mg of enoxaparin. LMWH has usually been employed in a low-dose (≤ 3400 anti-Xa units) or a high-dose (> 3400 anti-Xa units) fashion for VTE prophylaxis in general surgery. The FDA has approved only 40 mg (i.e., higher dose) of enoxaparin for VTE prophylaxis, and we agree the evidence more clearly supports the higher dose. The Cochrane systematic review did find three trials of LMWH compared with no treatment or placebo.[40] All three used higher doses of LMWH (3825 to 7500 anti-Xa units), and the pooled results revealed a statistically significant reduction in the odds of developing DVT (OR = 0.17; 95% CI: 0.05 to 0.54). This Cochrane analysis showed no difference between LDUH and LMWH in the pooled analysis of the three included trials. One of these three trials accounted for more than 85% of the weight in this analysis, and this trial compared 40 mg of enoxaparin daily with LDUH three times daily.[49] The ACCP acknowledges the benefit of higher doses (> 3400 anti-Xa units) for higher-risk patients.[1] This recommendation is derived from studies that showed a trend toward or a significant reduction in VTE in high-risk patients (i.e., patients with malignancy) with higher doses of LMWH.[50-52] Another study showed a trend toward more DVTs in patients with cancer when patients received low-dose LMWH (i.e., 20 mg of enoxaparin daily) compared with LDUH every 8 hours, whereas patients without cancer had similar outcomes regardless of treatment arm.[53] The meta-analysis by Mismetti and coworkers[41] found significantly fewer clinical PEs, albeit at the risk of more wound hematomas and major bleeding, with the use of high-dose LMWH. As a consequence of these findings, the ACCP guidelines recommend different doses of LMWH based on risk factors (discussed later). However, we feel that only the higher dose LMWH regimen should be used based on the numerous studies showing the ineffectiveness of the lower dose compared with other doses or agents.[50,51,53]

Nonheparin Pharmacologic Alternatives

The other pharmacologic options that have been studied are aspirin, dextran, warfarin, and fondaparinux. The two major trials supporting the use of aspirin are the Antiplatelet Trialists' Collaboration III (ATC III) and the PEP trial.[20] The ATC III combined 53 studies (22 involving general surgery) of various antiplatelet regimens for VTE prophylaxis. Although the pooled analysis for general surgery patients showed a significant reduction in DVT by 37% and all PE by 71%, along with a reduction in fatal PE by 71% in all surgical patients, the pooled analysis for all surgery patients did not show a significant impact on mortality. Though antiplatelet therapy had an impact on PE and fatal PE that was similar to that of LDUH reported in the two aforementioned meta-analyses, it had less influence on reducing rates of DVT and total mortality than LDUH did. More importantly, the antiplatelet regimens employed in the studies were very heterogeneous, with aspirin being the prophylactic agent in roughly one half of the trials and with aspirin dosing varying from as little as 250 mg/day to as much as 3900 mg/day. Regimens also employed other agents, such as dipyridamole, hydroxychloroquine, ticlopidine, and other nonsteroidal anti-inflammatory agents. We find it difficult to rely on the ATC III as proof of the efficacy of aspirin. The PEP trial[20] did not study general surgery patients, and extrapolating to general surgery patients therefore may be improper. Further issues with the PEP trial are discussed in later sections on joint arthroplasty and hip fracture. Dextran has been shown to reduce the rate of PE and fatal PE similar to LDUH, although it is less efficacious at reducing DVT rates.[35,55] Because of its cost, its intravenous route of administration, and its side effects, dextran has not been a highly used agent. Warfarin has been poorly studied in general surgery patients and, especially in light of its monitoring requirements, is not a recommended prophylactic agent in general surgery patients. Fondaparinux was shown to be not inferior to dalteparin in one study of high-risk abdominal surgery patients[56] but is not definitively recommended as a prophylactic regimen by any guidelines.

Mechanical Prophylaxis

The major nonpharmacologic options are GCS and IPC. The role of GCS has been investigated in a Cochrane systematic review, which combined studies in which GCS were used as prophylaxis in a variety of different clinical circumstances.[57] Only four of the seven trials that compared GCS with no treatment were in general surgical populations, with the remaining three investigating gynecologic, orthopedic, and neurosurgical populations. Nonetheless, this review demonstrated an odds ratio of 0.36 (95% CI: 0.26 to 0.49) in the rate of DVT with the use of thigh-high GCS compared with no treatment. GCS also enhanced the efficacy of other therapies, with an odds ratio of developing a DVT of 0.22 (95% CI: 0.15 to 0.34) by adding GCS to other therapies (which included dextran, LDUH, aspirin, and IPC). Unfortunately, very few studies have investigated the impact of GCS on rates of proximal DVT, PE, or mortality, which are more critical end points. Knee-high GCS are commonly employed in practice due to their better tolerance and easier fit, but these have not been as well studied as thigh-high GCS.[57] GCS require careful fitting to avoid complications and maximize benefits.[58] There have been few studies investigating the impact of IPC on rates of VTE. A meta-analysis pooled nine studies of IPC, five comparing IPC with placebo and four comparing IPC with LDUH.[35] In the 313 patients studied with IPC versus placebo, the odds ratio of developing a DVT with IPC was 0.43 (95% CI: 0.27 to 0.68). IPC also compared favorably with LDUH, demonstrating an odds ratio of developing a DVT of 0.48 (95% CI: 0.24 to 0.96) favoring IPC. However, there were only 190 patients in the four LDUH trials, and there were insufficient data on the outcomes for proximal DVT, PE, or mortality. The Cochrane review of heparins in colorectal surgery also looked at IPC and found only one qualified study, which did not show a significant reduction in the rate of DVT with the use of IPC compared with no treatment.[38] One study did show a significant reduction in PE rates by adding IPC to LDUH.[59] However, because of the relative paucity of data supporting IPC and GCS, most guidelines are cautious about recommending nonpharmacologic therapy as solo or first-line therapy, especially in higher-risk patients.

Populations at Risk

The question of which general surgery patients to treat is not well studied in the literature. Because most studies did not consistently define their study populations, the major guidelines do not agree on which patients should receive prophylaxis. The three major guidelines published since 2000, the International Consensus Statement,[3] the SIGN guidelines,[2] and the Sixth and Seventh ACCP Conference guidelines,[1,37] have somewhat conflicting recommendations for therapy. We will discuss the guidelines' prophylactic recommendations including which populations are at risk next.

CURRENT GUIDELINES

The SIGN guidelines recommend prophylaxis for all patients undergoing major general surgery who are at significant risk for VTE, a grade A recommendation. Although the study authors do list clinical risk factors for VTE (e.g., age, obesity, varicose veins, prior VTE, thrombophilia, hormonal therapy, pregnancy, immobility, general anesthesia) in part of their guidelines, they do not elucidate how many, if any, of these risk factors are required to prompt prophylaxis for patients undergoing major general surgery. Their grade A first-line recommendations are LDUH dosed at 5000 units every 8 to 12 hours or LMWH. In patients in whom these agents are contraindicated, the authors recommend the use of GCS or IPC, both grade A recommendations. They also make a grade A recommendation of GCS in addition to pharmacologic therapy for patients with multiple risk factors for VTE. In contrast to the other guidelines, the SIGN guidelines recommend aspirin as second-line prophylaxis after heparin products. The investigators make this grade A recommendation based on the ATC III and the PEP trials, of which we have previously discussed or will discuss the limitations. They list intravenous dextran as a possible alternative prophylaxis in high-risk patients undergoing major general surgery, another grade A recommendation.

The 2001 International Consensus Statement[3] takes a similar approach to the ACCP guidelines by first outlining which therapies are beneficial and then by recommending therapies by level of risk, which they define somewhat variably. The study authors classify their patient populations as low, moderate, or high risk. In the text, low-risk patients are defined as those undergoing minor surgery (i.e., operations other than intra-abdominal that last less than 45 minutes) without risk factors; moderate-risk patients as those older than 40 years and undergoing major surgery without risk factors, and high-risk patients as those undergoing major surgery and older than 60 years or with risk factors. The definitions in the accompanying table (Table VII in the article), however, differ from the text definitions and can be seen in Table 6-1 along with their therapeutic recommendations.

The Seventh ACCP Conference Guidelines[1] expand on this risk stratification scheme but in a way that we find even more cumbersome, confusing, and sometimes contradictory. The investigators divide their populations into low risk, moderate risk, higher risk, and highest risk.

Table 6-1. International Consensus Statement		
Risk Category	Definition	Therapeutic Recommendations
High	Major surgery (intra-abdominal surgery or operations lasting longer than 45 minutes) and > 60 years old Major surgery, 40-60 years old, and either cancer or history of DVT/PE Thrombophilia	Grade A: LDUH or LMWH Alternative grade A: IPC or GCS, or both Grade B: combined pharmacologic and mechanical methods
Moderate	Major surgery, 40-60 years old, without other risk factors (e.g., infectious disease, varicose veins, immobility) Minor surgery, > 60 years old Minor surgery, 40-60 years old, with history of DVT/PE or on estrogen therapy	Grade A: same as high risk Alternative grade A: same as high risk
Low	Major surgery, < 40 years old, without other risk factors (e.g., infectious disease, varicose veins, immobility) Minor surgery, 40-60 years old, without other risk factors	No data to guide therapy; some use GCS in addition to early ambulation

DVT, deep venous thrombosis; GCS, graded compression stockings; IPC, intermittent pneumatic compression; LDUH, low-dose unfractionated heparin; LMWH, low-molecular-weight heparin; PE, pulmonary embolism.
Adapted from Nicolaides AN, Breddin HK, Fareed J, et al: Prevention of venous thromboembolism. International Consensus Statement. Int Angiol 2001;20:1-37.

Although they have a table of 21 risk factors (Table 3 in the ACCP guidelines), they do not clarify whether these risk factors are equally weighted. They define their risk groups in the text and again in a table (Table 5 in the ACCP guidelines), but these definitions are not always internally consistent. The way the ACCP stratifies risk in the article is shown in Table 6-2. The authors' prophylaxis

Table 6-2. Comparison of ACCP Guidelines: Risk Category Definitions		
Risk Category	**ACCP Guidelines Text Definitions***	**ACCP Guidelines Table 5 Definitions***
Low	Minor surgery in patients < 40 years old with no additional risk factors	Minor surgery in patients < 40 years old with no additional risk factors
Moderate	Nonmajor surgery in patients 40-60 years old or with additional risk factors (undefined) Major surgery in patients < 40 years old	Minor surgery in patients with additional risk factors (undefined) Surgery in patients 40-60 years old with no additional risk factors (undefined)
Higher (text classification; *high* in table classification)	Nonmajor surgery in patients > 60 years old or with additional risk factors (undefined) Major surgery in patients > 40 years old or with additional risk factors (undefined)	Surgery in patients > 60 years old or 40-60 years old with additional risk factors (e.g., prior venous thromboembolism [VTE], cancer, hypercoagulability)
High (text classification; *highest* in table classification)	Patients with multiple risk factors (undefined)	Surgery in patients with multiple risk factors (e.g., > 40 years old, cancer, prior VTE) Hip or knee arthroplasty Hip fracture surgery Major trauma or spinal cord injury

*The American College of Chest Physicians (ACCP) defines risk groups somewhat differently in the text and a table of their guidelines.
Adapted from Geerts WH, Pineo GF, Heit JA, et al: Prevention of venous thromboembolism: The Seventh ACCP Conference on Antithrombotic and Thrombolytic Therapy. Chest 2004;126:338S-400S.

recommendations then vary by risk category, as seen in Table 6-3.

Although the intuitive rationale of giving more aggressive regimens to patients at higher risk (defined as increasing age, major versus minor surgery, and VTE risk factors) seems reasonable, their algorithm is contradictory at points. For example, how should a 45-year-old patient with a history of DVT undergoing a minor procedure be treated? When using the ACCP guidelines' Table 5 criteria, this patient would fit the highest-risk criteria, the second criterion for a high-risk patient (using the

Table 6-3. **Comparison of ACCP Guidelines: Prophylaxis Recommendations**

Risk Category	ACCP Guidelines Text Treatment Recommendations*	ACCP Guidelines Table 5 Recommendations*
Low	Early mobilization only	Early and aggressive mobilization
Moderate	LDUH (5000 U bid) (grade 1A) LMWH (≤ 3400 U daily) (grade 1A)	LDUH (q 12 hr) or LMWH (≤ 3400 U daily) or GCS or IPC
Higher (text classification; *high* in table classification)	LDUH (5000 U tid) (grade 1A) LMWH (> 3400 U daily) (grade 1A)	LDUH (q 8 hr) or LMWH (> 3400 U daily) or IPC
High (text classification; *highest* in table classification	Combined pharmacological (LDUH tid or high-dose LMWH) and mechanical (GCS and/or IPC) prophylaxis (grade 1C+)	LMWH (> 3400 U daily) or Fondaparinux or warfarin (goal INR of 2 to 3) or IPC/GCS + LDUH/LMWH
Patients at risk for bleeding	Properly fitted GCS or IPC (grade 1A)	No recommendations listed

*The American College of Chest Physicians (ACCP) defines risk groups somewhat differently in the text and a table of their guidelines.
GCS, graded compression stockings; INR, international normalized ratio; IPC, intermittent pneumatic compression; LDUH, low-dose unfractionated heparin; LMWH, low-molecular-weight heparin; PE, pulmonary embolism.
Adapted from Geerts WH, Pineo GF, Heit JA, et al: Prevention of venous thromboembolism: The Seventh ACCP Conference on Antithrombotic and Thrombolytic Therapy. Chest 2004;126:338S-400S.

Table 6-5 classification of high risk as between moderate and high risk), and the first definition of a moderate risk patient. Using the text definitions, this patient would be both higher risk and high risk. The ACCP guidelines, although the most expansive, may be hard to employ for general surgery patients.

OUR RECOMMENDATIONS

Our recommendations for how to manage general surgery patients borrow from the ACCP in that we recommend more aggressive treatment for higher-risk patients. However, we do not recommend the use of LDUH two times daily or LMWH at the lower dose (≤ 3400 units). Based on their lesser effectiveness, we also only recommend the use of nonpharmacologic approaches in patients who are at significant risk for bleeding or have contraindications for the use of heparins. Given the uncertainty about which patients clearly benefit but good evidence suggesting the benefits of heparins outweigh the risks, we favor setting the threshold for prophylaxis low. We define VTE risk factors as any of the following: age 40 years or older, major surgery (i.e., surgery lasting longer than 45 minutes), and history of VTE, cancer, hypercoagulability, obesity, varicose veins, or hormonal use. Our treatment recommendations for patients undergoing general surgery are as follows:

- Low-risk patients (< 40 years old, undergoing minor surgery without VTE risk factors) do not require any prophylaxis beyond early ambulation.
- Any high-risk patients (with at least one of our defined VTE risk factor) should receive prophylaxis with either LDUH three times daily or higher-dose LMWH (> 3400 units daily, which corresponds to 40 mg of enoxaparin daily).
- High-risk patients at significant risk for bleeding or who have contraindications to heparins should receive mechanical prophylaxis with IPC or thigh-high GCS.
- Patients who are at particularly increased risk (i.e., more than two VTE risk factors) should be considered for combined pharmacologic and mechanical prophylaxis.

6. What are the options for preventing venous thromboembolism in patients undergoing total hip replacement based on the available evidence?

BACKGROUND

Total hip replacement (THR) patients are generally at even higher risk for VTE than general surgery patient. Without prophylaxis, the rate of nonfatal PE has been reported to range from 3.2%[60] to 15.27%.[61] The rates of fatal PE in the same trials were 1.4%[60] to 2.3%.[61] Though more recent studies suggest lower rated[62] all guidelines recommend some form of prophylaxis for all THR patients.

EVIDENCE

LMWH and VKA

Multiple meta-analyses have established the superiority of LMWH and adjusted-dose VKA over placebo[63,64] and over LDUH[42,45,46,65,66] in total hip replacement (THR) in orthopedic surgery in general/in particular. The superiority of LMWH versus VKA is a matter of debate and depends on several factors, chief among them the timing of administration of prophylaxis. One meta-analysis that included more than 11,000 patients suggested that LMWH was superior to VKA for prophylaxis of VTE,[67] whereas an earlier meta-analysis found no significant difference in efficacy.[68] In a prospective, randomized, double-blind trial, dalteparin administered 2 hours preoperatively significantly reduced the incidence of proximal and symptomatic DVT when compared with warfarin. Although a statistically significant increase in centrally adjudicated major bleeding and blood transfusion was observed in the dalteparin group, the rates of wound hematoma and infection were comparable between the two groups.[69] An earlier study using very similar dosing schedules was less favorable; dalteparin caused a significant increase in bleeding at the surgical site but no significant reduction in proximal or symptomatic DVT.[70]

Aspirin

Little evidence supports the use of aspirin as sole prophylaxis in elective THR. The ATC III—a meta-analysis combining several thousand surgical patients receiving a wide variety of antiplatelet regimens, of which aspirin was a component in only slightly more than one half of patients included in the analysis—demonstrated a significant reduction in DVT and PE among all surgical patients. Among patients undergoing elective arthroplasty, the reduction in the rate of DVT was statistically significant, but the reduction in PE was not.[56] In another meta-analysis of 56 randomized, controlled trials, aspirin was the only modality that showed *no* significant reduction in the risk of all or proximal DVT.[71]

The PEP trial was a large, double-blind study performed from 1992 through 1998 that randomized 4088 patients undergoing elective hip and knee arthroplasty to 160 mg of aspirin or placebo, as well as other thromboprophylaxis "thought necessary" by the treating physician: LDUH in 18%, LMWH in 26%, and GCS in 30%.[20] Patients with a compelling indication or contraindication for the use of aspirin were excluded from the trial. Symptomatic DVT, nonfatal PE, and fatal PE were not significantly reduced at postoperative day 35 with the use of aspirin among patients undergoing joint arthroplasty. Fifteen DVTs occurred in the aspirin group and 19 DVTs in the placebo group, generating a hazard ratio of 0.78 (95% CI: 0.40 to 1.53). Similarly, 8 PEs were diagnosed in each group, generating a hazard ratio of 1.00 (95% CI: 0.37 to 2.66). There were 16 major bleeding events in the aspirin group requiring hematoma evacuation, compared with 8 events in the placebo group, a difference that did not reach statistical significance ($P = .1$). However, in their final analysis, the investigators asserted that the proportional effects of aspirin in elective joint arthroplasty "did not differ significantly" from those of hip fracture, despite the fact that a statistically significant benefit was shown for hip fracture patients but not in THR patients.

Fondaparinux

Fondaparinux has been compared with enoxaparin in several trials of patients undergoing THR, with generally favorable results. The first trial, published in 2001, was a study that utilized a number of doses of fondaparinux compared with enoxaparin 30 mg twice daily, both given postoperatively. It showed a statistically significant RRR of 82% in total VTE with 3 mg of fondaparinux compared with enoxaparin.[72] In the EPHESUS trial, 2309 hip arthroplasty patients were randomized to 2.5 mg of fondaparinux starting postoperatively or to 40 mg of once-daily enoxaparin starting preoperatively. Fondaparinux was associated with a statistically significant ARR in any (−5.1%; 95% CI: −8.0 to −2.6) and proximal (−1.8%; 95% CI: −3.7 to −0.5) DVT, but no difference in fatal and nonfatal PE, symptomatic DVT, or clinically significant major bleeding was observed between the two groups.[73] In another large, randomized trial, 2.5 mg of postoperatively administered fondaparinux showed little or no advantage over 30 mg of postoperatively administered enoxaparin. Although fondaparinux was associated with a statistically significant ARR of 2.5% in distal DVT + 2.6% in any DVT, no difference in VTE, proximal DVT, and fatal and nonfatal PE was observed between the two groups. In addition, there were actually fewer episodes of symptomatic VTE with the LMWH, though the rate of symptomatic VTE was much less than asymptomatic VTE and the authors thought this result was likely from chance.[74] A meta-analysis combining four large, randomized trials of fondaparinux versus enoxaparin showed a significant benefit to fondaparinux on the endpoints of VTE, any DVT, and any proximal DVT.[75] However, this meta-analysis combined studies of the patients with TKR and hip fracture patients. When restricting the meta-analysis to THR patients and to the more significant endpoints of proximal DVT, PE, death, and symptomatic DVT, the benefit of fondaparinux loses its statistical significance.[76]

Direct Thrombin Inhibitors

There is favorable evidence for the use of DTIs. Desirudin (Iprivask) was superior to enoxaparin 40 mg once daily in a large, multicenter, randomized trial from 1997 involving 2097 THR patients.[77] Later, five trials involving almost 10,000 patients undergoing hip and knee arthroplasty studied ximelagatran and mel agatran, with mixed results.[78-82] In the dose-ranging METHRO II study, 1900 patients undergoing hip and knee arthroplasty were randomized to various dosing combinations of melagatran and ximelagatran versus dalteparin.[79] Among THR patients, 3 mg of preoperatively administered melagatran followed by 24 mg of twice-daily ximelagatran was associated with an ARR of 13.6% (95% CI: 6.0 to 21.1) of total VTE at postoperative day 7 to 10. This dose was also associated with an increased incidence of "severe" bleeding, although the authors asserted that no bleeding led to re-operation and the study drug was continued in most patients. In another trial, 24 mg of twice-daily ximelagatran was compared with twice-daily enoxaparin, both started the morning after surgery in patients undergoing THR. Proximal DVT or PE, or both, occurred in 3.6% (28 of 782 patients) in the ximelagatran group and 1.2% (9 of 782) in the enoxaparin group, corresponding to a statistically significant ARR of 2.4% in favor of enoxaparin.[80] In the EXPRESS study, 2835 patients undergoing joint arthroplasty were randomized to another regimen of melagatran/ximelagatran compared with enoxaparin 40 mg daily. There was an ARR in major VTE, defined as proximal DVT, PE, and death where PE could not be ruled out, of 3.7% (95% CI: −5.6 to −1.8) with DTI in THR patients.[81] Severe bleeding was more frequent with DTI, occurring in 4.0% (37 of 915) in the melagatran/ximelagatran group, compared with 1.1% (10 of 942) in the enoxaparin group, but there was no significant difference in wound re-operation rates between the two groups. In METHRO III, 2788 patients undergoing joint arthroplasty were randomized to 3 mg of melagatran started 4 to 12 hours postoperatively, followed by 24 mg of twice-daily ximelagatran or 40 mg of once-daily enoxaparin started 12 hours preoperatively. Among THR patients, enoxaparin was associated with a statistically significant ARR in total VTE of 6% (95% CI: −10.1 to −2.0) but no difference in bleeding or major VTE, defined as proximal DVT, nonfetal PE, fetal PE, or unexplained death.[82]

Mechanical Prophylaxis

Few well-designed studies have examined mechanical prophylaxis with GCS, IPC and AVFP, which are more efficacious than placebo but less efficacious than pharmacologic prophylaxis.[1] In a meta-analysis of at least five trials, for example, warfarin was associated with a RRR in proximal DVT of 46% (95% CI: 25 to 82) compared with IPC.[68] In a later randomized trial from July 2004, 216 hip arthroplasty patients were randomized to LMWH or AVFP postoperatively after all patients had received perioperative LMWH prophylaxis.[36] AVFP significantly reduced total and proximal DVT, as well as postoperative drainage, oozing, bruising, and swelling, although about half of eligible patients reported at least some difficulty tolerating it. The superiority of one modality over another is unclear, although at least one randomized trial suggests that patients tolerate AVFP better than they do traditional IPC.[83]

Timing of Prophylaxis

Timing of prophylaxis has an impact on safety and efficacy. Thrombus formation begins perioperatively before hemostasis is achieved, so early thromboprophylaxis predictably results in less VTE but also more bleeding. No studies directly compare preoperatively and postoperatively administered LMWH. Comparisons of different drugs within the LMWH class are therefore indirect and somewhat misleading. Two meta-analyses have suggested that the timing of LMWH administration does not affect efficacy or safety,[84,85] whereas another meta-analysis has suggested that preoperative administration of LMWH is more efficacious than postoperative administration.[86] Because no studies have directly compared melagatran/ximelagatran or fondaparinux with similarly timed LMWH, any comparison of the efficacy and safety of the different drugs requires extrapolation of VTE rates from prior studies. Despite "perioperative" dosing schedules, the newer agents demonstrate an excellent safety profile. Some investigators have suggested that the optimal timing for thromboprophylaxis is 6 hours after surgery,[87] but the ACCP guidelines allow for a wider range.[1]

Timing of prophylaxis is often dictated by the choice of anesthesia. Whereas surgeons in Europe begin prophylaxis with LMWH 12 hours before surgery, surgeons in North America generally begin LMWH 12 hours after surgery. These different practice styles are in part based on dramatically different estimates of rates of spinal hematoma after spinal or epidural anesthesia with the use of enoxaparin: 1 in 2,250,000 in Europe versus 1 in 14,000 in the United States.[2] Mechanistically, however, a regimen of LMWH administered 12 hours before or after surgery does little to prevent thrombus formation, which likely begins perioperatively. The use of aspirin in conjunction with regional anesthesia does not seem to impart an increased risk of spinal hematoma.[20,88]

Duration of Prophylaxis

The duration of prophylaxis is also an evolving issue. There is a prolonged prothrombotic profile after THR,[89] and more than 75% of cases of VTE are diagnosed after discharge,[90] on average 17 days after surgery.[91] THR is associated with a 2.4% incidence of symptomatic VTE after 7 to 10 days of in-hospital prophylaxis.[92] Symptomatic VTE occurs more frequently with THR than total knee replacement (TKR), despite a higher overall incidence of VTE seen with the latter.[93]

Despite reviewing the same primary trials, meta-analyses have come to different conclusions regarding extended prophylaxis with LMWH. Three meta-analyses found a modest benefit and argue in its favor.[94-96] A later review found no statistically significant reduction in symptomatic VTE or PE and concluded that the benefit of extended prophylaxis had been "overstated,"[97] an opinion shared by other experts.[98] Looking at individual prospective trials, it seems that extending prophylaxis with once-daily enoxaparin for 3 to 4 weeks is associated with a statistically significant reduction in venographic VTE, with no compromise of safety.[99,100] The efficacy of VKA and LMWH may be similar in extended prophylaxis, but at least one study suggests that LMWH may be associated with less bleeding.[101]

CURRENT GUIDELINES

The Seventh ACCP Conference guidelines recommend several options (all grade 1A recommendations):

1. LMWH started 12 hours before surgery, 12 to 24 hours after surgery, or 4 to 6 hours after surgery at one half of the usual dose
2. Adjusted-dose VKA started preoperatively or on the evening after surgery with a target international normalized ratio (INR) range of 2 to 3
3. Fondaparinux started 6 to 8 hours after surgery

They recommend *against* the use of aspirin, LDUH, GCS, or IPC as the sole means of prophylaxis.[1] They suggest that prophylaxis be continued postoperatively for 10 days with LMWH, VKA, or fondaparinux (grade 1A) and be continued for 28 to 35 days with LMWH (grade 1A), VKA (grade 1A) or fondaparinux (grade 1C+).

The SIGN guidelines are far less stringent in their recommendations. They group hip and knee arthroplasty together and suggest that all patients undergoing major orthopedic surgery deserve mechanical or pharmacologic prophylaxis, or a combination of the two. They further suggest that patients undergoing THR can be "considered" for LDUH, LMWH, VKA adjusted to a target INR of 2 to 3, or aspirin (150 mg, once daily) that is started preoperatively and continued for 35 days.[2] They formally recommend prophylaxis for 7 to 15 days for all lower limb arthroplasty, which can be extended to 4 to 5 weeks in "very high-risk" patients.

OUR RECOMMENDATIONS
- Enoxaparin (30 mg SC every 12 hours or 40 mg SC every 24 hours) is one option with initiation 12 hours preoperatively or postoperatively, and extended for 28 to 35 days.
- VKA is another choice with the first dose given the night before or after surgery (INR goal of 2 to 3), and extended for 28 to 35 days.
- Fondaparinux (2.5 mg SC every 24 hours) is our final option with the first dose to be given 6 to 8 hours postoperatively and given for 2 weeks.
- Aspirin should *not* be used as sole prophylaxis.
- The use of melagatran/ximelagatran is promising, but FDA approval for these agents has not been granted, and they are unavailable for use in the United States.
- Mechanical prophylaxis has limited evidence supporting its use as sole prophylaxis. It should only be used when all pharmacologic options are contraindicated or in addition to pharmacologic agents in high risk patients (e.g., history of VTE or active malignancy). It is uncertain if there is any difference in efficacy & many GCS, IPC, or AVFP. Patient compliance is a very important factor in efficacy and is likely improved by patient education.
- Thromboprophylaxis should begin as soon before or after surgery as safely possible, according to the dosing parameters of the individual drugs and taking into consideration the means of anesthesia used.

7. What are the options for preventing venous thromboembolism in patients undergoing total knee replacement based on the available evidence?

BACKGROUND

TKR has been studied less extensively than THR, and many of the randomized trials and meta-analyses group these populations together. However, evidence from one should not be extrapolated to the other for several reasons.[3] First, the total DVT role is higher in TKR patients this is THR patients.[39] On the other hand, the role of proximal DVT is lower with TKR than with THR.[39] Lastly, there is generally greater concern for bleeding complications in TKR patients than THR patients.[37]

EVIDENCE

Ample evidence demonstrates the efficacy of LMWH and VKA over placebo in joint arthoplasty.[1] The superiority of one agent over the other is a matter of debate, but meta-analysis suggests that LMWH has superior efficacy compared with VKA,[102,103] with respective rates of proximal DVT of 5.9% and 10.2% with each agent and nonsignificant trend toward more bleeding with LMWH.[102]

The evidence for aspirin is limited in TKR. The PEP trial[22] and ATC III[56] were reviewed in some detail in Question 6 with our detailed critique of ATC III noted there. The former study showed no benefit to aspirin while the letter showed a benefit only on the rate of DVT without impacting PE rates.

Fondaparinux

Fondaparinux has compared favorably with enoxaparin. In a trial of 1049 consecutive TKR patients, the incidence of total VTE was 12.5% (45 of 361 patients) with fondaparinux and 27.8% (101 of 363) with enoxaparin, a statistically significant risk RRR of 55.2% (95% CI: 36.2 to 70.2) and ARR of 15.3% (95% CI: −22.3 to −9.3).[104] There was a significant difference in major bleeding episodes—11 with fondaparinux compared with 1 with enoxaparin—but no significant difference in death or rates of re-operation between the two groups. In the original trial, a statistically significant difference in proximal and symptomatic DVT was *not* seen between the two groups. However, when a composite of clinically significant end points (i.e., proximal DVT, symptomatic DVT, and PE) are considered, fondaparinux was statistically superior.[76] A cost-analysis was similarly favorable.[105]

Direct Thrombin Inhibitors

Melagatran and ximelagatran have been compared with LMWH[82,83,85,106] and VKA,[107,108] with inconclusive results. Because many of these trials examined hip and knee arthroplasty together, their results can be somewhat misleading. In METHRO II and METHRO III, rates of total VTE and bleeding complications did not significantly differ with melagatran/ximelagatran or dalteparin in the TKR subgroups.[79,82] In the EXPRESS trial, melagatran/ximelagatran resulted in a 4.9% ARR of major VTE (95% CI: −8.3 to −1.5) compared with once-daily enoxaparin, where major VTE was defined as proximal DVT, PE or death where PE could not be ruled out.[81] In a later, double-blind, multicenter trial involving 680 TKR patients, 24 mg of twice-daily ximelagatran starting the morning after surgery was compared with warfarin starting on the evening after surgery. Total VTE occurred in 19.2% (53 of 276) of patients assigned ximelagatran and 25.7% (67 of 261) of patients assigned warfarin, signifying a not statistically significant ARR of 6.5% (95% CI: −13.5 to 0.6). Although major bleeding was more frequent with ximelagatran, wound appearance, transfusion requirements, and re-operation rates were not significantly different.[107] In a larger study comparing 36 mg of twice-daily ximelagatran starting the morning after surgery and warfarin started the night before, use of the DTI resulted in an ARR in total VTE or death of 7.3% (95% CI: −12.3 to −2.8). There were no significant differences in safety with the higher dose.[108]

Mechanical Prophylaxis

The studies for mechanical prophylaxis are small, heterogeneous, and hindered by poor blinding.[1] As with pharmacologic prophylaxis, there are multiple variations of each modality that further complicate the direct comparison of various types of mechanical prophylaxis. One meta-analysis comprising 23 studies and 6001 patients found an incidence of DVT of 53% (1701 of 3214) with aspirin, 45% (541 of 1203) with warfarin, 29% (311 of 1075) with LMWH, and 17% (86 of 509) with IPC, statistically favoring both IPC and LMWH.[109] The analysis included several retrospective studies involving aspirin, and only 509 of the 6001 patients in the analysis used IPC, reflecting the small size of these trials. A randomized trial compared "asymmetric" IPC and "circumferential" IPC in 423 patients undergoing TKR and documented a very low incidence of total VTE of 6.9% (16 of 232) versus 15% (36 of 240), significantly in favor of the asymmetric design ($P = .007$).[110] GCS has been shown to be beneficial in general surgical patients[111] but seems to have limited benefit in orthopedic surgery based on available evidence.[1] Data for the AVFP are also mixed,[1] although evidence from two small trials supports its use.[111,112]

Timing of Prophylaxis

The decision about when to start prophylaxis is as significant with TKR as with THR, but most surgeons consider the consequence of postoperative bleeding to be greater in TKR than THR. No trials have examined LMWH given close to TKR, and the Seventh ACCP Conference guidelines do not stipulate the ideal timing of prophylaxis.[1] Fondaparinux and melagatran/ximelagatran are given closer to surgery than LMWH and are predictably associated with increased rates of bleeding, as discussed earlier.

Duration of Prophylaxis

The available evidence does not support extended prophylaxis beyond 7 to 10 days in TKR. Despite a higher overall incidence of postoperative VTE, symptomatic VTE and PE occur in approximately 1.4% of TKR patients treated with 7 to 10 days of in-hospital prophylaxis, which is approximately one half of the incidence after THR.[1] A disproportionate number of studies on extended prophylaxis focus exclusively on THR patients. In one randomized trial, 1195 adults undergoing THR and TKR were assigned 6 weeks of out-of-hospital prophylaxis with ardeparin sodium or placebo. The LMWH showed no benefit.[114] In another randomized trial the next year, extended out-of-hospital prophylaxis for 3 weeks with 40 mg of once-daily enoxaparin showed no benefit in TKR over placebo.[100] Meta-analysis combining these two studies was also unable to show a benefit to extended prophylaxis in TKR patients.[96]

CURRENT GUIDELINES

The Seventh ACCP Conference guidelines give the strongest recommendations for LMWH, adjusted-dose VKA with a target INR between 2 and 3, and fonda-parinux for 10 days (all grade 1A recommendations). IPC is given a grade 1B recommendation, reflecting perceived inconsistencies and methodologic flaws of the available evidence. They recommend *against* the use of aspirin (grade 1A), LDUH (grade 1A), or AVFP as sole prophylaxis (grade 1B).[1] The SIGN Guideline recommendations are discussed in Question 6.[2]

OUR RECOMMENDATIONS

- Enoxaparin (30 mg SC every 12 hours or 40 mg SC every 24 hours) is our first choice with initiation 12 hours preoperatively or postoperatively and extended for 7 to 10 days.
- VKA is an alternative and should be started the night before or after surgery with an INR goal of 2 to 3 and extended for 7 to 10 days.
- Fondaparinux (2.5 mg SC every 24 hours) is our last recommendation as sole prophylaxis and should be started 6 to 8 hours postoperatively for 7 to 10 days.
- The use of DTIs is promising, but melagatran/ximelagatran will not likely become available for use in the United States.
- Aspirin should *not* be used as sole prophylaxis.
- In patients at higher risk for VTE, particularly patients with a history of VTE or active malignancy, mechanical prophylaxis with IPC or AVFP should be strongly considered as an adjunct to pharmacologic therapy. Patient compliance is a very important factor in efficacy and is likely improved by patient education.
- Thromboprophylaxis should begin as soon before or after surgery as safely possible, according to the dosing parameters of the individual drugs and the means of anesthesia used.

8. What are the options for preventing venous thromboembolism in patients undergoing hip fracture surgery based on the available evidence?

BACKGROUND

Hip fracture surgery (HFS) is associated with significantly far higher rate of symptomatic DVT and PE than is elective joint arthroplasty, either as a direct consequence of the injury or reflective of the older and more debilitated nature of the population at risk.[1] The rate of fatal PE in the untreated population ranges from 1.4% to 7.5% within 3 months after fracture and is the fourth leading cause of death in this patient population.[1]

EVIDENCE

Heparins

Most studies exploring the role of LDUH and LMWH in HFS patients have shown no statistically significant benefit for either agent. However, most of these trials were small and flawed in numerous ways, including lack of placebo control, lack of blinding of any participants (i.e., patients, providers, and outcome assessors), and poor randomization. A Cochrane Database systematic review from 2002 included 31 trials with over 2900 patients and attempted to address the benefits and risks of these agents.[115] The reviewers concluded that LDUH and LMWH protected against lower limb DVT, with neither agent showing clear superiority over the other, but there was insufficient evidence to decide whether either agent prevented PE or death. However, we are not confident of the reviewers' findings.

The reviewers first attempted to show, through Analysis 01.01, that LDUH and LMWH reduce any DVT by pooling all studies they found. However, as the reviewers acknowledged, most of the studies in this analysis were of poor quality. They attempted to get around these issues by grading studies with a point scoring system and then selecting only "good quality" studies for Analysis 01.02. The reviewers claimed that no LMWH study met their standard even though the Jorgensen 1992 trial[116] actually did; nonetheless, this trial alone did not show a statistically significant benefit from LMWH on any DVT. Five LDUH trials met their standard, with the pooled results showing a benefit.

However, two of these trials, as reported by Gallus and colleagues in 1973[117] and Morris and Mitchell in 1977,[118] were still not placebo controlled and therefore subject to bias. Given that these two trials accounted for more than one third of the analysis, we are not confident that LDUH would still be superior to placebo if the analysis had been limited to placebo controlled trials. All trials in Analysis 01.02 used three times daily dosing of LDUH.

The reviewers then looked at the effect of LMWH and LDUH on DVT by location (proximal or distal) in Analyses 01.03 and 01.04. LMWH led to a statistically significant reduction in proximal DVT, but LDUH did not; conversely, LDUH led to a reduction in distal DVT, but LMWH did not. Nonetheless, the trials included in these analyses are all of lower quality than the standards the authors set for "good quality" or are not placebo controlled, making it difficult to rely on the analyses.

The reviewers next looked at studies that compared LDUH with LMWH. Although Analysis 05.01 suggests LMWH is superior to LDUH in preventing any DVT, Analysis 05.02 eliminates poor-quality trials and demonstrates no statistically significant difference between the two therapies, although there were fewer than 250 patients in Analysis 05.02.

Ultimately, we are not confident that LDUH or LMWH has been definitively shown to be of benefit in hip fracture patients. We therefore have little choice but to look at data on these agents for THR patients and extrapolate to the even higher-risk HFS population. Because LDUH has been shown to be inferior to LMWH in THR patients, we find it difficult to imagine LDUH would be effective in the higher-risk HFS population. We consider LDUH administered three times daily to be second-line therapy. We are uncertain of the benefit of LMWH in HFS patients but believe it may be a reasonable alternative given its utility in THR patients.

VKA

The evidence for VKA is limited.[1] One study comparing warfarin, aspirin, and placebo found that both aspirin and warfarin resulted in a statistically significant reduction in the combined endpoint of proximal DVT and PE; however, the overall incidence of this endpoint with each agent was still unacceptably high: 9.2% with warfarin and

10.6% with aspirin despite a daily dose of aspirin exceeding 1 gram during the study.[118]

Aspirin

The use of aspirin remains controversial,[120] despite favorable evidence from the PEP trial. The PEP trial was significantly larger and more methodologically sound than prior studies, randomizing more than 13,000 hip fracture patients to 160 mg of aspirin or placebo, as well as any other prophylaxis thought necessary by the treating physician.[20] Symptomatic DVT, proximal DVT, and fatal PE were all significantly reduced at day 35 with the use of aspirin—the only single trial we are aware of to demonstrate a statistically significant reduction in fatal PE. Symptomatic DVT occurred in 1.0% (69 of 6679) of patients assigned aspirin and 1.5% (97 of 6677) assigned placebo, corresponding to an RRR of 29% (95% CI: 3 to 48) and ARR of approximately 0.4% (95% CI: 0.04 to 0.8). Fatal PE occurred in approximately 0.3% (18 of 6679) assigned aspirin and approximately 0.6% (43 of 6,677) assigned placebo, corresponding to an RRR of 58% (95% CI: 27 to 76) and ARR of 0.4% (95% CI: 0.2 to 0.6). This difference represents a NNT of 267, or an absolute reduction in 4 total PEs per 1000 patients treated. However, there is some evidence that other forms of thromboprophylaxis eliminated the benefits of aspirin in the PEP trial. First, the subgroup of patients who received LMWH in addition to aspirin had no significant difference in the rate of symptomatic VTE (24 of 1761 on aspirin compared with 30 of 1663 with placebo), although this subgroup may have had inadequate power to detect a difference. Another notable finding was a rise in the rate of VTE in the placebo arm after the first postoperative week. The frequency of VTE was not statistically different between the aspirin and placebo arms during the first week. The difference only became statistically significant in the second postoperative week. This raises the likelihood that other prophylactic strategies, such as LMWH, might have eliminated the aspirin benefit in the first postoperative week but that after the likely discontinuation of the other prophylaxis at the end of the first week, the two groups began to diverge. Although there are few data regarding the benefit of extended prophylaxis in HFS patients, we suspect extended prophylaxis is beneficial in this population, and we feel that the positive outcomes of the aspirin arm of the PEP trial derive from the benefit of extended prophylaxis since aspirin was not protective in the first postoperative week. Regarding safety, fatal bleeding events occurred in roughly 0.2% of patients, regardless of treatment allocation. There was, however, a significant increase in postoperative bleeding that required blood transfusion—2.9% (197 of 6679) with aspirin and 2.4% (157 of 6677) with placebo, amounting to 6 events per 1000 patients treated—most of which were in a subgroup of patients receiving both aspirin and LDUH. There was no statistically significant difference in rates of wound hematoma or re-operation in the two groups. There was also, paradoxically, an increase in nonfatal and fatal myocardial infarction among patients receiving aspirin, which the investigators attributed to chance, misdiagnosis, and inadequate power. We, therefore, have significant reservations about the officacy of aspirin, despite the results of the PEP trial.

Fondaparinux

Fondaparinux has performed well in randomized trials.[121,122] The PENTHIFRA study assigned 1711 HFS patients to 2.5 mg of fondaparinux started 6 ± 2 hours postoperatively or 40 mg of once-daily enoxaparin started 12 ± 2 hours preoperatively. By day 11, 8.3% (52 of 626) of patients assigned fondaparinux and 19.1% (119 of 624) assigned enoxaparin were diagnosed with VTE, corresponding to an RRR of 56.4% (95% CI: 39.0 to 70.3) and ARR of 10.8% (95% CI: 6.6 to 15.3). Proximal DVT was also significantly reduced. Symptomatic VTE, however, was not.[121] Although minor bleeding occurred more frequently with fondaparinux, major bleeding, transfusion, or death from any cause was similar in the two groups.

Duration of Prophylaxis

There are few data for extended prophylaxis in HFS,[20,122] although some experts argue for its use.[123] In PENTHIFRA-PLUS, 656 patients were randomized to 2.5 mg of once-daily fondaparinux or placebo for approximately 3 weeks of extended prophylaxis after having completed 6 to 8 days of fondaparinux for in-hospital prophylaxis. The incidence of VTE was remarkably low with extended prophylaxis—1.4% (3 of 208) with fondaparinux versus 35.0% (77 of 220) with placebo—corresponding to a RRR of 95.9% (95% CI: 87.2 to 99.7) and an ARR of 33.6% (95% CI: 26.5 to 41.4). The rate of symptomatic VTE was only 0.3% (1 of 326) with extended thromboprophylaxis versus 2.7% (9 of 330) with placebo, which was also statistically significant. Major bleeding did not significantly differ between the two groups,[122] though there was a slight trend to more bleeding with fondaparinux (8 events vs. 2 with placebo).

We are confident that a head-to-head comparison of aspirin and a newer agent such as fondaparinux would demonstrate the venographic superiority of the latter, though we concede that such a finding may not translate into a reduction in symptomatic events. The PEP trial authors note in their discussion that "unfractionated and low-molecular-weight heparins produce greater reductions in venous thromboembolism than does aspirin."[20] The SIGN guidelines point out that fatal PE is the "most clinically relevant end point" and base their recommendations on the equivalence of aspirin with both LDUH and LMWH in the reduction of symptomatic VTE.[2] In more recent trials, however, fondaparinux has been shown to reduce dramatically the incidence of venographic and symptomatic events with RRRs significantly greater than those for aspirin. There are other issues of morbidity (e.g., post-phlebitic syndrome) that may swing the pendulum in favor of fondaparinux. One cost analysis, for example, suggests that the use of fondaparinux would reduce costs associated with recurrent VTE and post-phlebitic syndrome, particularly in patients undergoing HFS.[124] As with any clinical decision, the choice of thromboprophylaxis is not merely a question of efficacy and safety, but one of cost, convenience, and patient compliance. Aspirin remains an alternative for elderly and debilitated patients who may have contraindications to other agents, but it should not be viewed as a first-line agent.

Mechanical Prophylaxis

The data for mechanical prophylaxis are very limited. Many studies are small or methodologically flawed and must be interpreted with caution.[1] A 2000 Cochrane review showed a statistically significant ARR in DVT of 15% with mechanical prophylaxis when compared with placebo; however, the quality of the included trials was low, and there were significant problems with compliance.[115] One study of 304 patients with hip and pelvic fractures compared IPC with placebo and found a statistically significant ARR of 7% compared with placebo.[125] Other studies have suggested that AVFP is efficacious in this population, but these were small studies with little power to detect a statistically significant difference in their primary outcome.[126-128] There are no data to support the use of GCS in this population.[2]

CURRENT GUIDELINES

The Seventh ACCP Conference guidelines are nuanced in their recommendations. Their strongest recommendation (grade 1A) is reserved for fondaparinux, whereas LMWH (grade 1C+) and LDUH (grade 1B) receive more qualified recommendations. VKAs are not given a strong recommendation (grade 2B), reflecting the inconsistency of the available data. The use of mechanical prophylaxis is recommended where pharmacologic prophylaxis is contraindicated (grade 1C+). The guidelines recommend *against* the use of aspirin as sole prophylaxis (grade 1A).[1]

The SIGN guidelines, in contrast, gives a strong recommendation for the use of aspirin, suggesting 150 mg of aspirin started on admission and continued for 35 days unless contraindicated.[2] The SIGN guidelines reserve haparins for higher risk HFS patients or those unable to get aspirin or mechanical prophylaxis. The 1997 International consensus statement considered aspirin not the "method of choice," but they note that the PEP trial results were "awaited" at that time.[3]

The newer guidelines note the results of the PEP trial but ultimately decide that there are "too few comparative studies in this group to make secure recommendations."[129] They then go on to state that "the studies that exist are consistent with those from hip replacement patients from whom recommendations could be reasonably extrapolated." Their THR guidelines only consider warferin, LMWH, hirudin, and foot impulse technology as grade A recommendations.

OUR RECOMMENDATIONS

- Fondaparinux (2.5 mg SQ every 24 hours) started 6 hours postoperatively and continued for 2 weeks is our preferred choice, with strong consideration given to extending for 4 weeks.

- Enoxaparin (30 mg SC every 12 hours or 40 mg SC every 24 hours) started 12 hours preoperatively or postoperatively and continued for 2 weeks is a reasonable alternative. Extension of LMWH is of uncertain benefit but could be considered.
- LDUH (5000 units every 8 hours) started 12 hours preoperatively or postoperatively should be considered a second-line agent.
- In patients with contraindication to fondaparinux or heparin products or compelling indications for an antiplatelet drug, aspirin (160 mg PO) given every 24 hours starting postoperatively and continued for up to 5 weeks is an alternative second-line agent.
- In patients with higher risk of VTE, particularly patients with a history of VTE or active malignancy, mechanical prophylaxis with IPC or AVFP should be strongly considered as an adjunct. Patient compliance is a very important factor in efficacy and is likely improved by patient education.
- Thromboprophylaxis should begin as soon before or after surgery as safely possible, according to the dosing parameters of the individual drugs and the means of anesthesia used.
- Particularly for higher-risk patients, extended prophylaxis with fondaparinux for up to 4 weeks or aspirin for up to 5 weeks can be considered.

9. What are the options for preventing venous thromboembolism in trauma patients based on the available evidence?

BACKGROUND

Despite the high prevalence and obvious clinical and financial consequences of VTE in the trauma patient, few well-designed, randomized trials exist to guide recommendations. VTE remains a very common occurrence in this patient population, with overall rates of proximal DVT approaching 20%.[130] PE is the third leading cause of death in patients surviving more than 1 day after injury.[1] Thromboprophylaxis is further complicated because of underlying injuries that prevent or hinder the use of pharmacologic and mechanical prophylaxis, usually due to bleeding concerns or extensive lower extremity fractures. Increasing patient age, injury severity, and time from injury to initiation of prophylaxis are independently associated with large or obstructive VTE, but all trauma patients remain at high risk for VTE.[1] Consensus statements are often forced to extrapolate data from nontrauma and orthopedic studies, and even those studies that specifically focus on trauma patients are difficult to compare because of heterogeneity in the range, distribution, and severity of injury.

EVIDENCE
Pharmacologic and Mechanical Prophylaxis
The efficacy of pharmacologic and mechanical prophylaxis in this patient population has been called into question by two meta-analyses.[131,132] The latter analysis, which included randomized and nonrandomized trials, ultimately concluded that LDUH, LMWH, and mechanical prophylaxis are not significantly better than placebo or each other in the reduction of DVT and PE.[132] There are problems with the analysis beyond the small size and low quality of the included trials. In their comparison of LDUH with LMWH, the study authors used PE as the primary end point, despite the fact that the largest trial in this grouping had used total and proximal DVT as the primary end points and had found a statistically significant advantage of enoxaparin over LDUH on both of these outcomes.[133] Consequently, the shrinkage plot from the meta-analysis did not quite reach statistical significance (OR = 3.01; 95% CI: 0.59 to 15.49).

Few prospective trials compare mechanical and pharmacologic prophylaxis or different modalities of mechanical prophylaxis with each other. The meta-analysis by Velhamos and colleagues[132] included 691 patients in five trials comparing mechanical prophylaxis with placebo and 620 patients in four trials comparing mechanical prophylaxis with LDUH. Neither comparison generated a statistically significant difference. The largest randomized controlled trial of trauma patients randomized 487 consecutive patients with spine, pelvic, or lower extremity fractures to enoxaparin, IPC, or AVFP, depending on the nature and extent of their presenting injury. The incidence of DVT was 0.8% (1 of 120) with enoxaparin, 2.5% (5 of 199) with IPC, and 5.7% (3 of 53) with AVFP in the 76% (372 of 487) of patients available for analysis.[134] In a later study from 2003, the incidence of VTE did not significantly differ with the use of calf-length IPC or twice-daily enoxaparin though the rates of DVT were small in both arms. There were nonsignificant trends toward fever DVTs and more frequent minor bleeding episodes with enoxaparin but an equal number of major bleeding episodes in both groups, none of which required operative intervention.[135]

Compliance with mechanical prophylaxis can be problematic.[136] One study demonstrated a significantly higher rate of compliance with a new, battery-powered, miniaturized compression device,[137] but we know of no trials that examine its efficacy.

Vena Caval Filters

There is no evidence that vena caval filters (VCFs) reduce mortality in trauma patients,[138] although they do reduce the incidence of PE.[139] In a randomized trial of medical patients with proximal DVT, VCF insertion was associated with a reduction in PE at 12 days (1.1% versus 4.8%; OR = 0.22; 95% CI: 0.05 to 0.90). However, there was a concomitant increase in symptomatic DVT at 2 years (20.8% versus 11.6%; OR = 1.87: 95% CI: 1.10 to 3.20) in the patients who received VCF.[140] In a subsequent 8-year follow-up of 99% of these patients, the investigators found a continuation of this trend with an increased incidence of DVT (35.7% versus 27.5%; OR = 1.52; 95% CI: 1.02 to 2.27) and concomitant reduction in PE (6.2% versus 15.1%; OR = 0.37; 95% CI: 0.17 to 0.79) with VCF insertion.[141] There was no difference in mortality at either point of follow-up, although four of the five deaths in the no-filter group at 12 days were caused by PE. There are few prospective data for the use of temporary VCF, but at least one small, single-center, prospective study indicates that they are safe and efficacious but are removed in only a minority of cases at 150 days of follow-up.[142]

Routine Screening

The role of routine screening for asymptomatic VTE in trauma patients is a matter of debate.[142] Because most VTE is clinically asymptomatic and anticoagulation is frequently contraindicated in trauma patients, some authors have suggested that routine, noninvasive screening with ultrasonography may help stratify the management of patients at high risk for VTE. One well-designed study involving more than 200 trauma patients showed that surveillance venous duplex scanning does not affect outcome when used in conjunction with prophylaxis with enoxaparin.[143] A cost analysis from 1997 found that routine, twice-weekly screening with duplex ultrasonography in high-risk trauma patients admitted for at least 2 weeks was more cost effective than VCF in preventing VTE. The same analysis also concluded that enoxaparin was likely more cost-effective than duplex ultrasonography and VCF in this patient population.[145]

Duration of Prophylaxis

The ideal duration of prophylaxis is similarly a matter of debate. With the exception of hip fracture, no trials have specifically examined the role, efficacy, or safety of prolonged prophylaxis in trauma patients. It is likely that the risk of VTE extends beyond hospital stay because studies have found that VTE is often diagnosed after discharge.

CURRENT GUIDELINES

The Seventh ACCP Conference guidelines strongly recommend that all trauma patients with at least one risk factor for VTE receive thromboprophylaxis with LMWH, started as soon as considered safe (grade 1A) and continued until hospital discharge, including inpatient rehabilitation (grade 1C+). Extended prophylaxis with LMWH or VKA is given much more qualified recommendation (grade 2C) for patients with major impaired mobility. The use of IPC or GCS is recommended as monotherapy only in cases where pharmacologic thromboprophylaxis is contraindicated (grade 1B). The guidelines recommend against the use of IVC filters as primary prophylaxis (grade 1C).[1]

The SIGN guidelines similarly favor LMWH in patients with major lower extremity fractures and severe trauma but gives equally[2] strong recommendation for the sole use of mechanical prophylaxis with IPC and AVFP when pharmacologic prophylaxis is contraindicated. The sole use of aspirin is given weaker recommendation because of the lack of evidence.[2]

OUR RECOMMENDATIONS

- Enoxaparin (30 mg SC every 12 hours) should be started as soon as hemostasis allows and continued for at least the duration of the hospital stay.
- Mechanical prophylaxis should be considered as an alternative in all patients ineligible for pharmacologic prophylaxis, preferably with IPC, and at all times while the patient is not ambulatory.
- Screening with duplex ultrasonography can be considered at the time of presentation, but it should not be used instead of pharmacologic and mechanical prophylaxis.
- VCF should be reserved for high-risk patients with an absolute contraindication to mechanical and pharmacologic prophylaxis or with known proximal DVT and contraindications to anticoagulation.

10. What are the options for preventing venous thromboembolism in neurosurgery patients based on the available evidence?

BACKGROUND

The rate of DVT in untreated neurosurgical patients is similar to that seen in untreated general surgery patients. A pooled analysis by the Sixth ACCP Consensus Conference found a DVT rate of 22%, with a 5% proximal DVT rate.[37] Although this rate is pooled across different neurosurgical populations, the rate of VTE is even higher among patients with malignant brain tumors.[1] VTE is also likely a significant contributor to mortality rates in neurosurgical patients, with one autopsy series of consecutive postoperative deaths demonstrating that PE was present in 25% of patients, with PE representing the principal cause of death in almost 50% of patients with PE.[145]

EVIDENCE
Mechanical Prophylaxis

One of the major concerns with using DVT prophylaxis in neurosurgical patients is related to the bleeding complications of pharmacologic therapy. As a consequence, most reviews and guidelines encourage the use of non-pharmacologic therapy. The only trial we encountered that compared GCS with no treatment did demonstrate efficacy of GCS, but this was a small trial with only 161 patients in both arms.[147] Although the rate of all DVT in the GCS arm was 8.8% in this study, other studies that used GCS in the control arm suggest GCS is less efficacious, with rates of DVT as high as 26.3%[148] and 33%.[148] IPC has more data to support its use. A pooled analysis of the effects of IPC by the Sixth ACCP Consensus Conference demonstrated a DVT rate of only 7%, representing a 66% RRR compared with untreated controls.[37] Although the 1989 study by Turpie and colleagues[147] suggested no benefit of IPC over GCS, the evidence from the other studies pooled by the ACCP gives more credence to the efficacy of IPC.

Pharmacologic Prophylaxis

A meta-analysis performed in 2000 investigated the role of heparins as prophylactic agents in neurosurgical patients.[150] The only randomized, controlled trial of LDUH started preoperatively versus untreated controls showed a dramatic and statistically significant reduction in the rate of DVT from 34% to 6% with its use.[151] This trial, however, only had 50 patients in each arm and demonstrated a mild trend toward increased bleeding (2% to 4%, corresponding to one additional bleed). The three LMWH trials involved postoperative LMWH in combination with GCS or alone.[148,149,152] The meta-analysis showed a pooled reduction in DVT rates from 28.3% to 17.5%, which was statistically significant with an odds ratio of 0.54 (95% CI: 0.38–0.77). However, this was associated with a twofold increase in all bleeding rates from 3% to 6.1% (OR = 2.07; 95% CI: 1.10 to 3.87) and in major bleeding rates from 1.3% to 2.2% (OR = 1.68; 95% CI: 0.62 to 4.52), only the former of which reached statistical significance. Although there was a trend toward increased mortality with the use of LMWH, none of these deaths was attributed to study treatment, with most being attributed to nonhemorrhagic intracranial complications. It is unclear whether preoperative administration of heparin (LDUH or LMWH) affects the bleeding complications compared with postoperative administration. Several trials of preoperative LDUH[151,153-155] showed no significant increase in bleeding with preoperative LDUH, although these trials were observational only or had low power to detect differences between treatment arms. Nonetheless, the ACCP infers that LDUH is safe to use preoperatively in neurosurgical patients. In comparison, LMWH use has been associated with increased bleeding rates in a number of trials. The meta-analysis of randomized, controlled trials of LMWH found a statistically significant increase in all bleeding with the use of postoperative LMWH.[150] An unblinded trial by Dickinson and associates[156] showed significantly more bleeding with the use of preoperative LMWH, albeit at a dose of 30 mg given two times daily, compared with GCS. Although three prospective and retrospective observational trials (two early postoperative, one preoperative) of the use of LMWH have shown low rates of bleeding complications,[157-159] most guidelines recommend LMWH only postoperatively and with caution.

CURRENT GUIDELINES

The Seventh ACCP Conference guidelines recommend the routine use of prophylaxis in patients undergoing major neurosurgery, which is not defined, with a grade 1A recommendation of IPC with or without GCS.[1] The investigators consider perioperative LDUH (grade 2B recommendation) and postoperative LMWH (grade 2A) as acceptable alternatives and suggest combined pharmacologic and nonpharmacologic therapy for high-risk neurosurgery patients (presumably, although not explicitly, those with malignancy). The SIGN guidelines recommend GCS with or without IPC as grade A recommendations, viewing them as similarly effective.[2] The study authors also give LMWH a grade A recommendation but mention an increased risk of hemorrhage with its use. The 2001 International Consensus Statement succinctly states that a combination of LMWH and GCS is more effective than GCS alone without causing excessive bleeding.[3]

OUR RECOMMENDATIONS

We think that the Seventh ACCP Conference guidelines provide the soundest recommendations. All patients undergoing major neurosurgery should receive at least IPC, if not GCS in addition. If they have an underlying malignancy (and possibly if they have a history of VTE or thrombophilia), they should likely also receive postoperative LMWH. Although we believe the data showing the benefit of LDUH are weaker than for LMWH, we agree that LDUH three times daily is a reasonable prophylactic option.

- First-line prophylaxis for neurosurgical patients should be IPC with or without GCS. LDUH three times daily or postoperative LMWH are reasonable alternatives, but the latter may have a higher bleeding rate.
- Patients with two or more VTE risk factors (defined in the general surgery section) should be considered for combination pharmacologic and nonpharmacologic prophylaxis.

11. What are the options for preventing venous thromboembolism in patients with spinal cord injury based on the available evidence?

BACKGROUND
Spinal fracture and spinal cord injury (SCI) patients comprise a particularly high-risk subgroup of trauma patients in whom the risk of DVT is increased twofold and threefold, respectively.[139] The risk of VTE is highest 7 to -10 days after injury,[160] remains elevated throughout the rehabilitation period,[164] and decreases after 6 months.[161] Few trials have specifically examined prophylaxis in spinal cord injury patients, and those that have are generally underpowered to detect a difference. Clinicians are often forced to extrapolate from larger trials that include a heterogeneous patient population.

EVIDENCE
Heparin
The available data suggest that LMWH is superior to LDUH, as mentioned in the previous question regarding trauma patients. In a two-tiered, multicenter study looking at the acute and rehabilitative stages of spinal cord injury, investigators randomized 476 acute SCI patients to 5000 units of LDUH every 8 hours with concomitant calf- or thigh-length IPC or 30 mg of twice-daily enoxaparin.[161,164] Only 107 patients could be evaluated for the efficacy outcome during the acute phase study.[161] The incidence of VTE was not different between groups, but

nonfatal PE was significantly reduced at 2 weeks with the use of enoxaparin; nonetheless, the investigators concluded that the combination of LDUH and IPC is "generally similar" to enoxaparin.[162] In the second, rehabilitative phase of the study, 119 of 172 eligible patients were treated with 40 mg of once-daily enoxaparin or 5000 units of LDUH every 8 hours for up to 6 weeks, as determined by randomization during the first stage of the trial. There was a trend to fewer episodes of VTE with LMWH (8.5%) compared with LDUH (21.7%) but this was not statistically significant with an RRR of 0.67% (95% CI: 0.11 to 1.01). In addition, there was no statistically significant difference in DVT, nonfatal PE, fatal PE, bleeding, or death between the two groups. Symptomatic DVT was not quantified.[162] It appears that once-daily dosing of enoxaparin or dalteparin is as efficacious as LDUH every twice daily dosing of enoxaparin 30 mg preventing DVT and PE.[163,164]

Vitamin K Antagonists
Few trials have studied VKA as thromboprophylaxis for spinal cord injury. None of the trials were controlled or of high enough quality to justify its use in this clinical setting.[1]

Mechanical Prophylaxis
Few trials have directly compared pharmacologic and mechanical prophylaxis. GCS has not been studied in this population.[1] Some authorities suggest that monotherapy with mechanical prophylaxis is inappropriate for patients with SCI.[1] In one study, 120 head and spinal cord trauma patients were randomized to 40 mg of once-daily enoxaparin or IPC and followed with weekly screening duplex ultrasonography. There was no statistically significant difference in DVT or bleeding between the two groups despite early initiation of pharmacologic therapy.[166] However, the study was underpowered to detect a difference.

CURRENT GUIDELINES
The Seventh ACCP Conference guidelines recommend prophylaxis for all eligible patients (grade 1A) with LMWH alone (grade 1B) or the combined use of IPC and LDUH (grade 1B). They recommend against the use of LDUH, GCS, or IPC as sole prophylaxis (grade 1A) and against the use of VCF for primary prophylaxis (grade 1C).

Extended prophylaxis with LMWH or VKA during the rehabilitation phase is suggested (grade 1C), but the optimal duration of therapy is not addressed.[1]

The SIGN similarly recommend using LMWH. The guidelines also allow for the use of aspirin when LMWH is contraindicated.[2]

OUR RECOMMENDATIONS

- Enoxaparin (30 mg SC every 12 hours or 40 mg SC every 24 hours) or dalteparin (5000 units SC every 24 hours) should be started as soon as possible after injury and continued for at least 2 weeks.
- IPC in conjunction with LDUH (5000 units every 8 hours) can be employed as a second-line strategy, as can IPC alone in patients for whom pharmacologic prophylaxis is contraindicated.
- AVFP should be used when lower extremity injury precludes the use of IPC.
- Pharmacologic prophylaxis can be considered for up to 6 months, as the risk for thrombosis remains high for up to 6 months.

12. What are the options for preventing venous thromboembolism in gynecologic patients based on the available evidence?

BACKGROUND

Gynecologic surgery carries risks of VTE that are similar to those for general surgery. Pooled data from trials with untreated control arms show a DVT rate of 16% when prophylaxis is not used.[37] Other studies indicate DVT rates from 7% to 29% in general gynecologic surgery and up to 45% in patients with cancer.[166] Much like general surgery, the patient population ranges from relatively young patients undergoing low-risk procedures to patients with cancer undergoing major surgery.

EVIDENCE

Heparin

The therapy with the strongest data supporting its use is LDUH. Pooled data from studies demonstrate a RRR of 56% in the rate of DVT with the use of LDUH.[37]

A Cochrane review found an odds ratio of developing a DVT of 0.30 (95% CI: 0.12 to 0.77) with the use of LDUH in all gynecologic patients, an effect that was maintained in the subset with malignancy (OR = 0.30; 95% CI: 0.10 to 0.87).[167] Two of the three trials in the meta-analysis that showed a statistically significant reduction in DVT employed three times daily dosing of LDUH. This review also found no difference in the rate of DVT when LMWH was compared with LDUH. However, there were only four trials with a total enrollment of 596 patients that qualified for the analysis, making it less certain that these therapies are truly equivalent. The dose of LDUH employed in three of the four included trials was three times daily, whereas the LMWH dose used ranged from 1500 to 3000 anti-Xa units daily (with 4000 anti-Xa units corresponding to 40 mg of enoxaparin). The Seventh ACCP Conference guidelines raised concerns that, for cancer patients, LDUH two times daily might be inferior to LDUH three times daily or to LMWH at a daily dose of at least 4000 anti-Xa units.[1]

Warfarin
The Cochrane review pointed to very limited data on warfarin, which as a result is usually not employed for these patients.[167]

Mechanical Prophylaxis
The Sixth ACCP Conference guidelines report a 44% reduction in the rate of DVT with the use of IPC when data are pooled from studies, but relatively few patients have been studied with this modality.[37] A single study of 196 patients tested the efficacy of GCS in gynecologic patients.[168] There were no DVTs in the 104 patients who wore GCS, compared with four DVTs in the untreated control group. Despite the statistical significance of this finding, in our opinion, this study is too small to allow meaningful conclusions to be drawn.

CURRENT GUIDELINES
The major guidelines generally offer similar advice on how to manage gynecology patients. The SIGN guidelines recommend treating gynecology patients in the same manner as general surgery patients.[2] The 2000 American College of Obstetricians and Gynecologists (ACOG) guidelines divide

gynecology patients into three risk groups—low, moderate, and high—and offer treatment recommendations accordingly as shown in Table 6-4.[166]

The ACOG authors do qualify their recommendations. They acknowledge that it may not be worthwhile to use the more costly LMWH compared with LDUH, because the former has not been shown to be superior with regard to efficacy or bleeding risk. They also acknowledge that the use of GCS has not been as well studied in moderate-risk patients as LDUH. The authors also concede that IPC has not been as well investigated

Table 6-4. Summary of the ACOG Guidelines		
Risk Category	**Definition**	**Treatment Recommendations**
Low (< 3% risk of DVT)	Age ≤ 40 years and surgery lasting ≤ 30 minutes	Early mobilization (level C)
Moderate (10-40% risk of DVT)	Age > 40 and surgery of any duration without other clinical risk factors	• Thigh-high GCS (level A) or • IPC (level A) or • LDUH TID, first dose 2 hours preoperatively (level A) or • LMWH (2500 U daily of dalteparin, or 40 mg daily of enoxaparin), first dose 12 hours preoperatively (level A)
High (40-70% risk of DVT)	Age > 40 years plus risk factors (i.e., prior VTE, varicose veins, infection, malignancy, estrogen therapy, obesity, or prolonged surgery [not defined])	• LDUH tid (Level A) or • LMWH (5000 U daily of dalteparin or 40 mg daily of enoxaparin) (level A) or • IPC (level A)

ACOG, American College of Obstetricians and Gynecologists; DVT, deep venous thrombosis; GCS, graded compression stockings; IPC, intermittent pneumatic compression; LDUH, low-dose unfractionated heparin; LMWH, low-molecular-weight heparin; VTE, venous thromboembolism.
Adapted from American College of Obstetricians and Gynecologists (ACOG): Prevention of Deep Vein Thrombosis And Pulmonary Embolism. ACOG practice bulletin no. 21. Washington, DC, American College of Obstetricians and Gynecologists, 2000, pp 1-10.

in high-risk patients as LDUH or LMWH. They also suggest that combined pharmacologic and mechanical prophylaxis may be beneficial in high-risk patients, particularly patients undergoing radical vulvectomy with inguinal lymphadenectomy or pelvic exenteration for cancer.

The Seventh ACCP Conference guidelines[1] recommend a stepwise approach similar to that for general surgery. These guidelines are, however, more straightforward than the recommendations for general surgery patients. The study authors make a grade 1A recommendation of prophylaxis for all patients undergoing major surgery (not clearly defined although likely defined as nonlaparoscopic procedures lasting longer than 30 minutes). Their other recommendations are presented in Table 6-5.

OUR RECOMMENDATIONS
Our recommendations for how to manage gynecologic patients borrow from our recommendations for general

Table 6-5. Summary of ACCP Guidelines	
Patient Population	**Treatment Recommendations**
Benign disease undergoing procedure ≤ 30 minutes	Early ambulation (grade 1C+)
Patients with VTE risk factors (not defined) undergoing laparoscopic surgery	• LDUH (dosage not defined) (grade 1C) or • LMWH (dosage not defined) (grade 1C) or • IPC (grade 1C) or • GCS (grade 1C)
Major surgery for benign disease without additional risk factors	• LDUH (5000 U bid) (grade 1A) or • LMWH (= 3400 U daily) (grade 1C+) or • IPC (applied preoperatively) (grade 1B)
"Extensive" surgery for malignancy or patients with additional VTE risk factors (not defined)	• LDUH (5000 U tid) (grade 1A) or • LMWH (> 3400 U daily) (grade 1A) or • IPC (grade 1A) or • Combination pharmacologic (LDUH or • LMWH) and mechanical (GCS or IPC) prophylaxis (grade 1C)

GCS, graded compression stockings; IPC, intermittent pneumatic compression; LDUH, low-dose unfractionated heparin; LMWH, low-molecular-weight heparin; VTE, venous thromboembolism.
Adapted from Geerts WH, Pineo GF, Heit JA, et al: Prevention of venous thromboembolism: The Seventh ACCP Conference on Antithrombotic and Thrombolytic Therapy. Chest 2004;126:338S-400S.

surgery, because the scope of VTE risk and types and durations of surgery are often similar. We continue to recommend against the use of LDUH two times daily or LMWH at the lower dose (≤ 3400 units) based on the lack of evidence supporting their use. We also recommend the use of nonpharmacologic approaches only in patients who are at significant risk for bleeding or have contraindications for the use of heparins. Given the uncertainty about which patients clearly benefit but good evidence suggesting the benefits of heparins outweigh the risks, we favor setting the threshold for prophylaxis low. We use the same definitions of VTE risk factors as for general surgery patients. Our treatment recommendations for patients undergoing gynecologic surgery are as follows:

- Low-risk patients (those < 40 years and undergoing minor surgery without VTE risk factors) do not require any prophylaxis beyond early ambulation.
- Any high-risk patients (with at least one VTE risk factor) should receive prophylaxis with LDUH three times daily or higher-dose LMWH (> 3400 units daily).
- High-risk patients at significant risk for bleeding or who have contraindications to heparins should receive mechanical prophylaxis with IPC or thigh-high GCS.
- Patients who are at particularly increased risk (more than two VTE risk factors) should be considered for combined pharmacologic and mechanical prophylaxis.

Although we favor the previous algorithm, we think that following the ACOG or the ACCP guidelines is also reasonable.

13. What are the options for preventing venous thromboembolism in urologic patients based on the available evidence?

BACKGROUND
The data on VTE rates in urologic patients are 10 to 30 years old and may not apply to current patients.[1] However, the rate of symptomatic VTE depends on the nature of the procedure, with transurethral procedures carrying a lower risk of VTE than open procedures.[170,171]

Some have estimated the PE risk of open procedures at 0.4% to 2.7%, with fatal PE rates of 0.6%.[172]

EVIDENCE

The urologic literature is rather deficient in large, randomized, double-blind, placebo-controlled studies investigating the usefulness of prophylactic strategies. The Seventh ACCP Conference guidelines[1] identified only one study that met their requirements for inclusion, and our independent search did not reveal additional blinded, prospective studies. There have been numerous studies that were small, unblinded, observational, or retrospective, many of which give conflicting results. The ACCP guidelines chose to extend their recommendations from other abdominal surgical patients (i.e., general surgery and gynecology) with some modifications, which seems reasonable to us.

CURRENT GUIDELINES

The ACCP guidelines divide the urologic population into separate subgroups. Low-risk patients are those undergoing low-risk urologic procedures (e.g., transurethral procedures). Given the bleeding risk of heparins and the low likelihood of VTE in these patients, they recommend using only early ambulation as prophylaxis in this population (grade 1C+ recommendation). For patients undergoing major, open urologic procedures and who therefore carry a higher VTE risk, they recommend LDUH given twice or three times daily (grade 1A recommendation), although they allow for the use of IPC and/or GCS (grade 1B), or LMWH (grade 1C+). For urology patients who are at high risk for bleeding, they recommend use of nonpharmacologic therapy such as GCS and/or IPC (grade 1C+ recommendation). The ACCP offers a grade 1C+ recommendation of combination pharmacologic therapy and nonpharmacologic therapy for patients with multiple risk factors.

The SIGN guidelines[2] make a grade A recommendation for LDUH or LMWH in patients undergoing major or open urologic procedures who are at "significant risk of VTE (age > 40 years or other risk factors)." They allow for the use of IPC or GCS in patients with contraindications to LDUH or LMWH, a grade B recommendation. In patients undergoing transurethral resection of the prostate (TURP) who have multiple VTE risk factors, "antithrombotic prophylaxis with LDUH, LMWH, or GCS with or without IPC should be considered," which they regard as a grade C recommendation.

OUR RECOMMENDATIONS

Given the inadequacy of the literature, it is difficult to be certain of the best approach for urology patients. Given the similarity of the SIGN guidelines and the ACCP guidelines for this area, we believe it is reasonable to follow either of the guidelines. Our recommendations for patients undergoing urologic surgery are as follows:

- Patients undergoing low-risk urologic procedures, such as transurethral surgery, should receive only early ambulation as prophylaxis.
- Patients undergoing open urologic procedures should receive LDUH three times daily or LMWH, unless they are at increased risk for bleeding; IPC and GCS are reasonable alternatives for patients at high risk for hemorrhage.
- Consideration should be given to combined pharmacologic and nonpharmacologic therapy in patients with two or more VTE risk factors (defined in the general surgery section) who are undergoing open procedures.

14. What are the options for preventing venous thromboembolism in vascular surgery patients based on the available evidence?

BACKGROUND

The rate of VTE has been studied in vascular surgery in only small studies and using a variety of diagnostic tools. Studies using FUS to gauge DVT rates in vascular surgery patients not receiving prophylaxis have suggested rates in the 20% to 30% range.[172,173] Studies using Doppler ultrasound have generally shown marginally lower rates, although patients in many of these trials received prophylaxis or anticoagulation for other indications.[174-176]

EVIDENCE

There have been very few randomized, controlled trials of prophylactic regimens in vascular surgery patients.

One uncontrolled study demonstrated a distal DVT rate of only 2.5% by FUS (0% by ultrasound) using very high doses (8000 anti-Xa units daily) of LMWH with no bleeding complications in 40 vascular bypass patients.[177] Two other studies only compared two active treatment arms (LDUH versus LMWH) suggesting no difference in DVT or bleeding rates between the two therapies.[178,179] The remaining three showed limited benefit in various prophylactic regimens compared with control.[175,180,181] Belch and colleagues[180] showed a significant reduction in DVT rates with LDUH given two times daily (from 24% to 8%) but at a cost of increased bleeding complications (1 patient of 24 controls bled, compared with 8 of 25 treatment-arm patients). In this study, 2500 units of LDUH was administered preoperatively, followed by 5000 units two times daily postoperatively in those assigned to treatment. Killewich and coworkers[176] showed no difference between control and LDUH (5000 units two times daily) combined with calf-length IPC; however, the only end point was the proximal DVT rate, which was low (2%) in both arms of a study of only 100 patients. Spebar and associates[182] found no benefit of LDUH compared with no treatment in a small study of 43 patients.

Therefore, despite the evidence of a fairly high DVT rate (e.g., 28% DVT rate with a 6% proximal DVT rate[176]) in vascular surgery patients, there have been no trials definitively showing a benefit for prophylaxis over no prophylaxis in this population. The use of perioperative and postoperative antiplatelet agents and anticoagulants is common in vascular surgery patients, thereby raising further doubts about the additional benefit provided by prophylactic doses of anticoagulants.

CURRENT GUIDELINES

As a consequence of the lack of strong evidence supporting prophylaxis in vascular surgery patients, the Seventh ACCP Conference guidelines[1] recommend prophylaxis with LDUH or LMWH only in patients with thromboembolic risk factors (grade 1C+ recommendation); otherwise, the ACCP recommends no routine prophylaxis (grade 2B). The SIGN guidelines[2] make a grade C recommendation of LDUH or LMWH in "patients with critical limb ischemia or who are undergoing major peripheral vascular surgery (including amputation)."

OUR RECOMMENDATIONS

Our recommendations mirror those of the Seventh ACCP Conference guidelines. We recognize the difficulty of applying nonpharmacologic therapy in many vascular surgery patients, and we acknowledge the bleeding risk of pharmacologic therapy in this population. Given the paucity of evidence supporting prophylaxis, especially in light of the bleeding complications seen in one trial, the more cautious ACCP recommendations seem sounder to us.

- Patients with fewer than two VTE risk factors (defined in the general surgery section) should not receive routine prophylaxis, unless GCS and IPC are technically feasible.
- Patients with two or more VTE risk factors should receive LDUH three times daily or LMWH, although it is reasonable to use GCS and IPC if they are technically feasible.

15. What are the options for preventing venous thromboembolism in patients with laparoscopic surgery based on the available evidence?

BACKGROUND

The use of prophylaxis in patients undergoing laparoscopic surgery is controversial. Although patients undergoing "minimal access" surgery are mobilized more quickly and hospitalized for a shorter average stay than general surgery patients, laparoscopic surgery is not without risk. It is associated with longer operating times than some general surgical procedures,[183] and pneumoperitoneum and reverse Trendelenburg positioning have been shown to promote femoral venous stasis.[183-186] Nevertheless, a meta-analysis by Lindberg and coworkers[187] demonstrated an incidence of DVT of only 0.02% (though the PE rate was 0.06%) in more than 130,000 patients undergoing laparoscopy, all of whom had received prophylaxis for VTE.

EVIDENCE

There have been few well-designed, prospective, randomized trials examining the role of pharmacologic or mechanical prophylaxis. These studies have focused almost exclusively on laparoscopic cholecystectomy and have generally been small, heterogeneous, and given the low frequency of VTE in this particular population, underpowered to detect a treatment effect.

In a retrospective study, no clinically significant VTE developed in 569 patients receiving no prophylaxis after laparoscopic cholecystectomy, leading the study authors to question the need for routine prophylaxis.[188] In a very large, prospective study, symptomatic VTE developed in only 0.33% (8 of 2384) of patients undergoing laparoscopic surgery, of whom 100% received preoperative prophylaxis with nadroparin and 8.7% received GCS for a history of chronic venous insufficiency or DVT.[189] Later, 238 patients undergoing laparoscopic cholecystectomy were assigned nadroparin or placebo, followed by postoperative ultrasound screening. There was a nonsignificant trend to fewer DVTs with hadroparin but rates were low (3% or less) in each arm.[190] A study from Japan randomized 30 patients undergoing laparoscopic cholecystectomy to LMWH or placebo in conjunction with intraoperative IPC for all patients. Plasma levels of D-dimer were significantly higher in the placebo group at 24 hours postoperatively, the clinical significance of which is unclear.[191] Two other trials also showed exceptionally low rates of VTE in laparoscopic surgery with or without prophylaxis.[192,193]

Mechanical Prophylaxis

The evidence for mechanical prophylaxis is poor and must largely be extrapolated from other surgical populations.[1] IPC seemingly maintains peak flow velocity of the femoral vein during insufflation, based on one small study of 50 patients undergoing laparoscopic cholecystectomy.[186] GCS may have similar hemodynamic effects.[194]

Duration of Prophylaxis

Extended prophylaxis does not seem to be necessary. In the aforementioned study by Catheline and colleagues,[189] six of eight cases of DVT were diagnosed after hospital discharge, before postoperative day 10. An open-label, randomized trial—the first of its kind—found no role for extended prophylaxis in high-risk patients undergoing a variety of laparoscopic procedures. Patients considered high-risk were given dalteparin preoperatively and postoperatively and then discharged on dalteparin or nothing at all. Symptomatic DVT was rare in both groups at 3 months of follow-up, occurring in only 0.95% (1 of 105) of patients assigned no prophylaxis and 0% (0 of 104) of patients assigned dalteparin.[195]

CURRENT GUIDELINES

The Seventh ACCP Conference guidelines recommend "aggressive mobilization" for most patients (grade 1A), but they allow for the use of LDUH, LMWH, IPC, or GCS (grade 1C+) in patients with additional risk factors for VTE.[1]

The SIGN guidelines suggest prophylaxis for high-risk patient populations.[2] This classification of laparoscopic surgery as a low-risk procedure, although validated by some investigators,[196] has not been acknowledged by the Society of American Gastrointestinal Endoscopic Surgeons and the European Association for Endoscopic Surgery, both of whom recommend routine prophylaxis for all patients.[1] Some have taken an intermediate stance, suggesting a tailored approach based on individual risk for VTE.[197]

OUR RECOMMENDATIONS

- GCS or IPC should be used intraoperatively in all patients.
- Enoxaparin (30 mg SC every 12 hours or 40 mg SC daily), dalteparin (2500 to 5000 units SC every 24 hours), or LDUH (5000 units SC every 8 to 12 hours) started preoperatively and continued postoperatively until discharge can be considered in patients at high-risk for VTE.
- Prophylaxis should be continued until ambulation.
- Extended prophylaxis beyond hospital discharge is likely unnecessary.
- Patients should be educated about the signs and symptoms of VTE and instructed to return to the hospital for ultrasonography if they develop concerning signs or symptoms postoperatively.

REFERENCES

1. Geerts WH, Pineo GF, Heit JA, et al: Prevention of venous thromboembolism: The Seventh ACCP Conference on Antithrombotic and Thrombolytic Therapy. Chest 2004;126 (Suppl 3):338S-400S. IV

2. Scottish Intercollegiate Guidelines Network: Prophylaxis of Venous Thromboembolism: A National Clinical Guideline. SIGN publication no. 62, 2002. Available at http://www.sign.ac.uk/ Accessed February 10, 2005. **IV**

3. Nicolaides AN, Bergqvist D, Hill R, et al: Prevention of venous thromboembolism. International Consensus Statement. Int Angiol 1997;16:3-38. **IV**

4. Kakkar AK, Davidson BL, Haas K. On behalf of the Investigators Against Thromboembolism (INATE) Care Group. Compliance with recommended prophylaxis for venous thromboembolism: improving the use and rate of uptake of clinical practice guidelines. J Thromb Haemost 2004;2:221-227.

5. Murray DW, Britton AR, Bulstrode CJK: Thromboprophylaxis and death after total hip replacement. J Bone Joint Surg Br 1996;78:863-870. **I**

6. Salvati EA, Pellegrini VD, Sharrock NE, et al: Symposium: Recent advances in venous thromboembolic prophylaxis during and after total hip replacement. J Bone Joint Surg Am 2000;82:252-270. **V**

7. Ascani A, Radicchia S, Parise P, et al: Distribution and occlusiveness of thrombi in patients with surveillance detected deep vein thrombosis after hip surgery. Thromb Haemost 1996;75:239-241. **III**

8. Ciccone WJ 2nd, Fox PS, Neumyer M, et al: Ultrasound surveillance for asymptomatic deep venous thrombosis after total joint replacement. J Bone Joint Surg Am 1998;8:1167-1174. **III**

9. Wells PS, Lensing AW, Davidson BL, et al: Accuracy of ultrasound for the diagnosis of deep venous thrombosis in asymptomatic patients after orthopedic surgery: a meta-analysis. Ann Intern Med 1995;122:47-53. **I**

10. Rodgers A, MacMahon S: Systematic underestimation of treatment effects as a result of diagnostic test inaccuracy: implications for the interpretation and design of thromboprophylaxis trials. Thromb Haemost 1995;73:167-171. **V**

11. Lee AYY, Gent M, Julian JA, et al: Bilateral vs. Ipsilateral venography as the primary efficacy outcome in thromboprophylaxis clinical trials. J Thromb Haemost 2004;2:1752-1759. **III**

12. Bhandari M, Morrow F, Kulkarni AV, et al: Meta-analyses in orthopaedic surgery: A systematic review of their methodologies. J Bone Joint Surg Am 2001;83:15-24. **I**

13. Guyatt G, Schunemann HJ, Cook D, et al: Applying the grades of recommendation for antithrombotic and thrombolytic therapy: The Seventh ACCP Conference on Antithrombotic and Thrombolytic Therapy. Chest 2004;126(Suppl 3):179S-187S. IV

14. Girard P, Musset D, Parcut F, et al: High prevalence of detectable venous thrombosis in patients with acute pulmonary embolism. Chest 1999;116:903-908. III

15. Agnelli G: Prevention of venous thromboembolism in surgical patients. Circulation 2004;110 (Suppl 1):IV-4 to IV-12. V

16. Philbrick JT, Becker DM: Calf deep venous thrombosis: A wolf in sheep's clothing? Arch Intern Med 1988; 148:2131-2138. I

17. Lagerstedt CI, Olsson CG, Fagher BO, et al: Need for long-term anticoagulant treatment in symptomatic calf-vein thrombosis. Lancet 1985;2:515-518. II

18. Milne AA, Ruckley CV: Venous insufficiency following deep vein thrombosis. Vasc Med Rev1994;5:241-248. V

19. Wille-Jorgensen P, Jorgenson LN, Crawford C: Asymptomatic post-operative deep vein thrombosis and the development of post-thrombotic syndrome: A systematic review and meta-analysis. Thromb Haemost 2005; 93:236-241. I

20. Pulmonary Embolism Prevention (PEP) Trial Collaborative Group: Prevention of pulmonary embolism and deep vein thrombosis with low dose aspirin: Pulmonary Embolism Prevention (PEP) trial. Lancet 2000;355:1295-1302. II

21. Prevention of fatal postoperative pulmonary embolism by low doses of heparin: An international multicentre trial. Lancet 1975;12:45-51. II

22. Collins R, Scrimgeour A, Yusuf S, et al: Reduction in fatal pulmonary embolism and venous thrombosis by perioperative administration of subcutaneous heparin: Overview of results of randomized trials in general, orthopedic, and urologic surgery. N Engl J Med 1988;318:1162-1173. I

23. Hirsh J, O'Donnell M, Weitz JI: New anticoagulants. Blood 2005;105;453-463. V

24. Brody T, Larner J, Minneman K: Human Pharmacology: Molecular to Clinical, 3rd ed. St. Louis, Mosby, 1998. V

25. Gutt CN, Oniu T, Wolkener F, et al: Prophylaxis and treatment of deep vein thrombosis in general surgery. Am J Surg 2005;189:14-22. I

26. Bick RL, Haas S: Thromboprophylaxis and thrombosis in medical, surgical, trauma, and obstetric/gynecologic patients. Hematol Oncol Clin North Am 2003;17:217-258. V

27. Warkentin TE, Levine MN, Hirsh J, et al: Heparin-induced thrombocytopenia in patients treated with low-molecular-weight heparin or unfractionated heparin. N Engl J Med 1995;332:1330-1335. II

28. Anderson DR, Wilson SJ, Blundell J, et al: Comparison of a nomogram and physician-adjusted dosage of warfarin for prophylaxis against deep-vein thrombosis after arthroplasty. J Bone Joint Surg Am 2002;84: 1992-1997. III

29. Tan KT, Lip GY: Fondaparinux. Curr Pharm Des 2005;11:415-419. V

30. Di Nisio M, Middledorp S, Buller HR: Direct thrombin inhibitors. N Engl J Med 2005;353:1028-1040. V

31. Morris RJ, Woodcock JP: Evidence-based compression: prevention of stasis and deep vein thrombosis. Ann Surg 2004;239:162-171. V

32. Vanek VW. Meta-analysis of effectiveness of intermittent pneumatic compression devices with a comparison of thigh-high to knee-high sleeves. Am Surg 1998;11: 1050-1058. I

33. Charalambous C, Cleanthouos S, Trynfonidis M, et al: Foot-pump prophylaxis for deep venous thrombosis: rate of effective usage following knee and hip arthroplasty. Int Orthop 2003;27:208-210. III

34. Pitto RP, Hamer H, Heiss-Dunlop W, et al: Mechanical prophylaxis of deep-vein thrombosis after total hip replacement: a randomized clinical trial. J Bone Joint Surg Br 2004;86:639-642. II

35. Clagett GP, Reisch JS: Prevention of venous thromboembolism in general surgical patients: results of meta-analysis. Ann Surg 1988;208:227-240. I

36. Collins R, Scrimgoeur M, Yusuf S, et al: Reduction in fatal pulmonary embolism and venous thrombosis by perioperative administration of subcutaneous heparin. Overview of results of randomized trials in general, orthopedic, and urologic surgery. N Engl J Med 1988;318:1162-1173. I

37. Geerts WH, Heit J, Clagett GP, et al: Prevention of venous thrombosis. Chest 2001;119(Suppl 1): 132S-175S. IV

38. Wille-Jorgensen P, Rasmussen MS, Andersen BR, et al: Heparins and mechanical methods for thromboprophylaxis

in colorectal surgery. Cochrane Database Syst Rev 2004;(1):CD001217. I

39. Bergmann JF, Neuhart E: A multicenter randomized double-blind study of enoxaparin compared with unfractionated heparin in the prevention of venous thromboembolic disease in elderly in-patients bedridden for an acute medical illness. Thromb Haemost 1996;76:529-534. II

40. Samama MM, Cohen AT, Darmon JY, et al: A comparison of enoxaparin with placebo for the prevention of venous thromboembolism in acutely ill medical patients. N Engl J Med 1999;341:793-800. II

41. Mismetti P, Laporte S, Darmon JY, et al: Meta-analysis of low molecular weight heparin in the prevention of venous thromboembolism in general surgery. Br J Surg 2001;88:913-930. I

42. Nurmohamed MT, Rosendaal FR, Buller HR, et al: Low-molecular-weight heparin versus standard heparin in general and orthopedic surgery: A meta-analysis. Lancet 1992;340:152-156. I

43. Jorgensen LN, Wille-Jorgensen P, Hauch O: Prophylaxis of postoperative thromboembolism with low molecular weight heparins. Br J Surg 1993;80:689-704. I

44. Koch A, Bouges S, Ziegler S, et al: Low molecular weight heparin and unfractionated heparin in thrombosis prophylaxis after major surgical intervention: Update of previous meta-analysis. Br J Surg 1997;84: 750-759. I

45. Koch A, Ziegler S, Breitschwerdt H, et al: Low molecular weight heparin and unfractionated heparin in thrombosis prophylaxis: Meta-analysis based on original patient data. Thromb Res 2001;102:295-309. I

46. Leizorovicz A, Haugh MC, Chapuis FR, et al: Low molecular weight heparin in prevention of perioperative thrombosis. BMJ 1992;305:913-920. I

47. Palmer AJ, Schramm W, Kirchhof B, et al: Low molecular weight heparin and unfractionated heparin for prevention of thrombo-embolism in general surgery: A meta-analysis of randomised clinical trials. Haemostasis 1997;27:65-74. I

48. Breddin HK: Low molecular weight heparins in the prevention of deep-vein thrombosis in general surgery. Semin Thromb Hemost 1999;25(Suppl 3):83-89. I

49. Mcleod RS, Geerts WH, Sniderman K, et al, for the Canadian Colorectal Surgery DVT Prophylaxis

Trial: Subcutaneous heparin versus low-molecular-weight heparin as thromboprophylaxis in patients undergoing colorectal surgery. Results of the Canadian Colorectal DVT Prophylaxis Trial: A randomized, double-blind trial. Ann Surg 2001;233:438-444. **II**

50. Bergqvist D, Burmark US, Flordal PA, et al: Low molecular weight heparin started before surgery as prophylaxis against deep vein thrombosis: 2500 versus 5000 XaI units in 2070 patients. Br J Surg 1995;82:496-501. **II**

51. Wiig JN, Solhaug JH, Bilberg T, et al: Prophylaxis of venographically diagnosed deep vein thrombosis in gastrointestinal surgery: Multicentre trials 20 mg and 40 mg enoxaparin versus dextran. Eur J Surg 1995; 161:663-668. **II**

52. ENOXACAN Study Group: Efficacy and safety of enoxaparin versus unfractionated heparin for prevention of deep vein thrombosis in elective cancer surgery: A double-blind randomized multicentre trial with venographic assessment. Br J Surg 1997;84:1099-1103. **II**

53. Nurmohamed MT, Verhaeghe R, Haas S, et al: A comparative trial of a low molecular weight heparin (enoxaparin) versus standard heparin for the prophylaxis of postoperative deep vein thrombosis in general surgery. Am J Surg 1995;169:567-571. **II**

54. Antiplatelet Trialists' Collaboration: Collaborative overview of randomised trials of antiplatelet therapy-III: reduction in venous thrombosis and pulmonary embolism by antiplatelet prophylaxis among surgical and medical patients. BMJ 1994;308:235-246. **I**

55. Clagett GP, Anderson FA, Geerts W, et al: Prevention of venous thromboembolism. Chest 1998;114(Suppl 5): 531S-560S. **IV**

56. Agnelli G, Bergqvist D, Cohen AT, et al, on behalf of the PEGASUS investigators: Randomized clinical trial of postoperative fondaparinux versus perioperative dalteparin for prevention of venous thromboembolism in high-risk abdominal surgery. Br J Surg 2005;92: 1212-1220. **II**

57. Amaragiri SV, Lees TA: Elastic compression stockings for prevention of deep venous thrombosis. Cochrane Database Syst Rev 2000;(1):CD001484. **I**

58. Best AJ, Williams S, Crozier A, et al: Graded compression stockings in elective orthopaedic surgery. An assessment of the in vivo performance of commercially available stockings in patients having hip and knee arthroplasty. J Bone Joint Surg Br 2000;82:116-118. **III**

59. Ramos R, Salem BI, De Pawlikowski MP, et al: The efficacy of pneumatic compression stockings in the prevention of pulmonary embolism after cardiac surgery. Chest 1996;109:82-859. II

60. Charnley J. The long-term results or low-friction arthroplasty of the hip performed or a primary intervention. J Bone Joint Surg Br 1972;54:61-76.

61. Johnson R, Geen JR, Charnley J. Pulmonary embolism and its prophylaxis following the Charnley total hip replacement. Clin Orthop Relat Res (Clinical orthopaedics and Related Research) 1977;127:123-132.

62. Warwich D, Williams MH, Bennister GC. Death and thromboembolic disease after total hip replacement. A series of 1162 cases with no routine chemical prophylaxis. J Bone Joint Surg Br 1995;77:6-10.

63. Zufferey P, Laporte S, Quenet S, et al: Optimal low-molecular weight heparin regimen in major orthopaedic surgery: A meta-analysis of randomized trials. Thromb Haemost 2003;90:654-661. I

64. Mohr DN, Silverstein MD, Murtaugh PA, et al: Prophylactic agents for venous thrombosis in elective hip surgery: Meta-analysis of studies using venographic assessment. Arch Intern Med 1993;153:2221-2228. I

65. Anderson DR, O'Brien BJ, Levine MN, et al: Efficacy and cost of low-molecular-weight-heparin compared with standard heparin for the prevention of deep vein thrombosis after total hip arthroplasty. Ann Intern Med 1993;119:1105-1112. I

66. Planes A, Vochelle N, Mazas F, et al: Prevention of postoperative venous thrombosis: A randomized trial comparing unfractionated heparin with low molecular weight heparin in patients undergoing total hip replacement. Thromb Haemost 1988;60:407-410. II

67. Mismetti P, Laporte S, Zufferey P, et al: Prevention of venous thromboembolism in orthopedic surgery with vitamin K antagonists: A meta-analysis. J Thromb Haemost 2004;2:1058-1070. I

68. Freedman KB, Brookenthal KR, Fitzgerald RH, et al: A meta-analysis of thromboembolic prophylaxis following elective total hip arthroplasty. J Bone Joint Surg Am 2000;82:929-938. I

69. Hull RD, Pineo GF, Francis C, et al: Low-molecular-weight heparin prophylaxis using dalteparin in close proximity to surgery vs warfarin in hip arthroplasty patients: a double-blind, randomized comparison. Arch Intern Med 2000;160:2199-2207. II

70. Francis CW, Pellegrini VD, Totterman S, et al: prevention of deep-vein thrombosis after total hip arthroplasty: Comparison of warfarin and dalteparin. J Bone Joint Surg Am 1997;79:1365-1372. II

71. Imperiale TF, Speroff T: A Meta-analysis of methods to prevent venous thromboembolism following total hip replacement. JAMA 1994;271:1780-1785. I

72. Turpie AG, Gallus AS, Hoek JA, et al: A synthetic pentasaccharide for the prevention of deep-vein thrombosis after total hip replacement. N Engl J Med. 2001; 344:619-625. II

73. Lassen MR, Bauer KA, Eriksson BI, et al: Postoperative fondaparinux versus preoperative enoxaparin for prevention of venous thromboembolism in elective hip replacement surgery. Lancet 2002;359:1715-1720. II

74. Turpie AGG, Bauer KA, Eriksson BI, et al: Postoperative fondaparinux versus postoperative enoxaparin for prevention of venous thromboembolism after elective hip replacement surgery: A randomised double-blind trial. Lancet 2002;359:1721-1726. II

75. Turpie AGG, Bauer KA, Eriksson BI, et al: Fondaparinux vs enoxaparin for the prevention of venous thromboembolism in major orthopedic surgery: A meta-analysis of 4 randomized double-blind studies. Arch Intern Med 2002;162:1833-1840. I

76. Turpie AGG, Bauer KA, Eriksson BI, et al: Superiority of fondaparinux over enoxaparin in preventing venous thromboembolism in major orthopedic surgery using different efficacy end points. Chest 2004;126:501-508. II

77. Eriksson BI, Wille-Jorgensen P, Kalebo P, et al: A comparison of recombinant hirudin with a low-molecular-weight heparin to prevent thromboembolic complications after total hip replacement. N Eng J Med 1997;337:1329-1335. II

78. Eriksson BI, Arfwidsson AC, Frison L, et al: A dose-ranging study of the oral direct thrombin inhibitor ximelagatran, and its subcutaneous form, melagatran, compared with dalteparin in the prophylaxis of thromboembolism after hip or knee replacement: METHRO I. MElagatran for THRombin inhibition in Orthopaedic surgery. Thromb Haemost 2002;87:231-237. II

79. Eriksson BI, Bergqvist D, Kalebo P: Ximelagatran and melagatran compared with dalteparin for prevention of venous thromboembolism after total hip or knee replacement: The METHRO II randomised trial. Lancet 2002;360:1441-1447. II

80. Colwell CW Jr, Berkowitz SD, Davidson BL, et al: Comparison of ximelagatran, an oral direct thrombin inhibitor, with enoxaparin for the prevention of venous thromboembolism following total hip replacement: a randomized double-blind study. J Thromb Haemost 2003;1:2119-2130. **II**

81. Eriksson BI, Agnelli G, Cohen AT, et al: The direct thrombin inhibitor melagatran followed by oral ximelagatran compared with enoxaparin for the prevention of venous thromboembolism after total hip or knee replacement: The EXPRESS study. J Thromb Haemost 2003;1:2490-2496. **II**

82. Eriksson BI, Agnelli G, Cohen AT, et al: Direct thrombin inhibitor melagatran followed by oral ximelagatran in comparison with enoxaparin for prevention of venous thromboembolism after total hip or knee replacement: the METHRO III study. Thromb Haemost 2003;89: 288-296. **II**

83. Robertson KA, Bertot AJ, Wolfe MW, et al: Patient compliance and satisfaction with mechanical devices for preventing deep venous thrombosis after joint replacement. J South Orthop Assoc 2000;9:182-186. **II**

84. Strebel N, Prins M, Agnelli G, Buller HR: Preoperative or postoperative start of prophylaxis for venous thromboembolism with low-molecular-weight heparin in elective hip surgery? Arch Intern Med 2002;162: 1451-1456. **I**

85. Kearon C, Hirsh J: Starting prophylaxis for venous thromboembolism postoperatively. Arch Intern Med 1995;155:366-372. **I**

86. Hull RD, Brant RF, Pineo GF, et al: Preoperative vs postoperative initiation of low-molecular-weight heparin prophylaxis against venous thromboembolism in patients undergoing elective hip replacement. Arch Intern Med 1999;159:137-141. **I**

87. Raskob GE, Hirsh J: Controversies in timing of the first dose of anticoagulant prophylaxis against venous thromboembolism after major orthopedic surgery. Chest 2003;124(Suppl 6):379S-385S. **V**

88. Burger W, Chemnitius JM, Kneissl GD, et al: Low-dose aspirin for secondary cardiovascular prevention—Cardiovascular risks after its perioperative withdrawal versus bleeding risks with its continuation—Review and meta-analysis. J Intern Med 2005;257:399-414. **I**

89. Arnesen H, Dahl OE, Aspelin T, et al: Sustained prothrombotic profile after hip replacement

surgery: the influence of prolonged prophylaxis with dalteparin. J Thromb Haemost 2003;1:971-975. **II**

90. White RH, Gettner S, Newman JM, et al: Predictors of rehospitalization for symptomatic venous thromboembolism after total hip arthroplasty. N Engl J Med 2000;343:1758-1764. **III**

91. White RH, Romano PS, Zhou H, et al: Incidence and time course of thromboembolic outcomes following total hip or knee arthroplasty. Arch Intern Med 1998;158: 1525-1531. **III**

92. Kearon C: Duration of venous thromboembolism prophylaxis after surgery. Chest 2003;124(Suppl 6): 386S-392S. **V**

93. Douketis JD, Eikelboom JW, Quinlan DJ, et al: Short-duration prophylaxis against venous thromboembolism after total hip or knee replacement. Arch Intern Med 2002;162:1465-1471. **I**

94. Cohen AT, Bailey CS, Alikhan R, et al: Extended thromboprophylaxis with low molecular weight heparin reduces symptomatic venous thromboembolism following lower limb arthroplasty. Thromb Haemost 2001;85:940-941. **I**

95. Hull RD, Pineo GF, Stein PD, et al: Extended out of hospital low-molecular-weight heparin prophylaxis against deep venous thrombosis in patients after elective hip arthroplasty. Ann Intern Med 2001; 135:858-869. **I**

96. Eikelboom JW, Quinlan DJ, Douketis JD: Extended-duration prophylaxis against venous thromboembolism after total hip or knee replacement: A meta-analysis of the randomized trials. Lancet 2001;358:9-15. **I**

97. O'Donnell M, Linkins LA, Kearon Clive, et al: Reduction of out-of-hospital symptomatic venous thromboembolism by extended thromboprophylaxis with low-molecular weight heparin following elective hip arthroplasty. Arch Intern Med 2003;163:1362-1366. **I**

98. Heit JA: Low-molecular-weight heparin: The optimal duration of prophylaxis against postoperative venous thromboembolism after total hip or knee replacement. Thromb Res 2001;101:V163-V173. **V**

99. Bergqvist D, Benoni G, Bjorgell O, et al: Low-molecular-weight heparin (enoxaparin) as prophylaxis against venous thromboembolism after total hip replacement. N Engl J Med 1996; 335:696-700. **II**

100. Comp PC, Spiro TE, Friedman RJ, et al: Prolonged enoxaparin therapy to prevent venous thromboembolism after primary hip or knee replacement. J Bone Joint Surg Am 2001;83:336-345. II

101. Samama CM, Vray M, Barre J, et al: Extended venous thromboembolism prophylaxis after total hip replacement: A comparison of low-molecular-weight heparin with oral anticoagulant. Arch Intern Med 2002;162: 2191-2196. II

102. Brookenthal KR, Freedman KB, Lotke PA, et al: A meta-analysis of thromboembolic prophylaxis in total knee arthroplasty. J Arthroplasty 2001;16:293-300. I

103. Howard AW, Aaron SD: Low molecular weight heparin decreases proximal and distal deep venous thrombosis following total knee arthroplasty. Thromb Haemost 1998;79:902-906. I

104. Bauer KA, Eriksson BI, Lassen MR, et al: Fondaparinux compared with enoxaparin for the prevention of venous thromboembolism after elective major knee surgery. N Engl J Med 2001;345:1305-1310. II

105. Dranitsaris G, Kahn SR, Stumpo C, et al: Pharmacoeconomic analysis of fondaparinux versus enoxaparin for the prevention of thromboembolic events in orthopedic surgery patients. Am J Cardiovasc Drugs 2004;4:325-333. I

106. Heit JA, Colwell CW, Francis CW, et al: Comparison of the oral direct thrombin inhibitor ximelagatran with enoxaparin as prophylaxis against venous thromboembolism after total knee replacement: A phase 2 dose-finding study. Arch Intern Med 2001;161:2215-2221. II

107. Francis CW, Davidson BL, Berkowitz SD, et al: Ximelagatran versus warfarin for the prevention of venous thromboembolism after total knee arthroplasty: A randomized, double-blind trial. Ann Intern Med 2002;137:648-655. II

108. Francis CW, Berkowitz SD, Comp PC, et al: Comparison of ximelagatran with warfarin for the prevention of venous thromboembolism after total knee replacement. N Engl J Med 2003;349:1703-1712. II

109. Westrich GH, Haas SB, Mosca P, Peterson M: Meta-analysis of thromboembolic prophylaxis after total knee arthroplasty. J Bone Joint Surg Br 2000;82: 795-800. I

110. Lachiewicz PF, Kelley SS, Haden LR: Two mechanical devices for prophylaxis of thromboembolism after total

knee arthroplasty. J Bone Joint Surg Br 2004;86: 1137-1141. II

111. Wells PS, Lensing AWA, Hirsh J: Graduated compression stockings in the prevention of postoperative venous thromboembolism. Arch Intern Med 1994;154:67-72. I

112. Westrich GH, Sculco TP: Prophylaxis against deep venous thrombosis after total knee arthroplasty. Pneumatic plantar compression and aspirin compared with aspirin alone. J Bone Joint Surg Am 1996;78: 826-834. II

113. Wilson NV, Das SK, Kakkar VV, et al: Thrombo-embolic prophylaxis in total knee replacement. J Bone Joint Surg Br 1992;74:50-52.

114. Heit JA, Elliott CG, Trowbridge AA, et al: Ardeparin sodium for extended out-of-hospital prophylaxis against venous thromboembolism after total hip or knee replacement. Ann Intern Med 2000;132: 853-861. II

115. Handoll HH, Farrar MJ, McBirnie J, et al: Heparin, low molecular weight heparin and physical methods for preventing deep vein thrombosis and pulmonary embolism following surgery for hip fractures. Cochrane Database Syst Rev 2000;(2): CD000305. I

116. Jorgensen PS, Knudsen JB, Broeng L, et al: The thromboprophylactic effect of a low-molecular-weight heparin (Fragmin) in hip fracture surgery. A placebo-controlled study. Clin Orthop Relat Res 1992;278:95-100. II

117. Gallus AS, Hirsh J, Tuttle RJ, et al: Small subcutaneous doses of heparin in prevention of venous thrombosis. N Engl J Med 1973;288:545-551. II

118. Morris GK, Mitchell JRA: Preventing venous thromboembolism in elderly patients with hip fractures: studies of low-dose heparin, dipyridamole, aspirin, and flurbiprofen. BMJ 1977;1:535-537. II

119. Powers PJ, Gent M, Jay RM, et al: A randomized trial of less intense postoperative warfarin or aspirin therapy in the prevention of venous thromboembolism after surgery for fractured hip. Arch Intern Med 1989; 149:771-774. II

120. Cohen AT, Skinner JA, Kakkar VV: Antiplatelet treatment for thromboprophylaxis: A step forward or backwards? BMJ 1994;309:1213-1215. V

121. Eriksson BI, Bauer KA, Lassen MR, et al: Fondaparinux compared with enoxaparin for the prevention of venous thromboembolism after hip-fracture surgery. N Engl J Med 2001;345:1298-1304. II

122. Eriksson BI, Lassen MR: Duration of prophylaxis against venous thromboembolism with fondaparinux after hip fracture surgery. Arch Intern Med 2003;163:1337-1342. II

123. Bergqvist D: Assessment of the risk and the prophylaxis of venous thromboembolism in surgical patients. Pathophysiol Haemost Thromb 2003;33:358-361. V

124. Annemans L, Minjoulat-Rey MC, De Knock M, et al: Cost consequence analysis of fondaparinux versus enoxaparin in the prevention of venous thromboembolism after major orthopaedic surgery in Belgium. Acta Clin Belg 2004;59:346-357. I

125. Fisher CG, Blachut PA, Salvian AJ, et al: Effectiveness of pneumatic leg compression devices for the prevention of thromboembolic disease in orthopaedic trauma patients: A prospective, randomized study of compression alone versus no prophylaxis. J Orthop Trauma 1995;9:1-7. II

126. Anglen JO, Bagby C, George R: A randomized comparison of sequential-gradient calf compression with intermittent plantar compression for prevention of venous thrombosis in orthopedic trauma patients. Am J Orthop 1998;27:53-58. II

127. Stranks GJ, MacKenzie NA, Grover ML, et al: The A-V impulse system reduces deep-vein thrombosis and swelling after hemiarthroplasty for hip fracture. J Bone Joint Surg Br 1992;74:775-778. II

128. Kennedy JG, Soffe KE, Rogers BW, et al: Deep vein thrombosis prophylaxis in hip fractures: a comparison of the arteriovenous impulse system and aspirin. J Trauma 2000;48:268-272. II

129. Nicolaides AN, Breddin HK, Fareed J, et al: Prevention of venous thromboembolism: international consensus statement. Int Angiol 2000;20:1-37. IV

130. Geerts WH, Code KI, Jay RM, et al: A prospective study of venous thromboembolism after major trauma. N Engl J Med 1994;331:1601-1606. III

131. Upchurch GR Jr, Demling RH, Davies J, et al: Efficacy of subcutaneous heparin in prevention of venous thromboembolic events in trauma patients. Am Surg 1995;61:749-755. I

132. Velmahos GC, Kern J, Chan LS, et al: Prevention of venous thromboembolism after injury: An evidence-based report. Part I. Analysis of risk factors and evaluation of the role of vena caval filters. J Trauma 2000;49: 132-139. **I**

133. Geerts W, Jay RM, Code KI, et al: A comparison of low-dose heparin with low-molecular-weight heparin as prophylaxis against venous thromboembolism after major trauma. N Engl J Med 1996;335:701-707. **II**

134. Knudson MM, Morabito D, Paiement GD, et al: Use of low molecular weight heparin in preventing thromboembolism in trauma patients. J Trauma 1996;41:446-459. **II**

135. Ginzburg E, Cohn SM, Lopez J, et al: Randomized clinical trial of intermittent pneumatic compression and low molecular weight heparin in trauma. Br J Surg 2003;90:1338-1344. **II**

136. Cornwell EE 3rd, Chang D, Velmahos G, et al: Compliance with sequential compression device prophylaxis in at-risk trauma patients: A prospective analysis. Am Surg 2002;68:470-473. **III**

137. Murakami M, McDill TL, Cindrick-Pounds L, et al: Deep venous thrombosis prophylaxis in trauma: improved compliance with a novel miniaturized pneumatic compression device J Vasc Surg 2003;38:923-927. **II**

138. McMurtry AL, Owings JT, Anderson JT, et al: Increased use of prophylactic vena cava filters in trauma patients failed to decrease overall incidence of pulmonary embolism. J Am Coll Surg 1999;189:314-320. **III**

139. Velmahos GC, Kern J, Chan LS, et al: Prevention of venous thromboembolism after injury: An evidence-based report. Part II. Analysis of risk factors and evaluation of the role of vena caval filters. J Trauma 2000;49: 140-144. **I**

140. Decousus H, Leizorovicz A, Parent F, et al: A Clinical trial of vena caval filters in the prevention of pulmonary embolism in patients with proximal deep-vein thrombosis. N Engl J Med 1998;338:409-415. **II**

141. The PREPIC Study Group: Eight-year follow-up of patients with permanent vena cava filters in the prevention of pulmonary embolism. Circulation 2005;112: 416-422. **II**

142. Grande WJ, Trerotola SO, Reilly PM, et al: Experience with the recovery filter as a retrievable inferior vena cava filter. J Vasc Interv Radiol 2005;16:1189-1193. **III**

143. Knudson MM, Ikossi DG: Venous thromboembolism after trauma. Curr Opin Crit Care 2004;10:539-548. Ⓥ

144. Schwarcz TH, Quick RC, Minion DJ, et al: Enoxaparin treatment in high-risk trauma patients limits the utility of surveillance venous duplex scanning. J Vas Surg 2001;34:447-452. Ⓘ︎Ⓘ︎Ⓘ︎

145. Brasel KJ, Borgstrom DC, Weigelt JA: Cost-effective prevention of pulmonary embolus in high-risk trauma patients. J Trauma 1997;42:456-460. Ⓘ

146. Agnelli G: Prevention of venous thromboembolism after neurosurgery. Thromb Haemost 1999;82: 925-930. Ⓥ

147. Turpie AG, Hirsh J, Gent M, et al: Prevention of deep vein thrombosis in potential neurosurgical patients: A randomized trial comparing graduated compression stockings alone or graduated compression stockings plus intermittent pneumatic compression with control. Arch Intern Med 1989;149:679-681. Ⓘ︎Ⓘ

148. Nurmohamed MT, van Riel AM, Henkens CM, et al: Low molecular weight heparin and compression stockings in the prevention of venous thromboembolism in neurosurgery. Thromb Haemost 1996;75:233-238. Ⓘ︎Ⓘ

149. Agnelli G, Piovella F, Buoncristiani P, et al: Enoxaparin plus compression stockings compared with compression stockings alone in the prevention of venous thromboembolism after elective neurosurgery. N Engl J Med 1998;339:80-85. Ⓘ︎Ⓘ

150. Iorio A, Agnelli G: Low-molecular-weight and unfractionated heparin for prevention of venous thromboembolism in neurosurgery: A meta-analysis. Arch Intern Med 2000;160:2327-2332. Ⓘ

151. Cerrato D, Ariano C, Fiacchino F: Deep venous thrombosis and low-dose heparin prophylaxis in neurosurgical patients. J Neurosurg 1978;49:378-381. Ⓘ︎Ⓘ

152. Melon E, Keravel Y, Gaston A, et al: Deep venous thrombosis prophylaxis by low molecular weight heparin in neurosurgical patients [abstract]. Anesthesiology 1987;75:A214. Ⓘ︎Ⓘ

153. Wen DY, Hall WA: Complications of subcutaneous low-dose heparin in neurosurgical patients. Surg Neurol 1998;50:521-525. Ⓘ︎Ⓘ︎Ⓘ

154. MacDonald RL, Amidei C, Lin G, et al: Safety of perioperative subcutaneous heparin for prophylaxis of venous thromboembolism in patients undergoing craniotomy. Neurosurgery 1999;45:245-251. Ⓘ︎Ⓘ︎Ⓘ

155. Constantini S, Kanner A, Friedman A, et al: Safety of perioperative minidose heparin in patients undergoing brain tumor surgery: A prospective, randomized, double-blind study. J Neurosurg 2001;94:918-921. **II**

156. Dickinson LD, Miller LD, Patel CP, et al: Enoxaparin increases the incidence of postoperative intracranial hemorrhage when initiated preoperatively for deep venous thrombosis prophylaxis in patients with brain tumors. Neurosurgery 1998;43:1074-1081. **II**

157. Gerlach R, Scheuer T, Beck J, et al: Risk of postoperative hemorrhage after intracranial surgery after early nadroparin administration: Results of a prospective study. Neurosurgery 2003;53:1028-1035. **III**

158. Gerlach R, Raabe A, Beck J, et al: Postoperative nadroparin administration for prophylaxis of thromboembolic events is not associated with an increased risk of hemorrhage after spinal surgery. Eur Spine J 2004;13:9-13. **III**

159. Kleindienst A, Harvey HB, Mater E, et al: Early antithrombotic prophylaxis with low molecular weight heparin in neurosurgery. Acta Neurochir (Wien) 2003;145:1085-1091. **III**

160. Spinal Cord Injury Thromboprophylaxis Investigators: Prevention of venous thromboembolism in the acute phase after spinal cord injury: A randomized multi-center trial comparing low-dose heparin plus intermittent pneumatic compression with enoxaparin. J Trauma 2003;54:1116-1126. **II**

161. Lamb GC, Tomski MA, Kaufman J, et al: Is chronic spinal cord injury associated with increased risk of venous thromboembolism? J Am Paraplegia Soc 1993;16:153-156. **III**

162. Spinal Cord Injury Thromboprophylaxis Investigators: Prevention of venous thromboembolism in the rehabilitation phase after spinal cord injury: Prophylaxis with low-dose heparin or enoxaparin. J Trauma 2003;54:1111-1115. **II**

163. Hebbeler SL, Marciniak CM, Crandall S, et al: Daily vs twice daily enoxaparin in the prevention of venous thromboembolic disorders during rehabilitation following acute spinal cord injury. J Spinal Cord Med 2004;27:236-240. **II**

164. Chiou-Tan FY, Garza H, Chan KT, et al: Comparison of dalteparin and enoxaparin for deep venous thrombosis prophylaxis in patients with spinal cord injury. Am J Phys Med Rehabil 2003;82:678-685. **II**

165. Kurtoglu M, Yanar H, Bilsel Y, et al: Venous thromboembolism prophylaxis after head and spinal trauma: intermittent pneumatic compression devices versus low molecular weight heparin. World J Surg 2004;28:807-811. II

166. American College of Obstetricians and Gynecologists (ACOG): Prevention of Deep Vein Thrombosis And Pulmonary Embolism. ACOG practice bulletin no. 21. Washington, DC, American College of Obstetricians and Gynecologists, 2000, pp 1-10. IV

167. Oates-Whitehead RM, D'Angelo A, Mol B: Anticoagulant and aspirin prophylaxis for preventing thromboembolism after major gynaecological surgery. Cochrane Database Syst Rev 2003;(4): CD0003679. I

168. Turner GM, Cole SE, Brooks JH: The efficacy of graduated compression stockings in the prevention of deep vein thrombosis after major gynaecological surgery. Br J Obstet Gynaecol 1984;91:588-591. II

169. White RH, Zhou H, Romano PS: Incidence of symptomatic venous thromboembolism after different elective or urgent surgical procedures. Thromb Haemost 2003;90:446-455. III

170. Donat R, Mancey-Jones B: Incidence of thromboembolism after transurethral resection of the prostate (TURP): A study on TED stocking prophylaxis and literature review. Scand J Urol Nephrol 2002;36:119-123. III

171. Kibel AS, Loughlin KR: Pathogenesis and prophylaxis of postoperative thromboembolic disease in urological pelvic surgery. J Urol 1995;153:1763-1774. V

172. Angelides NS, Nicolaides AN, Fernandes J, et al: Deep venous thrombosis in patients having aorto-iliac reconstruction. Br J Surg 1977;64:517-518. III

173. Hartsuck JM, Greenfield LJ: Postoperative thromboembolism. A clinical study with I125-fibrinogen and pulmonary scanning. Arch Surg 1973;107: 733-739. III

174. Passman MA, Farber MA, Marston WA, et al: Prospective screening for postoperative deep venous thrombosis in patients undergoing infrainguinal revascularization. J Vasc Surg 2000;32:669-675. III

175. Killewich LA, Aswad MA, Sandager GP, et al: A randomized, prospective trial of deep venous thrombosis prophylaxis in aortic surgery. Arch Surg 1997;132:499-504. II

176. Hollyoak M, Woodruff P, Muller M, et al: Deep venous thrombosis in postoperative vascular surgical patients: A frequent finding without prophylaxis. J Vasc Surg 2001;34:656-660. **III**

177. Gossetti B, Irace L, Gattuso R, et al: Prevention of deep venous thrombosis in vascular surgical procedures by LMW-heparin. Int Angiol 1988;7(Suppl):25-27. **III**

178. Farkas JC, Chapuis C, Combe S, et al: A randomized controlled trial of a low-molecular-weight heparin (enoxaparin) to prevent deep-vein thrombosis in patients undergoing vascular surgery. Eur J Vasc Surg 1993;7:554-560. **II**

179. Speziale F, Verardi S, Taurino M, et al: Low molecular weight heparin prevention of post-operative deep vein thrombosis in vascular surgery. Pharmatherapeutica 1988;5:261-268. **II**

180. Belch JJ, Lowe GD, Pollack JG et al: Low dose heparin in the prevention of deep-vein thrombosis after aortic bifurcation graft surgery. Thromb Haemost 1980;42:1429-1433. **II**

181. Spebar MJ, Collins GJ, Rich NM, et al: Perioperative heparin prophylaxis of deep venous thrombosis in patients with peripheral vascular disease. Am J Surg 1981;142:649-650. **II**

182. Caprini JA, Arcelus JI: Prevention of postoperative venous thromboembolism following laparoscopic cholecystectomy. Surg Endosc 1994;8:741-747. **V**

183. Wazz G, Branicki F, Taji H, et al: Influence of pneumoperitoneum on the deep venous system during laparoscopy. JSLS 2000;4:291-295. **III**

184. Holzheimer RG: Laparoscopic procedures as a risk factor of deep venous thrombosis, superficial ascending thrombophlebitis and pulmonary embolism—Case report and review of the literature. Eur J Med Res 2004;9:417-422. **V**

185. Rahr H, Fabrin K, Larsen J: Coagulation and fibrinolysis during laparoscopic cholecystectomy. Thromb Res 1999;93:121-127. **III**

186. Schwenk W, Bohm B, Fugener A, et al: Intermittent pneumatic sequential compression (ISC) of the lower extremities prevents venous stasis during laparoscopic cholecystectomy: A prospective randomised study. Surg Endosc 1998;12:7-11. **II**

187. Lindberg F, Bergqvist D, Rasmussen I: Incidence of thromboembolic complications after laparoscopic

cholecystectomy: Review of the literature. Surg Laparosc Endosc 1997;7:324-331. **III**

188. Blake AM, Toker SI, Dunn E: Deep venous thrombosis prophylaxis is not indicated for laparoscopic cholecystectomy. JSLS 2001;5:215-219. **III**

189. Catheline JM, Capelluto E, Gaillard JL: Thromboembolism prophylaxis and incidence of thromboembolic complications after laparoscopic surgery. Int J Surg Invest 2000;2:41-47. **III**

190. Schaepkens Van Riempst JT, Van Hee RH, Weyler JJ: Deep venous thrombosis after laparoscopic cholecystectomy and prevention with nadroparin. Surg Endosc 2002;16:184-187. **II**

191. Okuda Y, Kitajima T, Egawa H, et al. A combination of heparin and an intermittent pneumatic compression device may be more effective to prevent deep-vein thrombosis in the lower extremities after laparoscopic cholecystectomy. Surg Endosc 2002;16:781-784. **III**

192. Bounamedux H, Didier D, Polat O, et al. Antithrombotic prophylaxis in patients undergoing laparoscopic chole-cystectomy. Thromb Res 1997;86:271-273.

193. Bacz I, Schreider B, Kohler T, et al. Prevention of thromboembolism in minimal invasive interventions and brief inpatient treatment. Results of a multicenter, prospective, randomized, controlled study with a low weight heparin. [German] Chirung 1997;68:1275-1280.

194. Wilson YG, Allen PE, Skidmore R, et al: Influence of compression stockings on lower-limb venous haemodynamics during laparoscopic cholecystectomy. Br J Surg 1994;81:841-844. **III**

195. Tincani E, Piccoli M, Turrini F: Video laparoscopic surgery: Is out-of-hospital thromboprophylaxis necessary? J Thromb Haemost 2005;3:216-220. **II**

196. Bergqvist D, Lowe G: Venous thromboembolism in patients undergoing laparoscopic and arthroscopic surgery and in leg casts. Arch Intern Med 2002;162:2173-2176. **V**

197. Zacharoulis D, Kakkar AK: Venous thromboembolism in laparoscopic surgery. Curr Opin Pulm Med 2003;9:356-361. **V**

7

Anticoagulation Management in the Surgical Patient

John Evans and Gary Crooks

1. Which surgical procedures have not been associated with an increased bleeding risk in patients therapeutic on oral anticoagulation?

Search Date: April 2005

Search Strategy: *A search of PubMed, from 1990 to 2005, with the terms "surgical procedures, operative" (MeSH) AND "anticoagulants" (MeSH) AND "perioperative care" (MeSH); 301 citations found. Titles and abstracts were scanned with relevant citations selected. Bibliographies of all relevant citations were reviewed.*

Many patients undergoing surgery are chronically on anticoagulation medications. The risks of thromboembolism posed by discontinuation of anticoagulation therapy must be weighed against the risks of excessive bleeding posed by the continuation of anticoagulation in the perioperative period.

Neither the search strategy nor a systematic review by Dunn and colleagues[1] of patients receiving oral anticoagulants and undergoing surgical procedures yielded any randomized, controlled clinical trials comparing continuation of anticoagulation perioperatively with discontinuing perioperative anticoagulation altogether or with bridging with other anticoagulants such as heparins. Following the best evidence published to date, this systematic review examining management of patients receiving long-term oral anticoagulation with warfarin and undergoing various surgical procedures found that there was no increased risk of major bleeding for single and multiple dental extractions, joint and soft tissue injections and arthrocenteses, cataract surgery, and esophagogastroduodenoscopy or colonoscopy without biopsy when the procedures were conducted on patients with an international normalized ratio (INR) in the therapeutic range.[1] Although the review reported increased rates of bleeding in patients on therapeutic warfarin who underwent cutaneous surgery and genitourinary procedures, there are reports of many dermatologic procedures being conducted safely while on therapeutic anticoagulation.[2]

2. Which patients who require interruption of warfarin anticoagulation perioperatively should receive bridging therapy, and what is the optimal method of bridging?

Search Date: April 2005

Search Strategy: A search of PubMed, from 1990 to 2005, with the terms "bridging" and "anticoagulants" (MeSH); 31 citations found. Titles and abstracts were scanned with relevant citations selected. Bibliographies of all relevant citations were reviewed.

A systematic review of perioperative management of patients receiving oral anticoagulation with warfarin found that the observed rates of arterial thromboembolism and stroke in patients in whom anticoagulation was discontinued perioperatively are greater than the predicted time-adjusted rates for persons not receiving anticoagulation.[1] This risk is weighed against the increased risk of major bleeding associated with anticoagulation in the perioperative period, estimated to be 2% to 4% with major surgery,[1] and the consequences of each adverse outcome. In some patients, the risk of thromboembolism outweighs the increased risk of hemorrhage, justifying the use of unfractionated heparin (UFH) or low-molecular-weight heparin (LMWH) as bridging therapy. Unfortunately, no randomized, controlled trials have been conducted to identify which populations would benefit from perioperative bridging anticoagulation therapy, nor are there randomized, controlled trials comparing outcomes with different bridging strategies. There is no consensus among expert opinions or clinical practice recommendations regarding which patients should be anticoagulated with bridging therapy and how the bridging should be done. Although randomized, controlled trials are lacking, retrospective studies suggest that bridging with LMWH is a safe and cost-effective alternative to UFH.[3-5]

ACC/AHA RECOMMENDATIONS

The American College of Cardiology/American Heart Association (ACC/AHA) Foundation Guide to Warfarin Therapy[6] states that warfarin can be stopped 4 to 5 days preoperatively in most patients, thereby leaving them unprotected for 2 to 3 days preoperatively. However, this period can be reduced by withholding anticoagulation for only 2 days preoperatively and administering 2.5 mg of oral vitamin K 2 days before surgery. This guide suggests that heparin can be given to further limit the time a patient is unprotected from therapeutic anticoagulation. The guidelines recommend that preoperative prophylactic doses of heparin (5000 units of UFH or 3000 anti-Xa units of LMWH, where 4000 anti-Xa units corresponds to 40 mg of enoxaparin given subcutaneously every 12 hours) can be given for patients at moderate risk for thromboembolism and restarted 12 hours postoperatively along with warfarin unless the patient is at high risk for postoperative bleeding. These same guidelines suggest that for high-risk patients, treatment should be initiated with therapeutic doses of UFH or LMWH, with discontinuation 5 hours before surgery in the case of intravenous UFH or 24 hours before surgery for subcutaneous UFH or LMWH. Although there is no consensus regarding which patients should be considered high risk, Kearon and coworkers[7] reserve the use of bridging anticoagulation with intravenous UFH for patients with acute venous thromboembolism or acute arterial embolism within the previous month.

OUR RECOMMENDATIONS

Based on these recommendations, we suggest bridging anticoagulation in patients with acute venous or arterial embolism. Given the possibility that observed rates of embolism after surgery may be higher than the rates in patients untreated with anticoagulation, it is also reasonable to bridge with UFH or LMWH in patients with venous thromboembolism in the past 3 months, recurrent venous thromboembolism, or atrial fibrillation with previous embolism. Although it may be reasonable to use bridging anticoagulation in patients with mechanical heart valves, no definitive studies provide evidence on which to base this decision, and LMWH has not been approved by the U.S. Food and Drug Administration (FDA) for this indication.

3. What is the role of vena caval filters in the patient with acute deep venous thrombosis?

Search Date: April 2005

Search Strategy: *A search of PubMed, from 1990 to 2005, with the terms "vena cava filters" (MeSH) and "venous thrombosis" (MeSH); 407 citations reviewed. Titles and abstracts were scanned, with relevant citations selected. Bibliographies of all relevant citations were reviewed.*

The only widely accepted indications for inferior vena cava filter placement in patients with acute venous thromboembolism are absolute contraindications to anticoagulants or documented failure of anticoagulant therapy.[8,9] A systematic review of the literature concluded that there is no definitive evidence to support any alternative indications for vena caval interruption in patients with acute deep venous thrombosis (DVT).[10] Although there are several randomized, controlled trials evaluating the role of vena caval filter as prophylaxis against DVT and pulmonary embolism, there is only one randomized, controlled clinical trial evaluating the role of vena caval filters in patients who have already been diagnosed with a proximal DVT.[11] Although this trial did show a statistically significant reduction in risk of pulmonary embolism with placement of a vena caval filter from 4.8 to 1.1% (OR = 0.22; 95% CI: 0.05 to 0.90), no statistically significant impact on mortality was demonstrated. The placement of a vena caval filter was associated with a statistically significant increase in the rate of recurrent DVT at 2 years: 20.8% in the filter group compared with only 11.6% in the no filter group (OR = 1.87; 95% CI: 1.10 to 3.20).

No consensus recommendations regarding the placement of vena caval filter exist. Due to a lack of evidence on which to base recommendations and because "the reports do not use consistent standards, definitions, or techniques, making it difficult to compare outcomes and determine the relative efficacy and safety of the available devices," the Vena Cava Filter Consensus Conference was only able to establish reporting standards for indications for filter placement in an effort to make future review of the question more clear.[12] We recommend that venal filter filters be placed in surgical patients diagnosed with acute DVT's only when anticoagulation is contraindicated or is known to have failed.

4. Is there any indication for thrombophilia evaluation in a patient with an isolated postoperative deep venous thrombosis?

Search Date: April 2005

Search Strategy: A search of PubMed, from 1990 to 2005, with the terms "thrombophilia, diagnosis (MeSH) OR thrombophilia, epidemiology" (MeSH)) AND "venous thrombosis" (MeSH); 324 citations found. Titles and abstracts were scanned with relevant citations selected. Bibliographies of all relevant citations were reviewed.

There have been no randomized, controlled trials indicating that the identification of a condition predisposing to thrombophilia in patients with postoperative DVT has any impact on the treatment or outcome. According to the guidelines written by the Haemostasis and Thrombosis Task Force of the British Committee for Standards in Haematology,[13] "There is no evidence that the detection of a heritable thrombophilic defect is useful in guiding clinical decision-making in relation to the choice of anticoagulant or to the intensity or duration of anticoagulant therapy to treat a thrombotic event." As with any patient with a new DVT, age-appropriate cancer screening is appropriate.

5. Should an upper extremity deep venous thrombosis be treated differently from a proximal deep venous thrombosis of the lower extremity?

Search Date: April 2005

Search Strategy: A search of PubMed, from 1990 to 2005, with the terms "upper extremity" (MeSH) AND "venous thrombosis" (MeSH); 223 citations found. Titles and abstracts were scanned, with relevant citations selected. Bibliographies of all relevant citations were reviewed.

The major risks of upper extremity DVT include pulmonary embolism (PE) and post-thrombotic sequelae.[14,15] The incidence of PE in patients with an untreated upper extremity DVT has been reported to be as high as 36%,[14] although estimates average as low as 12%.[16] Given this risk, patients with DVT of the upper extremity are typically treated in the same manner as patients with proximal lower extremity DVT.

Treatment modalities include limb elevation, graduated compression arm sleeve, anticoagulation, catheter-directed thrombolysis, suction thrombectomy, angioplasty, vein stenting, surgical thrombectomy, thoracic outlet decompression, and superior vena cava filter.[17] Unfortunately, no systematic reviews or randomized, controlled clinical trails have been conducted to evaluate differences in treatment modalities. There is, however, general agreement that in patients without contraindication, anticoagulation is the cornerstone of therapy.[17]

6. Is postoperative atrial fibrillation an indication for anticoagulation?

Search Date: April 2005

Search Strategy: A search of PubMed, from 1990 to 2005, with the terms "postoperative atrial fibrillation" and "anticoagulants" (MeSH); 5 citations found. Titles and abstracts were scanned, with relevant citations selected. Bibliographies of all relevant citations were reviewed.

No randomized, controlled trials evaluating the use of anticoagulants in treating postoperative atrial fibrillation have been conducted. Although patients with postoperative atrial fibrillation are excluded in the clinical guidelines for the management of newly detected atrial fibrillation from American Academy of Family Physicians and American College of Physicians,[18] it is reasonable to follow the ACC/AHA/ESC Guidelines for the Management of Patients with Atrial Fibrillation.[19] These guidelines state that the weight of evidence or opinion favors administration of antithrombotic medication in patients who develop postoperative atrial fibrillation as recommended for nonsurgical patients because the incidence of postoperative stroke in these patients is 1.2 to 1.4%.[20]

Recommendations following these guidelines include anticoagulation with warfarin if atrial fibrillation persists for 48 hours or longer. Warfarin should be titrated to a goal INR of 2.0 to 3.0 and be continued for 4 weeks after restoration of sinus rhythm. In nonsurgical patients without significant risk factors for stroke (e.g., patients younger than 65 with no cardiovascular disease) or with contraindications to anticoagulation, aspirin (325 mg daily) may be used to reduce the risk of stroke,[21,22] and there is consensus in the belief that this risk reduction can be extrapolated to surgical patients.[19] There is a lack of evidence and a lack of consensus opinion regarding the use of heparin until the INR is therapeutic in patients most at risk.

7. Is there an advantage to a particular route (oral, subcutaneous, intramuscular, or intravenous) of vitamin K administration in reversal of anticoagulation?

Search Date: April 2005

Search Strategy: A search of PubMed, from 1990 to 2005, with the terms "vitamin K" (MeSH) AND "anticoagulants OR antagonists and inhibitors" (MeSH); 19 citations found. Titles and abstracts were scanned, with relevant citations selected. Bibliographies of all relevant citations were reviewed.

Vitamin K is available as oral tablets or in ampules for administration. Intramuscular administration is not recommended because it may form a depot at the injection site and cause a hematoma to form (according to product information). Subcutaneous administration has been unpredictable and unreliable.[23-25] Intravenous vitamin K can reverse warfarin anticoagulation in 4 to 6 hours, whereas oral vitamin K works over the course of 24 hours.[26]

Although there are no randomized, controlled clinical trials comparing outcomes with intravenous versus oral vitamin K to reverse anticoagulation, oral vitamin K is generally preferred unless very rapid reversal is required.[6] However, if gastrointestinal absorption is impaired, the intravenous route should be used. There is a risk of anaphylaxis with intravenous vitamin K. Oral doses of 1 to 2 mg are usually sufficient to reduce the INR, but if the INR is particularly high, 5 mg may be required. Doses of 0.5 to 1 mg of intravenous vitamin K are used for partial INR reversal; 5 to 10 mg given intravenously can normalize the INR.[27] Large doses pose the risk of some resistance to re-anticoagulation.

REFERENCES

1. Dunn AS, Turpie AG: Perioperative management of patients receiving oral anticoagulants: A systematic review. Arch Intern Med 2003;163:901-908. I

2. Billingsley EM: Intraoperative and postoperative bleeding problems in patients taking warfarin, aspirin, and nonsteroidal anti-inflammatory agents. Dermatol Surg 1997;23:381-383. VI

3. Douketis JD, Johnson JA, Turpie AG: Low-molecular-weight heparin as bridging anticoagulation during interruption of warfarin: Assessment of a standardized periprocedural anticoagulation regimen. Arch Intern Med 2004; 64:1319-1326. V

4. Spyropoulos AC, Frost FJ, Hurley JS, Roberts M: Costs and clinical outcomes associated with low-molecular-weight heparin vs unfractionated heparin for perioperative bridging in patients receiving long-term oral anticoagulant therapy. Chest 2004;125:1642-1650. III

5. Amorosi SL, Tsilimingras K, Thompson D, et al: Cost analysis of "bridging therapy" with low-molecular weight versus unfractionated heparin during temporary interruption of chronic anticoagulation. Am J Cardiol 2004;93: 509-511. V

6. Hirsh J, Fuster V, Ansell J, et al: American Heart Association/American College of Cardiology foundation guide to warfarin therapy. Circulation 2003;107: 1692-1711. IV

7. Kearon C, Hirsh J: Management of anticoagulation before and after elective surgery. N Engl J Med 1997; 336:1506-1511. V

8. Hyers TM, Agnelli G, Hurd RD, et al: Antithrombotic therapy for venous thromboembolic disease. Chest 2001;119(Suppl):176S-193S. IV

9. Geerts WH. Heit JA, Clagett JP, et al: Prevention of venous thromboembolism. Chest 2001;119(Suppl): 132S-175S. IV

10. Girard P, Stern JB, Parent F: Medical literature and vena cava filters: So far so weak. Chest 2002;122:963-967. V

11. Decousus H, Leizorovicz A, Parent F, et al: A clinical trial of vena caval filters in the prevention of pulmonary embolism in patients with proximal deep-vein thrombosis: Prevention du Risque d'Embolie Pulmonaire par Interruption Cave Study Group. N Engl J Med 1998;338:409-415. II

12. Vena Cava Filter Consensus Conference: Recommended reporting standards for vena caval filter placement and patient follow-up. J Vasc Surg 1999;30:573-579. IV

13. Haemostasis and Thrombosis Task Force, British Committee for Standards in Haematology: Investigation and management of heritable thrombophilia. Br J Haematol 2001;114:512-528. IV

14. Prandoni P, Polistena I, Bernardi E, et al: Upper extremity deep venous thrombosis: Risk factors, diagnosis and complications. Arch Intern Med 1997;157:57-62. VI

15. Lindblad B, Tengborn L, Bergqvist D: Deep vein thrombosis of the axillary subclavian veins: Epidemiologic data, effects of different types of treatment and late sequelae. Eur J Vasc Surg 1988;2:161-165. VI

16. Horattas MC, Wright DJ, Fenton AH, et al: Changing concepts of deep venous thrombosis of the upper extremity—report of a series and review of the literature. Surgery 1988;104:561-567. VI

17. Hylton V, Goldhaber Z: Upper extremity deep vein thrombosis. Circulation 2002;106:1874-1880. V

18. Snow V, Weiss KB, LeFevre M, et al: Management of newly detected atrial fibrillation: A clinical practice guideline from the American Academy of Family

Physicians and the American College of Physicians. Ann Intern Med 2003;139:1009-1017. IV

19. Fuster V, Ryden LE, Cannon DS, et al: ACC/AHA/ESC guidelines for the management of patients with atrial fibrillation. J Am Coll Cardiol 2001;38:1231-1265. IV

20. Crystal E, Connolly SJ, Sleik K, et al: Interventions on prevention of postoperative atrial fibrillation in patients undergoing heart surgery: A meta-analysis. Circulation 2002;106:75-80. I

21. Stroke Prevention in Atrial Fibrillation Investigators: Stroke prevention in atrial fibrillation study: Final results. Circulation 1991;84:527-539. II

22. Laupacis A, Albers G, Dalen J, et al: Antithrombotic therapy in atrial fibrillation. Chest 1998;114(Suppl): 579S-589S. IV

23. Raj G, Kumar R, McKinney WP: Time course of reversal of anticoagulant effect of warfarin by intravenous and subcutaneous phytonadione. Arch Intern Med 1999;159:2721-2724. II

24. Whitling AM, Bussey HI, Lyons RM: Comparing different routes and doses of phytonadione for reversing excessive anticoagulation. Arch Intern Med 1998;158:2136-2140. III

25. Crowther MA, Douketis JD, Schnur T, et al: Oral vitamin K lowers the international normalized ratio more rapidly than subcutaneous vitamin K in the treatment of warfarin-associated coagulopathy. Ann Intern Med 2002;137:251-254. III

26. Watson HG, Baglin T, Laidlaw SL, et al: A comparison of the efficacy and rate of response to oral and IV vitamin K in the reversal of over-anticoagulation with warfarin. Br J Haematol 2001;115:145-149. III

27. Warkentin TE, Crowther MA: Reversing anticoagulants both old and new. Can J Anesth 2002;49:S11-S25. V

8

Hematologic Issues in Medical Consultation

Daniel I. Steinberg and Nadia Ahmad

1. In patients with sickle cell disease undergoing surgery, does routine preoperative transfusion reduce morbidity or mortality?

Search Date: January 2006

Search Strategy: *PubMed search of "sickle cell anemia AND transfusion AND surgery," limited to English and humans; 283 citations found, with titles and abstracts reviewed for relevancy; 25 citations selected and reviewed in detail, with all bibliographies reviewed.*

Surgery is common in patients with sickle cell disease. Many sickle cell patients who undergo surgery have a significant preexisting anemia that does not cause symptoms. Although hotly debated, the best preoperative transfusion strategy for these patients is unclear. No high-quality randomized trials have examined the effect of transfusion compared with no transfusion in patients with sickle cell disease undergoing surgery.

Although one randomized, controlled trial from Saudi Arabia studied the effect of transfusion compared with no transfusion, the trial was inconclusive. The study authors did not report the baseline characteristics of the patients, information about allocation concealment, blinding, or whether analysis was based on intention to treat.[1] A meta-analysis by the Cochrane Collaboration found the methodology of this trial too vague to allow interpretation of the results. This meta-analysis found insufficient high-quality evidence to make any recommendation about the effect of routine blood transfusions before surgery in people with sickle cell disease.[2]

There is a lack of randomized, controlled trials addressing this issue, probably because routine preoperative transfusion in this population makes good sense physiologically and has long been viewed as the standard of care. However, a survey in the United Kingdom examining the management of 114 patients with sickle cell disease undergoing diverse types of operations found wide variations in practice, with 43% of patients receiving no transfusions before surgery. In this survey, multivariable logistic regression analysis found that preoperative transfusion could increase or decrease the risk of postoperative complications (odds ratio [OR] for postoperative complications, 1.7; 95% CI, 0.5 to 6).[3] Other nonrandomized trials have had various results, with some researchers concluding that withholding transfusion may be safe for patients undergoing low-risk surgery,[4] others finding that nontransfused patients had higher rates of painful crisis and acute chest syndrome,[5] and still others finding that perioperative transfusion led to lower rates of postoperative sickle events.[6]

The wide variation in practice and inconsistency in nonrandomized trial results set the stage for a high-quality randomized, controlled trial of preoperative transfusion compared with no transfusion.

Different preoperative transfusion strategies have been compared. The most important randomized, controlled trial assessing this issue compared an aggressive preoperative transfusion strategy (i.e., designed to maintain a hemoglobin level of 10 g/dL and to decrease the hemoglobin S level to less than 30%) with a conservative strategy (i.e., designed only to maintain a hemoglobin of 10 g/dL) in 551 patients with homozygous sickle cell disease confirmed by electrophoresis.[7] Cholecystectomy; ear, nose, and throat procedures; and orthopedic procedures were the most common operations performed. The aggressive strategy resulted in an increase in transfusion-related hemolysis and the development of new alloantibodies, without any clear effect on the frequency of acute chest syndrome, painful crisis, postoperative infection, or death, suggesting that there may be no advantage to achieving a lower percentage of hemoglobin S before surgery. The wide confidence intervals include the possibility of a reduction or increase in these outcomes (Table 8-1).

Although quite tempting when considered physiologically, the effect of preoperative blood transfusion in

Table 8-1. Effects of Transfusion Strategies in a Randomized Trial of 604 Surgical Procedures in Patients with Sickle Cell Disease

Outcome	Aggressive Transfusion Group (Hgb >10 g/dL and hemoglobin S < 30%)	Conservative Transfusion Group (Hgb > 10g/ dL only)	Odds Ratio (95% CI)
Death	0.66%	0%	4.95 (0.24 to 103)
Postoperative infection	7%	5%	1.49 (0.76 to 2.94)
Acute chest syndrome	11%	10%	1.10 (0.65 to 1.86)
Painful crisis	5%	7%	0.69 (0.35 to 1.67)
New alloantibody	10%	5%	2.34 (1.22 to 4.49)
Hemolysis (delayed or immediate)	6%	1%	4.97 (1.67 to 14.78)

Adapted from Riddington C, Williamson L: Preoperative blood transfusions for sickle cell disease. Cochrane Database Syst Rev 2001;3:CD003149.

sickle cell patients compared with no transfusion is still unclear. Many observational studies have been done and have had conflicting results. A randomized, controlled trial is necessary to help settle the issue.

It appears that an aggressive preoperative transfusion strategy causes more transfusion-related complications than a conservative strategy, without conferring any clear benefit. Until better evidence is available, it seems prudent that clinicians adopt a conservative transfusion strategy for most patients. Withholding routine preoperative transfusion altogether may be reasonable in selected cases, although this remains a matter of clinical judgment and individual patient circumstances, and it requires further study in randomized, controlled trials.

2. How should thrombotic thrombocytopenic purpura be diagnosed?

Search Date: January 2006

Search Strategy: PubMed search of "thrombotic thrombocytopenic purpura," field, abstract/title, limits: clinical trial and humans; 57 citations found, 18 selected and reviewed. Bibliographies of all citations were searched. Separate search of thrombotic thrombocytopenic purpura, limit: review; 5 recent reviews selected and reviewed, with bibliographies searched. Search included the American College of Physicians PIER and the guidelines of the American Society of Hematology.

Without an objective, gold standard test, the diagnosis of thrombotic thrombocytopenic purpura (TTP) has always rested on clinical criteria. TTP was originally defined in the 1960s as the pentad of thrombocytopenia, microangiopathic anemia, neurologic abnormalities, renal abnormalities, and fever.[8] However, the frequencies of clinical findings in TTP have varied widely among case series. Fever was documented in 26% of patients in one series and in 98% of patients in another series. The frequency of neurologic abnormalities has varied from 63% to 92% across case series. Renal abnormalities have shown similar variations[8-10] (Table 8-2).

A more modern and practical definition of TTP is one that mimics the inclusion criteria from a randomized, controlled trial that demonstrated the benefits of plasma exchange and plasma infusion in TTP. Specifically, clinicians should diagnose TTP and consider treatment of a patient who presents with a platelet count less than 100,000, who has microangiopathic hemolytic anemia as evidenced by schistocytes on a peripheral blood smear, and who has no identifiable cause for the thrombocytopenia or the anemia (e.g., disseminated intravascular coagulation, carcinoma, eclampsia).[10] This definition has been adopted by hematologists, with thrombocytopenia and anemia referred to as primary diagnostic criteria and with neurologic and renal manifestations and fever viewed as common features but not essential to the diagnosis of TTP[11] (see Table 8-2).

Although TTP can have many different causes and crossover between TTP and other syndromes such as

Table 8-2. Diagnosis of Thrombotic Thrombocytopenic Purpura

Essential Diagnostic Criteria*

Thrombocytopenia (platelet count < 100,000)
Microangiopathic hemolytic anemia (i.e., schistocytes on peripheral blood smear)
No alternative explanation for the previous two criteria

Other Clinical Features[†]

Renal abnormalities (59% to 88%)
Neurologic abnormalities (63% to 92%)
Fever (26% to 98%)
Weakness[‡]
Nausea, vomiting, diarrhea, abdominal pain[‡]
ADAMTS13 deficiency or presence of ADAMTS13 inhibitor[§]

Presence of all three criteria alone is sufficient to establish a presumptive diagnosis of thrombotic thrombocytopenic purpura/hemolytic uremic syndrome (TTP/HUS) and to begin treatment with plasma exchange or plasma infusion.
[†]*Considered common but not essential for diagnosis.*
[‡]*Prevalence of these findings in TTP/HUS is unclear.*
[§]*The role of ADAMTS13 testing in the diagnosis of TTP remains unclear.*
Adapted from George JN: How I treat patients with thrombotic thrombocytopenic purpura–hemolytic uremic syndrome. Blood 2000;96:1223-1229; George JN: Thrombotic thrombocytopenic purpura: A syndrome that keeps evolving. J Clin Apher 2004;19:63-65.

hemolytic uremic syndrome (HUS) exists, these differences do not affect the initial diagnosis and management. In the major randomized, controlled trial to examine plasma exchange and plasma infusion, survival rates for patients with or without renal failure were similar, making precise determination of the clinical syndrome (i.e., TTP or TTP/HUS) unnecessary before beginning treatment.[12]

Deficiency of and the presence of an inhibitor to the von Willebrand cleaving protease ADAMTS13 (a disintegrin and metalloprotease, with thrombospondin-1–like domains) is a proposed cause of TTP. However, data are conflicting about the utility of ADAMTS13 testing in the diagnosis of TTP. One prospective, cohort trial found that the ADAMTS13 level did not correlate with a diagnosis of plasma exchange–responsive TTP.[13] The authors of this trial and an international expert on TTP[14] agree that the decision to initiate plasma exchange should be based on the presence of the clinical diagnostic criteria of thrombocytopenia, microangiopathic hemolytic anemia, and lack of immediately discernable alternative cause for these two conditions.

Thrombocytopenia and microangiopathic hemolytic anemia are nonspecific findings, and patients initially thought to have TTP/HUS are occasionally diagnosed with other conditions. The high mortality rate for untreated TTP/HUS mandates that clinicians begin treatment as soon as TTP/HUS is suspected. However, to identify alternative disease states that require specific treatments other than plasma exchange and to avoid unnecessary exposure to the risks of plasma exchange, clinicians should, when clinically indicated, continue to search for an alternative diagnosis even after treatment for TTP/HUS has been initiated. If an alternative cause is found, plasma exchange can be stopped. Examples of diseases that have become apparent only after plasma exchange was started include Rocky Mountain spotted fever, cytomegaloviral sepsis, disseminated aspergillosis, metastatic lung or pancreatic cancer, acute lymphocytic leukemia, malignant hypertension, and heparin-induced thrombocytopenia.[11]

Because TTP can be a tricky diagnosis to confirm, in part because other serious conditions can mimic it, and because treatment typically requires involvement of a hematologist, the medical consultant should seek early consultation with an experienced hematologist when the diagnosis of TTP is suspected.

3. In patients with thrombotic thrombocytopenic purpura, how effective are various interventions such as plasma exchange and other treatments?

Search Date: January 2006

Search Strategy: *PubMed search of "thrombotic thrombocytopenic purpura," field, abstract/title, limits: clinical trial and humans; 57 citations found, 18 selected and reviewed. Bibliographies of all citations were searched. Separate search of thrombotic thrombocytopenic purpura, limit: review; 5 recent reviews selected and reviewed, with bibliographies searched. Search included the American*

College of Physicians PIER and the guidelines of the American Society of Hematology.

Before treatment was available, mortality rates for TTP were 80% to 90%. Numerous case series and observational studies have documented consistently large reductions in mortality with plasma exchange compared with no treatment.[15] It is therefore unlikely that a randomized, controlled trial of plasma exchange versus placebo will ever be performed.

PLASMA EXCHANGE AND PLASMA INFUSION

The superiority of plasma exchange compared with simple plasma infusion was established in a randomized, controlled trial by Rock and associates in 1991.[10] Patients were included if they had a platelet count less than 100,000; microangiopathic hemolytic anemia, as evidenced by schistocytes on a peripheral smear; and no identifiable alternative cause for the thrombocytopenia or anemia. A total of 102 patients were given plasma exchange with fresh frozen plasma (FFP) or plasma infusion with FFP.

Platelet response, defined as a platelet count greater than 150,000 in the absence of new neurologic deficits, was better in the plasma exchange group at 9 days (absolute increase in the percentage of patients with a response of 21.5%; 95% CI, 2.9% to 38.2%) and at 6 months (absolute increase in platelet response of 29%; 95% CI, 10.7% to 45.4%).

The mortality rate was lower for the plasma exchange group at 9 days (ARR for death with plasma exchange of 12%; 95% CI, 2% to 24%). Although not statistically significant, a trend toward reduction in mortality at 6 months was found (absolute risk reduction [ARR] for death with plasma exchange of 15%; 95% CI, −2.5% to 32.5%). The study authors also performed a survival analysis that found a statistically significant mortality reduction at 6 months.

The goal for treating patients with TTP should be to institute plasma exchange with FFP as soon as possible. The mortality rate for patients given only plasma infusion in the Rock trial was 37%, far lower than the mortality rates of 80% to 90% for patients who receive no treatment. If plasma exchange is not immediately available, plasma infusion with FFP should be started until plasma exchange can be arranged.

Although there is crossover between TTP and HUS, this should not affect initial management. Survival rates of patients with or without renal failure in the Rock trial were similar, making precise determination of the clinical syndrome (i.e., TTP or TTP/HUS) before treatment unnecessary.[10]

Complications of plasma exchange should be considered. In 71 consecutive patients treated with plasma exchange for suspected TTP/HUS, 15% developed line infections, 10% developed thrombosis (i.e., catheter obstruction or venous thrombosis), and 4% had complications of pneumothorax or bleeding from the line insertion. Complications resulted in two deaths.[11,16] Although plasma exchange and large-bore line insertion carry some risk, because of the rapid and high mortality for untreated TTP, treatment is still mandatory.

ASPIRIN AND DIPYRIDAMOLE

No high-quality trials have been done to determine the independent value of aspirin or dipyridamole in TTP. One small, observational trial found an 87.5% response rate in patients treated with plasma exchange, Solu-Medrol, and intravenous dipyridamole.[17] One randomized trial of patients with TTP receiving plasma exchange and methylprednisolone compared aspirin and dipyridamole with no antiplatelet agents.[18] Although a weak, non–statistically significant trend toward lower mortality rates in the antiplatelet arm was found (ARR of 10.6%; 95% CI, −3.3% to 25.3%), the true benefit of these two antiplatelet agents in TTP remains unclear.

In the Rock trial discussed earlier, aspirin and dipyridamole were given to all patients as background therapy for at least 2 weeks. The most rigorous application of the Rock trial findings would be to administer aspirin and dipyridamole to patients receiving plasma exchange or plasma infusion.

FRESH FROZEN PLASMA VERSUS CRYOSUPERNATANT

Although FFP has traditionally been used in plasma exchange and transfusion, the use of cryosupernatant (i.e., cryoprecipitate poor plasma [CPP]) as replacement fluid has been studied. There is some evidence that von Willebrand factor multimers may be responsible for TTP, and using fluid from which these have been removed, such as CPP, may be more effective than FFP. In one observational trial, 95% of patients with TTP treated by plasma exchange with CPP were alive at 1 month.[19] The first randomized, controlled trial to directly compare plasma exchange using FFP or CPP was underpowered to determine any differences in effect, with wide and overlapping confidence intervals for all outcomes.[20] For example, the mean platelet level on day 13 of therapy was 171,000/µL (range, 87,000 to 199,000/µL) for the FFP group and 160,000/µL (range, 73,000 to 189,000/µL) for the CPP group. The absolute reduction of mortality with CPP was 1.64% (95% CI of −28% to 32%), leaving open the possibility that CPP may be harmful. Unfortunately, the second randomized, controlled trial on the topic was similarly underpowered, finding the absolute risk reduction in mortality for the CPP group to be 4.7%, but with a wide 95% CI of −10.6% to 22.5%.[21] The true effect of CPP compared with FFP as replacement fluid in plasma exchange remains unknown. Larger trials are needed.

GLUCOCORTICOIDS

Although oral and intravenous glucocorticoids have been used alone and as background therapy with apparent success in observational studies, there are no randomized or high-quality cohort trials of steroids versus placebo in patients receiving plasma exchange. However, many expert clinicians are in favor of a trial of steroids in patients not responding to plasma exchange.[15]

SPLENECTOMY

Splenectomy has not been studied rigorously enough to draw conclusions about its effectiveness in managing TTP. In one review of 33 patients with relapsing or exchange-refractory disease who underwent splenectomy, the 10-year relapse-free survival rate was 70% (95% CI, 50% to 83%).[22] However, this was a retrospective trial with no placebo comparison group, and the reduced rate of relapse could very well have been the natural course of TTP in these patients, without an effect from the intervention.

Splenectomy should be reserved as a last resort in selected patients who are not responding to extended attempts at plasma exchange and glucocorticoids. Randomized trials are needed to determine the effectiveness of splenectomy in treating patients with TTP.

IMMUNOSUPPRESSIVE AGENTS: RITUXIMAB, VINCRISTINE, AND CYCLOPHOSPHAMIDE

Antibodies to ADAMTS13 are found in 33% to more than 90% of idiopathic TTP patients,[23,24] supporting the view that TTP may be an autoimmune disease in some patients. Although numerous immunosuppressant drugs have been tested, most studies are small, retrospective, and of poor quality, producing results that are unclear.

Isolated case reports and small, retrospective series have reported apparent success with rituximab in patients with TTP.[25] Taken together, these reports indicated possible success with rituximab in 25 of 26 cases of TTP. In September 2005, the first prospective, cohort trial of rituximab in 11 patients with refractory and relapsing ADAMTS13-deficient TTP reported that all patients achieved clinical remission at 6 months of follow-up.[25] However, the sample size was small, and there was no control group. Interpretation and application of the results are further complicated by the fact that patients had received various treatments before the rituximab, including vincristine, splenectomy, cyclosporine, and others.

In a prospective cohort of 23 patients with acquired TTP, 7 of 8 patients who received vincristine in addition to plasma exchange had an increase in ADAMTS13 activity and platelet count.[26] There was no control group, and the background therapy varied widely among the trial participants, making useful interpretation of the results extremely difficult.

Numerous case reports of cyclophosphamide in the treatment of TTP have been reported, although it is impossible to make conclusions about the drug's effectiveness because patients and background therapies varied widely. No clinical trials of cyclophosphamide in the treatment of TTP have been conducted.

Although the use of immunosuppressive drugs in TTP is an exciting prospect, enthusiasm for their use seems to be ahead of the available evidence, and they should be reserved only for selected refractory cases. Because most immunosuppressive drugs are tested in TTP patients who undergo testing for ADAMTS13 deficiency, another question is how effective these drugs may be in a population of TTP patients who have not been tested for deficiency of or antibodies against ADAMTS13. Immunosuppressive therapy should be administered under the supervision of a hematologist with the knowledge that their use is not evidence based at this point. Some might argue that in a disease such as refractory TTP, for which few good options exist, the use of unproven drugs can be justified. This may be so, but without rigorous trials, clinicians cannot be sure that they are not inflicting more harm than good when employing untested treatments. If possible, the patient should be involved in the decision-making process and advised of the risks, benefits, and uncertainties that surround the use of immunosuppressive drugs in the treatment of TTP.

In summary, patients who present with a platelet count less than 100,000, schistocytes on a peripheral smear, and no other cause for these findings should be considered to have TTP and treated as soon as possible with aspirin, dipyridamole, and plasma exchange with FFP. Plasma infusion, although less effective than plasma exchange, can be used temporarily until plasma exchange can be instituted. Many patients require extended courses of plasma exchange, and the catheter should be left in until the platelet count and results of the peripheral smear are stable for at least a few days. Expert consultation by an experienced hematologist is mandatory because of the high mortality rate for TTP and the fact that these cases often involve treatment modalities that have not been rigorously evaluated, leading to complicated risk-benefit decisions that often are based more on clinical experience than on solid evidence (Table 8-3).

4. How is heparin-induced thrombocytopenia diagnosed?

Search Date: January 2006

Search Strategy: *PubMed Search of "heparin-induced thrombocytopenia" AND "diagnosis or recognition or*

Table 8-3. Summary of Evidence for Interventions in Thrombotic Thrombocytopenic Purpura/Hemolytic Uremic Syndrome

Intervention	Evidence	Comments
Plasma exchange vs. no treatment	Observational studies report mortality reductions of 80% or more with plasma exchange.	Randomized trials are considered unethical and are unlikely to be done.
Plasma exchange vs. plasma infusion	Survival analysis of randomized, controlled trials (RCTs) found reduced mortality at 6 months for plasma exchange.	Background therapy included aspirin and dipyridamole for all patients.
Aspirin and/or dipyridamole vs. placebo	No high-quality evidence of effect	Were used as background in only RCT of plasma exchange vs. plasma infusion
Corticosteroids vs. placebo	No high-quality evidence	Used by experts in patients who do not respond to plasma exchange
Splenectomy vs. no splenectomy	No high-quality evidence	Considered a last resort by experts
Cryosupernatant vs. fresh frozen plasma (FFP) as replacement fluid	Observational data support cryosupernatant vs. placebo; RCTs are indeterminate in comparing the two.	Confidence intervals in both RCTs include possibility that cryosupernatant could be more harmful than FFP
Vincristine, rituximab, and cyclophosphamide	Small, uncontrolled, cohort trials and case reports; true effects still unknown	Considered by experts in certain cases refractory to plasma exchange

detection or identification or laboratory," limited to title, English; 65 citations found. Relevant citations were selected, and bibliographies were reviewed for additional references.

Heparin-induced thrombocytopenia (HIT) is an immune-mediated disorder caused by immunoglobulin G (IgG) antibodies that bind to platelet factor 4 (PF4). The PF4 becomes immunogenic when it binds to heparin. The PF4/heparin complex then binds to Fc receptors on platelets, resulting in platelet activation, thrombin generation, and platelet aggregation.[27]

HIT is diagnosed by combining clinical evidence of heparin-related thrombocytopenia and thrombosis with laboratory evidence of antiplatelet factor 4/heparin, platelet-activating IgG antibodies. The diagnosis of HIT requires clinical and laboratory findings because each criterion can be present in isolation in other disease states or can be clinically insignificant in certain cases. The American College of Chest Physicians (ACCP) recommendation on which patients should be evaluated for possible HIT is shown in Box 8-1.[28]

Thrombocytopenia is often the first sign that raises suspicion of HIT. The ACCP recommends that routine platelet count monitoring be based on the prevalence of HIT in different patient groups (Table 8-4). These are weak recommendations (ACCP grade 2C) because no prospective

---

Box 8-1. Recommendations for Evaluating Patients for Heparin-Induced Thrombocytopenia

For patients receiving heparin or for those who have received heparin within the previous 2 weeks, we recommend excluding a diagnosis of heparin-induced thrombocytopenia (HIT) if the platelet count falls by 50% or more or a thrombotic event occurs between days 4 to 14 after initiation of heparin, even if the patient is no longer receiving heparin therapy when thrombosis or thrombocytopenia has occurred. This is an American College of Chest Physicians recommendation, grade 1C (i.e., intermediate strength recommendation that may change when stronger evidence is available).

Table 8-4. Estimates of Baseline Prevalence and Risk of Clinical Heparin-Induced Thrombocytopenia in Various Patient Populations and ACCP Recommendations for Platelet Monitoring

Patient Population	Prevalence of HIT	Platelet Monitoring
Postoperative orthopedic patients receiving UFH	5%	At least every other day between postoperative days 4 and 14 or until UFH is stopped, whichever occurs first
Postoperative cardiac surgery patients receiving UFH	2% to 3%	
Other postoperative patients receiving prophylactic UFH	Less than 1%	
Medical patients receiving therapeutic-dose UFH (IV or SQ) for the treatment of venous or arterial thrombosis	1%	
Postoperative orthopedic patients receiving LMWH	1%	Every 2-3 days from day 4 to 14 or until heparin is stopped, whichever occurs first
Medical and obstetric patients receiving prophylactic-dose UFH	0.1% to 1.0%	
Postoperative patients receiving LMWH* (excluding postoperative orthopedic patients)		
Postoperative or critical care patients receiving UFH flushes		
Medical and obstetric patients receiving LMWH after first receiving UFH	Less than 0.01%	Routine platelet monitoring not suggested

* Risk in this group is closer to 0.1%,
ACCP, American College of Chest Physicians; HIT, heparin-induced thrombocytopenia; LMWH, low-molecular-weight heparin; UFH, unfractionated heparin.
Adapted from Hassell K: The management of patients with heparin-induced thrombocytopenia who require anticoagulant therapy. Chest 2005;127(Suppl):1S-8S.

studies have been done comparing the effect of different platelet monitoring strategies on clinical outcomes.

The diagnosis of HIT is most accurately made by applying the principles of Bayes' theorem. In this diagnostic decision-making model, the clinician must first estimate the clinical probability of disease (i.e., pretest probability). This is then combined with the results of diagnostic testing to yield a posttest probability of disease.

STEP ONE: DETERMINING THE PRETEST PROBABILITY OF HEPARIN-INDUCED THROMBOCYTOPENIA

Estimation of a patient's pretest probability of HIT is based on a number of factors: the baseline prevalence of HIT in that patient population, the magnitude and temporal features of the thrombocytopenia, the patient's signs and symptoms, the presence or absence of alternative diagnosis, and the physician's clinical judgment and experience.

The baseline prevalence of HIT provides an anchoring point from which to start building an estimate of pretest probability. Data on the prevalence of HIT come mainly from retrospective studies and are summarized in Table 8-4.

After determining a patient's baseline risk of HIT, the clinician should determine whether the magnitude and timing of the thrombocytopenia fits with one of the three types of HIT. In *typical-onset HIT*, which affects two thirds of HIT patients, the platelet count begins to fall 5 to 10 days after starting heparin. Thrombocytopenia, defined as a drop in platelets of 50% or more from baseline or an absolute platelet count of less than 150,000, usually occurs about 7 to 14 days after beginning heparin. About 25% to 30% of patients experience *rapid-onset HIT*, in which the platelet count falls immediately after beginning heparin. This form of HIT occurs in patients who have been recently exposed to heparin (within approximately the past 100 days) and is thought to represent platelet activation in patients who have residual circulating HIT antibodies that formed after the first heparin exposure.[28-30] In *delayed-onset HIT*, occurring in only about 3% to 5% of patients, the platelet count falls several days after heparin exposure.[31-33]

Although thrombocytopenia is often defined as a platelet level of less than 150,000, the most recent ACCP guideline states that a relative thrombocytopenia is a more reliable marker of possible HIT. This is because many patients have very low baseline platelet counts, and postoperative patients often experience an absolute thrombocytopenia that recovers in a few days. However, clinicians must assess each situation independently, and the ACCP states that "no single definition of thrombocytopenia is appropriate in all clinical situations."[28]

The signs and symptoms of HIT are not specific and should raise suspicion of HIT mainly in patients who exhibit thrombocytopenia consistent with HIT. These signs and symptoms are listed with their frequencies (where available) in Table 8-5.

Alternative causes for a patient's thrombocytopenia must be considered. Common causes of thrombocytopenia include a laboratory error, platelet clumping, perioperative

---

Table 8-5. **Clinical Manifestations of Heparin-Induced Thrombocytopenia**

Thrombocytopenia ≥ 50% from baseline (95%)*

Thrombosis (35% to 75%)

   Deep vein thrombosis

   Pulmonary embolism

   Venous limb gangrene

   Adrenal hemorrhagic necrosis

   Cerebral vein thrombosis

   Arterial thrombosis (limb > stroke > myocardial infarction > other)

Skin necrosis and erythematous plaques (10% to 20%)†

Acute systemic reactions (25%)‡

Decompensated disseminated intravascular coagulation

*Rarely, a patient may have an exposure to heparin that is consistent with heparin-induced thrombocytopenia (HIT) and have multiple clinical findings but only mild thrombocytopenia (< 50% drop from baseline). HIT should be excluded in this case with laboratory testing.
†Occurs in patients receiving subcutaneous heparin injections.
‡Seen when patients who have already formed HIT antibodies receive a bolus of heparin.
Adapted from Warkentin TE: New approaches to the diagnosis of heparin-induced thrombocytopenia. Chest 2005;127(Suppl):35S-45S.

hemodilution, sepsis, multiorgan dysfunction syndrome, post-transfusion purpura, and immune thrombocytopenia caused by drugs, such as quinine, quinidine, rifampin, vancomycin, clopidogrel, ticlopidine, sulfa drugs, and glycoprotein IIb/IIIa inhibitors.

Clinicians must then combine all of the previous information and make an estimate of the pretest probability of HIT for the patient. An international expert on HIT supports the Four Ts system for estimating the pretest probability of HIT (Table 8-6). This clinical prediction rule is based mainly on the clinical experience of experts and on the findings of observational studies and has not been prospectively validated. However, it is a helpful way to summarize and combine the information that is used to determine the pretest probability of HIT.

STEP TWO: LABORATORY TESTING FOR HEPARIN-INDUCED THROMBOCYTOPENIA

After the pretest probability of HIT has been determined, a diagnostic test is then obtained. The two best studied laboratory tests are the platelet serotonin release assay (SRA) and the solid-phase PF4/heparin enzyme immunoassay (EIA).

In the SRA, platelets are "washed," making them very sensitive to HIT serum or plasma. The positivity of the test is measured by the percent of serotonin release from the sensitized platelets after exposure to HIT antibodies. This test is sensitive but labor intensive, and it is performed in only a few reference laboratories.[27]

Two PF4/heparin EIAs are available. Both are antigen assays that detect HIT antibodies. The commercially available PF4/polyanion EIA test detects many antibodies, including IgA, IgM, and IgG, and some nonpathogenic antibodies, limiting the test's specificity. A PF4/heparin EIA that detects only IgG HIT antibodies is more specific but less widely available. A positive result in both tests is expressed as absorbance in optical density (OD) units, with a higher OD number indicating a more strongly positive test.[27]

Positive and negative likelihood ratios for the SRA and EIA have been reported for post–cardiac surgery[27,28] and post–orthopedic surgery[34] patients (Tables 8-7 and 8-8). Diagnostic test properties depend heavily on the

Table 8-6. The Four Ts Approach to Estimating the Pretest Probability of Heparin-Induced Thrombocytopenia

Clinical Feature	2 Points*	1 Point	No Points
Thrombocytopenia	> 50% platelet fall to nadir ≥ 20,000	30%-50% platelet fall, or nadir of 10,000 to 19,000	< 30% platelet fall, or nadir < 10,000
Timing† of the onset of platelet fall or other sequelae of HIT	Days 5-10, or ≤ day 1 with recent heparin (past 30 days)	> Day 10 or timing unclear, or < day 1 with recent heparin (past 31-100 days)	< day 4 (no recent heparin)
Thrombosis or other sequelae systemic	Proven new thrombosis; skin necrosis; or acute systemic reaction after IV UFH bolus	Progressive or recurrent thrombosis; lesions; erythematous skin suspected but not proven thrombosis	None
Other causes of platelet drop	None evident	Possible	Definite

* Points (0, 1, or 2) are assigned for each of four categories, with a maximum score of 8. A pretest probability score of 6 to 8 indicates a high probability (> 80%), 4 or 5 indicates an intermediate probability, and 0 to 3 indicates a low probability (< 5%).
† First day of immunizing heparin exposure considered day zero.
HIT, heparin-induced thrombocytopenia; IV, intravenous; UFH, unfractionated heparin.
From Warkentin TE: Heparin-induced thrombocytopenia diagnosis and management. Circulation 2004;110:e454-e458.

population that they are derived in, and whether these tests can be directly applied to other patient groups, such as general medical patients, is unclear.

Table 8-7. Operating Characteristics of Laboratory Tests Used in the Diagnosis of Heparin-Induced Thrombocytopenia in Patients after Cardiac Surgery

Diagnostic Test	Test Result	Likelihood Ratio For Diagnosis of HIT
Serotonin release assay	Serotonin release ≥ 90%	20
	Serotonin release ≥ 80%	10
	Serotonin release < 80%	0.05
PF4/heparin EIA for IgG HIT antibodies	Optical density 2 ≥ 2.0 units	20
	Optical density ≥ 1.0 units	4.8
	Optical density < 1.0 units	0.15

EIA, enzyme immunoassay; HIT, heparin-induced thrombocytopenia.
Calculated by the author from data in Warkentin TE: New approaches to the diagnosis of heparin-induced thrombocytopenia. Chest 2005;127(Suppl):35S-45S.

STEP THREE: COMBINING PRETEST PROBABILITY WITH DIAGNOSTIC TEST RESULTS

The pretest probability of HIT can be combined with the appropriate likelihood ratio by using a commonly available graphic nomogram or one of the many available online Bayes' theorem calculators. Five case studies using the data in Tables 8-7 and 8-8 can illustrate Bayes' theorem in practice and highlight common dilemmas in the diagnosis of HIT.

Table 8-8. Operating Characteristics of Laboratory Tests Used in the Diagnosis of Heparin-Induced Thrombocytopenia in Patients after Orthopedic Surgery Receiving Unfractionated and Low-Molecular-Weight Heparin

Diagnostic Test	Test Result	Likelihood Ratio For Diagnosis of HIT
Serotonin release assay	Serotonin release > 90% (all pts)	100
	Serotonin release of 20% to 50% (all pts)	30 to 40
	Serotonin release > 20% in pts treated with UFH	20
	Serotonin release > 20% in pts. treated with LMWH	33
	Serotonin release < 20% in pts treated with UFH or with LMWH	0
PF4/heparin EIA for IgG HIT Antibodies	Optical density > 2.0 units (all pts)	100
	Optical density of 0.5 to 0.75 (all pts)	15 to 20
	Optical density > 0.40 in pts treated with UFH	9
	Optical density > 0.40 in pts treated with LMWH	16.6
	Optical density < 0.40 in pts treated with UFH or LMWH	0

EIA, enzyme immunoassay; HIT, heparin-induced thrombocytopenia; LMWH, low-molecular-weight heparin; pts, patients; UFH, unfractionated heparin.
Likelihood ratios were calculated by the author from data in Warkentin TE, Greinacher A: Heparin-induced thrombocytopenia: Recognition, treatment, and prevention. The seventh ACCP Conference on Antithrombotic and Thrombolytic Therapy. Chest 2004;126(Suppl):311S-337S and Warkentin TE, Sheppard JA, Moore JC, et al: Laboratory testing for the antibodies that cause heparin-induced thrombocytopenia: How much class do we need? J Lab Clin Med 2005;146:341-346.

Case 1. *A patient receiving prophylactic doses of low-molecular-weight heparin (LMWH) after orthopedic surgery is estimated to have an 80% pretest probability of HIT. The patient has a strongly positive SRA test, with serotonin release greater than 20% (LR = 33). The posttest probability of HIT is 99%, confirming the diagnosis.*

Case 2. *A post–cardiac surgery patient with a 10% pretest probability of HIT has a strongly negative SRA test result (LR = 0.05). The posttest probability of HIT is only 0.5%, and the diagnosis can be excluded with reasonable certainty.*

Case 3. *A post–cardiac surgery patient with an 80% pretest probability has a strongly negative SRA test result (LR = 0.05). The posttest probability of HIT is 16.6%. The negative SRA test result has lowered the chance of HIT, although not enough to exclude it, and further testing is needed. At this point, the patient could undergo a PF4 EIA IgG test, with 16.6% becoming the new pretest probability of HIT heading into this second test. If the PF4 EIA test is strongly negative (LR = 0.15), the posttest probability of HIT would be 2.9%. Whether this posttest probability is low enough to confidently exclude the possibility of a serious disease such as HIT is unclear. Until long-term follow-up studies of patients with posttest probabilities in this range document that untreated patients do not suffer adverse outcomes, how to handle disease probabilities in this range will remain a matter of clinical judgment.*

Case 4. *A post–cardiac surgery patient has a 10% pretest probability of HIT but has a weakly positive PF4 EIA test result (LR = 4.8), resulting in a posttest probability of 35%. This intermediate posttest probability can neither exclude nor confirm a diagnosis of HIT. Further testing is needed.*

Case 5. *A post-orthopedic surgery patient receiving unfractionated heparin prophylaxis has a 90% pretest probability of HIT and a strongly negative PF4 EIA IgG test result, with an optical density of less than*

0.40 (LR = 0). The posttest probability of HIT is zero, and the diagnosis can be confidently excluded. It is postulated that in rare cases, HIT may be caused by IgM or IgA antibodies. If so, even a perfectly sensitive test for IgG antibodies could miss the rare case of HIT. Whether HIT could be caused by IgM or IgA antibodies and whether these should be tested for in suspected cases is being debated and requires further study.

CONCLUSION

The workup for possible HIT can be initiated by the medical consultant. The first and most important step is to estimate the pretest probability of disease. However, because highly specialized laboratory testing is required and the interpretation of these tests and resultant *posttest* probabilities can be difficult, early consultation with a hematologist experienced in the diagnosis of HIT is mandatory. Prospectively validated clinical prediction rules are needed to help estimate pretest probability, and the various laboratory tests for HIT need to be rigorously studied in the general medical population.

5. How effective are alternative anticoagulants for the treatment of heparin-induced thrombocytopenia in patients not undergoing cardiac surgery or percutaneous coronary intervention?

Search Date: January 2006

Search Strategy: *PubMed search of "heparin induced thrombocytopenia" in title/abstract, limited to English and humans and limited to meta-analysis (9 citations), clinical trials (65 citations) or review articles of past three years (125 citations). Abstracts were reviewed, and bibliographies of selected citations were reviewed, including review of the American College of Chest Physicians recent guidelines on anticoagulation.*

HIT is an immune-mediated adverse reaction to heparin in which IgG antibodies bind to heparin. This complex binds to PF4. The heparin/IgG/PF4 complex then binds to the Fc receptor on platelets, triggering platelet activation and thrombosis.

Studies of alternative anticoagulants have examined outcomes in two populations: patients with HIT without evidence of thrombosis (HIT) and patients with HIT and evidence of thrombosis (HITTS). This review addresses the treatment of HIT and HITTS in the general medical and surgical populations. Evidence on the role of alternative anticoagulants in patients with HIT who require certain procedures (e.g., cardiopulmonary bypass, percutaneous coronary intervention) are not addressed in this review.

INITIAL MANAGEMENT OF SUSPECTED OR CONFIRMED HEPARIN-INDUCED THROMBOCYTOPENIA WITH OR WITHOUT EVIDENCE OF THROMBOSIS

The first step in the diagnosis and treatment of HIT involves estimating the pretest probability of disease (see Question 4). Validated clinical prediction rules have not yet been developed, and the ideal treatment threshold for starting an alternative anticoagulant in suspected HIT remains unknown. Experts agree that treatment should be initiated before laboratory confirmation of HIT is obtained, whether the patient has evidence of thrombosis or not, but they differ in their recommendations about when to initiate treatment. One expert advocates starting treatment at a "low/moderate" level of suspicion.[35] The ACCP recommends waiting until HIT is "strongly suspected" before administering an alternative anticoagulant.[28] No prospective studies have examined whether initiating treatment at low, intermediate, or high pretest probability levels affects the clinical outcomes of patients with HIT.

Experts and the evidence do agree that when HIT is suspected, discontinuing heparin therapy alone is not sufficient (Box 8-2). An alternative anticoagulant must be started immediately, at the time heparin therapy is stopped. A high-quality systematic review found that when patients with HIT had heparin therapy discontinued but no alternative anticoagulation started, the risk of new thrombosis was 18.6% to 51.6%, with the highest risk in orthopedic patients.[36]

ALTERNATIVE ANTICOAGULANTS

No randomized, controlled trials have compared alternative anticoagulants with no treatment in patients with

> **Box 8-2. Initial Management of Strongly Suspected or Confirmed Heparin-Induced Thrombocytopenia with or without Thrombosis**
>
> - Discontinue heparin or low-molecular-weight heparin therapy.
> - Initiate treatment immediately with a direct thrombin inhibitor. Do not wait for the results of heparin-induced thrombocytopenia (HIT) antibody testing.
> - Test for hit antibodies if appropriate
> - Order doppler ultrasonography of the legs, even if there are no signs of deep venous thrombosis.*
> - Do not give warfarin. If warfarin has been given, give vitamin K.†
> - Avoid prophylactice platelet transfusion.‡
> - Obtain a hematology consult and pharmacokinetics support.
>
> *American College of Chest Physicians (ACCP) grade 1C,* grade 2C,† and grade 2C ‡ recommendations.*

HIT or HITTS. Because cohort trials have found that untreated patients with HIT have at least a 20% to 50% risk of developing thrombosis[36] and that treatment reduces this risk, it is unlikely that randomized trials of treatment with alternative anticoagulants versus no treatment in HIT will be performed.

Four alternative anticoagulants are most commonly used for the treatment of HIT: argatroban, lepirudin, bivalirudin, and danaparoid. Danaparoid was withdrawn from the U.S. market in 2002 but is approved for use in Canada and Europe.[28]

The pharmacokinetics of the alternative anticoagulants is provided in Table 8-9. Clinicians should consult their hospital's pharmacy for the most recent and accurate dosing and monitoring information.

ARGATROBAN
Patients with Heparin-Induced Thrombocytopenia
Two cohort trials have evaluated argatroban in patients with HIT. These trials used prospective enrollment of patients to the active arm and compared them with historical controls. In both trials, HIT was defined as a platelet count less than

Table 8-9. Pharmacokinetics of Common Alternative Anticoagulant Drugs for the Treatment of Heparin-Induced Thrombocytopenia

Drug	Mechanism	Dosing	Monitoring	Elimination (Half-Life)
Argatroban	Direct thrombin inhibitor	Infusion rate of 2 µg/kg/min; no bolus.	Activated partial thromboplastin time (aPTT)	Hepatobiliary (40–50 min)
Lepirudin	Direct thrombin inhibitor	Bolus,* 0.4 mg/kg in certain circumstances; infusion rate,† 0.1 to 0.15 mg/kg/hr	aPTT	Renal (80 min)
Bivalirudin	Direct thrombin inhibitor	Infusion rate, 0.15–2.0 mg/kg/hr; no bolus	aPTT	Enzymatic (80%), renal (20%); half-life (25 min)
Danaparoid	Factor Xa inhibitor	Weight-based bolus,‡ then stepwise increasing intravenous infusion	Anti-Xa levels	Renal (24 hr)

*Avoidance of bolus may reduce accumulation of drug in patients with undiagnosed renal failure and may lower the incidence of anaphylaxis.
†There is suggestion that a lower infusion rate of 0.1mg/kg/hr may lower bleeding complications.
‡Danaparoid is not approved for use in the United States; consult a local pharmacy for dosing and monitoring information.
Adapted from Warkentin TE, Greinacher A: Heparin-induced thrombocytopenia: Recognition, treatment, and prevention. The seventh ACCP Conference on Antithrombotic and Thrombolytic Therapy. Chest 2004;126(Suppl):311S-337S.

100×10^9/L or a 50% reduction in count after heparin therapy with no alternative explanation. Exclusion criteria for both trials were an unexplained activated partial thromboplastin time (aPTT) more than two times the control value; a documented coagulation disorder or bleeding diathesis unrelated to HITTS; a lumbar puncture within the past 7 days; or a history of previous aneurysm, hemorrhagic stroke, or recent (within 6 months) thrombotic stroke unrelated to HITTS.

In the first study, argatroban reduced the composite end point of death, amputation, or new thromboembolic event in patients with HIT by a relative risk reduction of 34% (95% CI, 7% to 60%). The absolute risk reduction was 13.2% (95% CI, 2.7% to 23.2%), and the number needed to treat to prevent one composite outcome was 8 (95% CI, 4 to 37). New thrombotic events were common (22.4%) in the untreated historical control group. The relative risk reduction of new thrombotic events was 64% (95% CI, 28% to 99%), with an absolute risk reduction of 14.3% (95% CI, 6.3% to 22.4%) and a number needed to treat of 7 (95% CI,, 4 to 16).[37,38]

In the second study, the relative risk reduction of the same composite end point was 28% (95% CI, −0.3% to 48%). Although this barely missed statistical significance, the confidence interval indicates a likely benefit for argatroban, especially considering the positive results of the first trial. In this trial, the incidence of new thrombosis in untreated historical control patients was high (23%). The relative risk reduction of new thrombotic events was 75% (95% CI, 42% to 100%), with an absolute risk reduction of 17% (95% CI, 9.6% to 25.2%) and a number needed to treat of 6 (95% CI, 4 to 10).[37,39]

Reductions in the composite outcome of death, amputation, or new thrombotic event in both trials seem to result largely from the reduction in new thrombotic events, because the individual outcomes of death and amputation did not reach statistical significance in either study.

Patients with Heparin-Induced Thrombocytopenia and Evidence of Thrombosis

The studies of argatroban in HIT discussed previously also included patients with HITTS. For the composite end point of death, amputation, or new thromboembolic event, both trials were indeterminate, although a trend toward benefit is seen. In the first study, the relative risk reduction was 22.6% (95% CI, −6.4% to 49.8%).[38] The second trial found similar results, with a relative risk reduction of 27% (95% CI, −1.1% to 52.5%).[39] The effect of argatroban on the individual outcomes of death and amputation could not be determined, with wide confidence intervals in both trials.

Argatroban did show benefit in reducing new thrombotic events in patients with HITTS. The first trial found a relative risk reduction of 44% (95% CI, 3.6% to 89%), with an absolute risk reduction of 15.3% (95% CI, 1.2% to 31%) and a number needed to treat of 7 (95% CI, 3 to 80).[38] The second trial found a relative risk reduction of 62% (95% CI, 25% to 100%), with an absolute risk reduction of 21.6% (95% CI, 8.6% to 36.6%) and a number needed to treat of 5 (95% CI, 3 to 12).[39]

Bleeding Risk with Argatroban

The bleeding risk with argatroban in these studies was unclear, with wide confidence intervals around all outcomes. In both trials, major bleeding was defined as intracranial bleeding, retroperitoneal bleeding, bleeding into a prosthetic joint, bleeding that caused a drop in hemoglobin of 2 g/dL or more, or bleeding that required transfusion of 2 or more units of blood. Bleeding not meeting these criteria was classified as minor. For both trials, bleeding events were calculated for the combined group of HIT and HITTS patients.[40] In the first trial, major bleeding occurred in 6.91% of the argatroban group. There was an absolute risk increase in major bleeding with argatroban of 0.17% (95% CI, −4.8% to 4.6%) and an absolute risk reduction in minor bleeding of 0.14% (95% CI, −8.6 to 9.0%).[38] In the second trial, the incidence of major bleeding in the argatroban group was 5.7%. The absolute risk reduction in bleeding with argatroban was 1.2% (95% CI, −2.6% to 6.2%) for major bleeding and 6.1% (95% CI, −2.1% to 14.6%) for minor bleeding[39] (Table 8-10).

LEPIRUDIN

Patients with Heparin-Induced Thrombocytopenia and Risk of Bleeding with Lepirudin

A meta-analysis of three prospective cohort trials of lepirudin in the treatment of HIT was published in 2005.[41] All trials compared patients with a laboratory-confirmed

Table 8-10. Summary of the Effects of Argatroban in Patients with HIT or HITTS

Study and Design	Patient Group	Outcome	RRR (95% CI)	ARR or ARI (95% CI)	NNT (95% CI)
Lewis et al,[38] 2001 Multicenter, prospective, cohort with historical controls	HIT without thrombosis	Death, amputation, or new thrombosis	34% (7% to 60%)	ARR = 13.2% (2.7% to 23.2%)	8 (4 to 37)
		New thrombosis	64% (28% to 99%)	ARR = 14.3% (6.3% to 22.4%)	7 (4 to 16)
	HIT with thrombosis (HITTS)	Death, amputation, or new thrombosis	22.6% (−6.4% to 49.8%)	NS*	NS*
		New thrombosis	44% (3.6% to 89%)	ARR = 15.3% (1.2% to 31%)	7 (3 to 80)
	HIT or HITTS (all patients)	Major bleeding†	—‡	ARI = 0.17% (−4.8% to 4.6%)	NS*
Lewis et al,[39] 2003	HIT without thrombosis	Death, amputation, or new thrombosis	28% (−0.3% to 48%)	NS*	NS*

Multicenter, prospective, cohort with historical controls		New thrombosis	75% (42% to 100%)	ARR = 17% (9.6% to 25.2%)	6 (4 to 10)
	HIT with thrombosis (HITTS)	Death, amputation or new thrombosis	27% (-1.1% to 52.5%)	NS*	NS*
		New thrombosis	62% (25% to 100%)	ARR = 21.6% (8.6% to 36.6%)	5 (3 to 12)
	HIT or HITTS (all patients)	Major bleeding⁻	—‡	1.2% (-2.6% to 6.2%)	NS*

*When results were not statistically significant (NS), only one measurement of outcome was calculated, based on available data.
† Major bleeding was defined as intracranial bleeding, retroperitoneal bleeding, bleeding into a prosthetic joint, bleeding that caused a drop in hemoglobin of 2g/dL or more, or bleeding that required transfusion of 2 or more units of blood.
‡Calculations could not be made with certainty based on original data (e.g., data not available, number of subjects unclear).
ARI, absolute risk increase; ARR, absolute risk reduction; HIT, heparin-induced thrombocytopenia; HITTS, HIT and evidence of thrombosis; NNT, number needed to treat; RRR, relative risk reduction.

clinical diagnosis of HIT (i.e., platelet count drop to ≥ 100,000 or decrease by ≥ 50% from baseline, with or without development of thrombosis during heparin therapy) with historically matched controls who did not receive anticoagulation with an alternative agent. The pooled data (N = 403) included patients from different populations, including internal medicine (41.7%), orthopedic surgery (15.9%), cardiovascular surgery (10.7%), trauma surgery (7.4%), and other groups (24.3%).

A Kaplan-Meier analysis of the data found that lepirudin reduced the combined end point of death, amputation, or new thrombosis by a relative risk reduction of 43%, with a number needed to treat of 4.5 (P = .0473). This effect largely resulted from a reduction in new thrombosis, which occurred in 32.1% of the control group and in 11.9% of the lepirudin group (relative risk reduction [RRR] = 63%, number needed to treat [NNT] = 4.9, P = .0008). The effect of lepirudin on the individual outcomes of death and amputation was unclear. Major bleeding (defined as fatal bleeding, permanently disabling or life-threatening bleeding, intracranial bleeding, or bleeding that required surgery or transfusion) was common in the lepirudin group (29.4%) as opposed to historical controls (9.1%), with a number needed to harm of 4.9 (P = .014). The study authors suggest that the rate of bleeding, which almost offsets the benefits of lepirudin, may be reduced by lowering the starting dose of lepirudin to 0.1 mg/kg/hr. The aPTT level should be measured every 4 hours until two consecutive measurements are in the therapeutic range before switching to once-daily monitoring.

Patients with Heparin-Induced Thrombocytopenia and Evidence of Thrombosis

A high-quality systematic review[36] found that lepirudin reduced the combined outcome of death, amputation, or further thrombosis by a relative risk reduction of 53% (95% CI, 28% to 70%), with a number needed to treat of 3.9 (95% CI, 3 to 8). Further thrombotic events were reduced by a relative risk reduction of 60% (95% CI, 20% to 81%) (Table 8-11).

Argatroban versus Lepirudin

No clinical trials have directly compared argatroban and lepirudin in patients with HIT or HITTS. The ACCP

Table 8-11. Summary of the Effects of Lepirudin in the Treatment of HIT and HITTS

Study and Design	Patient Group	Outcome	Effect of Lepirudin*
Lubenow et al,[41] 2005 Meta-analysis of three prospective cohort studies with historical controls (HAT-1, HAT-2, HAT-3)	Patients with HIT	Death, amputation, or new thrombotic event	RRR = 43% NNT = 4.5 (P = .047)
		New thrombotic events	RRR = 63% NNT = 4.9 (P = .0008)
		Major bleeding†	NNH = 4.9 (P = .014)
Hirsh et al,[36] 2004 Systematic review of HAT-1 and HAT-2 trial data	Patients with HITTS	Death, amputation or further thrombosis	RRR = 53% (95% CI, 28% to 70%) NNT = 3.9 (95% CI, 3 to 8)
		Further thrombosis	RRR = 60% (95% CI, 20% to 81%)

*Reported measures of effect vary based on data available in studies cited
†Major bleeding was defined as intracranial bleeding, retroperitoneal bleeding, bleeding into a prosthetic joint, bleeding that caused a drop in hemoglobin of 2g/dL or more, or bleeding that required transfusion of 2 or more units of blood.
HAT, Heparin-Associated Thrombocytopenia trials; HITS, HIT and evidence of thrombosis; NNT, number needed to treat; RRR, relative risk reduction.

recommends that the choice of drug be based on individual patient characteristics, local expertise with a particular drug, and available pharmacokinetic knowledge and support. In general, because of elimination routes, argatroban is preferred in patients with impaired renal function and lepirudin in patients with compromised liver function.

DANAPAROID

The most relevant evidence regarding danaparoid comes from a cohort trial that compared danaparoid with lepirudin in patients with HIT and HITTS.[42]

Patients with Heparin-Induced Thrombocytopenia

Time-to-event analysis found that in patients with HIT, danaparoid increased the combined end point of death, amputation, and new thrombotic event compared with lepirudin (hazard ratio for danaparoid 2.9; 95% CI, 1.1 to 7.6). This result should be interpreted with caution because it was a nonrandomized, cohort trial, and the effect of danaparoid could not be determined for any of the individual outcomes (i.e., death, amputation, or thrombotic event), with very wide confidence intervals around all results.

Patients with Heparin-Induced Thrombocytopenia and Evidence of Thrombosis

The effect of danaparoid compared with lepirudin on the combined end point could not be determined. The precise event rates used in the time-to-event analysis are unclear, but the confidence intervals are likely very to be wide ($P = .913$). Danaparoid resulted in an absolute risk increase in new thrombosis of 1.5% (95% CI, −6.8% to 12.9%), although the confidence interval was wide, and the true effect of danaparoid remains unclear.

Bleeding Risk of Danaparoid versus Lepirudin

Time-to-event analysis found bleeding to be much less common in the danaparoid group (hazard ratio for danaparoid = 0.2 [95% CI, 0.07 to 0.8]). Based on this trial, conclusions about the relative efficacy of danaparoid and lepirudin cannot be made with certainty. However, the incidence of bleeding does appear to be lower with danaparoid.

Danaparoid does not cross the placenta, and it is unknown whether argatroban or lepirudin do so.[43]

Lepirudin may have a role in the treatment of pregnant women with HIT, although this remains to be rigorously studied.

BIVALIRUDIN

Case series indicate a possible role for bivalirudin in the treatment of HIT and HITTS. However, because of the variation among patients in these case series and the lack any controlled cohort trials, the effectiveness of bivalirudin in treating HIT or HITTS remains unclear. The ACCP recommends that for patients with HIT or HITTS not undergoing cardiac surgery, lepirudin or argatroban be used instead of bivalirudin, assigning bivalirudin a weak (grade 2C) recommendation. Theoretical advantages to bivalirudin include its combined renal and hepatobiliary clearance and its short half-life compared with the other direct thrombin inhibitors (see Table 8-9). In certain circumstances (i.e., patients at very high risk for bleeding or patients with severe liver and kidney dysfunction), these characteristics may make bivalirudin an attractive option, although little evidence exists to support its use.

CONCLUSIONS

When HIT or HITTS is suspected, heparin or low-molecular-weight heparin should be stopped and treatment with an alternative anticoagulant should begin immediately. Delaying the start of alternative anticoagulation after discontinuing heparin is associated with an increase in thrombotic events in patients with HIT. Although no direct comparative evidence exists, argatroban and lepirudin have been proved to be effective in treating HIT and HITTS in cohort trials.

In patients with renal failure or in whom renal function is unknown or unstable, argatroban is a reasonable first choice because it undergoes hepatobiliary clearance. Lepirudin undergoes renal clearance and should be considered first in patients with compromised liver function. The incidence of major bleeding is 5% to 7% in patients treated with argatroban and about 29% in patients receiving lepirudin. Expert opinion is that bleeding with lepirudin may be reduced by lowering the infusion rate to 0.1mg/kg/hr and closely following the aPTT until steady therapeutic levels are achieved. Little reliable evidence exists for the use of danaparoid or bivalirudin in the treatment of patients with HIT or HITTS not undergoing cardiac surgery or catheterization, although each drug has special characteristics that may make it attractive for use in specific circumstances. Consultation with a hematologist and pharmacokinetics support are recommended for the management of HIT.

6. Does red blood cell transfusion improve mortality in critically ill patients?

Search Date: March 2006

Search Strategy: *Medline search of "red cell transfusion and critically ill patients," limits: humans and English; 12 citations found, 6 selected and reviewed. Bibliographies of all citations were searched, including a search of UpToDate.*

Anemia is common in critically ill patients admitted to intensive care units. In a prospective, cross-sectional study by Vincent and colleagues, 63% of intensive care unit (ICU) patients had hemoglobin levels less than 12 g/dL, and 29% had levels less than 10 g/dL.[44] The transfusion rate in this population is also high, ranging from 37% in the study of Vincent and coworkers[44] to 85% in a retrospective chart review by Corwin and colleagues.[45] However, the clinical effects of various degrees of anemia in the critically ill and the appropriateness of red blood cell (RBC) transfusions in anemic ICU patients are unclear.

Corwin and associates[45] found that in 28% of patients transfused, there was no clear indication for transfusion or that the sole indication was a low hematocrit level of approximately 27 g/dL. Moreover, in the remaining 72% who did have other indications for transfusion, the pre-transfusion hematocrit levels were also approximately 27 g/dL. These findings support the well-conceived theory of the *transfusion trigger*; more often than not, the decision to transfuse red blood cells is triggered by a predetermined hemoglobin or hematocrit level rather than an evidence-based indication.

To be fair, there are sound physiologic principles that help to explain the effects of anemia in the critically ill and support RBC transfusion in this population. Factors that contribute to anemia in the ICU include sepsis; overt or occult blood loss, including phlebotomy; decreased erythropoietin production caused by *EPO* gene suppression by inflammatory mediators; and an immune-associated functional iron deficiency.[44-46] The resultant low hemoglobin concentration is thought to be deleterious because it adds to the oxygen debt (i.e., difference between oxygen use and oxygen delivery), thereby hindering tissue perfusion.[47]

Oxygen delivery (Do_2) is determined by the equation Do_2 = cardiac output × arterial oxygen content. The arterial oxygen content consists of hemoglobin-bound oxygen and, to a lesser extent, dissolved oxygen. Therefore, Do_2 = cardiac output × [(1.39 × [Hb] × arterial oxygen saturation) + (Pao_2 × 0.0031)]. Normally, the rate of oxygen delivery exceeds consumption by a factor of four. If the intravascular volume is maintained and the cardiovascular status is not impaired, oxygen delivery will be adequate as long as the hematocrit is above 10 g/dL. Increased cardiac output and a rightward shift of the oxygen-hemoglobin curve leading to increased oxygen extraction can compensate for the decrease in arterial oxygen content. These predictions were confirmed in a study in which healthy resting humans underwent isovolemic hemodilution to a hemoglobin of 5 g/dL, at which point only 3 of the 55 volunteers showed electrocardiographic changes suggesting myocardial ischemia.[48]

In critically ill patients, however, compensatory mechanisms may be limited, and oxygen use may become pathologically dependent on oxygen delivery. Intravascular volume may not be maintained, and the patient's cardiovascular status may be impaired. Oxygen demand may also be high because it is influenced by muscle activity, temperature, heart rate, sympathetic activity, and overall metabolic state. Moreover, elevated arterial lactate concentrations may change the slope of the oxygen extraction ratio. An elevated arterial lactate, an oxygen extraction ratio of greater than 0.3, and a Do_2 of less than 10 to 12 mL/kg/min are each indicators of poor tissue perfusion, and it is thought that attempts should be made to increase Do_2 by red cell transfusion, improvement of oxyhemoglobin saturation, or augmentation of cardiac output.

The previous reasoning appears grounded in sound physiologic principles and is widely accepted. However, red cell transfusion is not without risk. In addition to the commonly discussed risks of allergic reaction and infection, RBC transfusion poses immunomodulatory risks and microcirculatory complications.[49] There is also evidence suggesting that "old" stored blood lacks the expected oxygen carrying capacity and does not consistently improve tissue oxygenation.[50] Given these risks, it is important to establish whether transfusion provides a true mortality benefit in the critically ill.

The only multicentered, randomized, controlled clinical trial addressing the mortality benefit of RBC transfusions in the ICU is the Transfusion Requirements in Critical Care (TRICC) trial by Hebert and coworkers.[49] The TRICC trial compared a restrictive transfusion strategy that maintained hemoglobin levels between 7 and 9 g/dL to a liberal strategy that maintained hemoglobin levels between 10 and 12 g/dL. From November 1994 to November 1997, the trial enrolled 838 critically ill patients from 22 tertiary level ICUs and 3 community ICUs in Canada. Patients were clinically euvolemic after initial treatment and were followed for 60 days to assess the primary end points of all-cause 30-day mortality and severity of organ dysfunction. The study investigators were not blinded, and the analysis was by intention to treat. Overall, 30-day mortality rates were similar in both groups (18.7% in the restrictive group versus 23.3% in the liberal group, $P = .11$). However, certain subgroups within the restrictive strategy group had lower mortality rates: patients with APACHE scores less than 20 (8.7% versus 16.1%, $P = .03$) and patients younger than 55 years (5.7% versus 13%, $P = .02$). The secondary end point of mortality rate during hospitalization was also lower for the restrictive group (22.2% versus 28.1%, $P = .05$), as were the mortality rates in the ICU and at 60 days, with the latter two lacking statistical significance. Overall, transfusions were reduced by 54% in the restrictive group, with a third of the patients never receiving a transfusion.[49]

In 2002, Vincent and colleagues[44] demonstrated an association between RBC transfusion and mortality in ICUs through a prospective, observational, cross-sectional study that enrolled 3534 patients from 146 western European ICUs over a 2-week period in November 1999. The study divided subjects into two well-balanced groups of transfused and nontransfused patients, matching patients from each group according to their propensity to receive a transfusion and thereby controlling for confounding variables. The overall mortality rate and the ICU mortality rate were significantly different in the two groups: 29% in the transfused group versus 14.9% in the nontransfused group ($P < .001$) and 18.5% in the transfused group versus 10.1% in the nontransfused group ($P < .001$), respectively. Moreover, mortality rates were higher for the transfused patients at all levels of organ dysfunction, except for the most severe. A dose-response relationship was observed; each additional unit of RBC transfused correlated with a higher mortality.[44] These findings are similar to those of an earlier retrospective chart review by Corwin and colleagues,[45] in which a low-transfusion group receiving 1 to 5 units of RBCs in the ICU was compared with a high-transfusion group receiving more than 5 units. An increased rate of transfusion was associated with more prolonged mechanical ventilation, longer ICU stay, and increased mortality.[45] Although the studies by Vincent and colleagues[44] and Corwin and associates[45] suggest an association between transfusion and mortality in ICUs, they do not imply causality. It is not possible to conclude whether higher rates of transfusions resulted in increased mortality or patients received higher rates of transfusions because they were sicker. However, given the findings of the TRICC trial, it appears that a lower hemoglobin goal and fewer RBC transfusions are at least equivalent to, if not better than, a higher hemoglobin goal in critically ill patients.

It may not, however, be appropriate to generalize these findings to the entire ICU population. When early goal-directed therapy (EGDT) in septic shock was evaluated by Rivers and colleagues[51] in 2001, a significant mortality benefit was demonstrated. Part of the EGDT protocol required maintaining hemoglobin levels greater than 10 g/dL if the central venous oxygen saturation was less than 70%. The mean hematocrit in the control group was significantly lower than the EGDT group (30.1 g/dL versus 32.1 g/dL, $P < .001$).[51] It is therefore likely that subgroups of critically ill patients exist that may benefit from higher hemoglobin goals. Among these subgroups may be patients with septic shock and perhaps patients with cardiovascular disease. More definitive studies are required to examine the role of blood transfusion and its mortality benefit in subpopulations of critically ill patients.

The evidence supporting an optimal hemoglobin level and the benefit of RBC transfusion in critically ill patients is limited, with one large, randomized, controlled trial providing most of the evidence and a series of retrospective and prospective observational studies hinting at associations. Given the available data, most critically ill patients probably do not derive a benefit from higher hemoglobin levels and likely can be safely transfused when levels fall below 7 g/dL. This approach may also improve their survival by limiting their exposure to the potentially immunosuppressive and microcirculatory complications of RBC transfusion. However, certain subgroups of patients, including those with early sepsis and low mixed venous oxygen saturation levels and those with acute coronary syndromes, likely should be transfused for hemoglobin levels less than 10 g/dL, at least until further data are available. Regardless of the hemoglobin level, patients should be transfused when signs and symptoms of anemia develop. In the critically ill patient, just as in any other patient, an accelerated heart rate and dyspnea are better indications for transfusion than the traditional transfusion trigger of an absolute hemoglobin level.[52]

REFERENCES

1. Al-Jaouni SK, Al-Muhayawi SM, Qari MH, Nawas MA: The safety of avoiding transfusion preoperatively in patients with sickle cell hemoglobinopathies [abstract]. Blood 2002;100(Pt2):21b. (II)

2. Riddington C, Williamson L: Preoperative blood transfusions for sickle cell disease. Cochrane Database Syst Rev 2001;3:CD003149. (I)

3. Buck J, Casbard A, Llewelyn C, et al: Preoperative transfusion in sickle cell disease: A survey of practice in England. European Journal of Hematology 2005;75:14-21. (VI)

4. Fu T, Corrigan NJ, Quinn CT, et al: Minor elective surgical procedures using general anesthesia in children with sickle cell anemia without pre-operative blood transfusion. Pediatr Blood Cancer 2005;45:43-47. III

5. Haberkern CM, Neumayr LD, Orringer EP, et al: Cholecystectomy in sickle cell anemia patients: Perioperative outcome of 364 cases from the National Preoperative Transfusion Study. Blood 1997;89: 1533-1542. III

6. Weiner SJ, Miller ST, Koshy M, et al: Surgery and anesthesia in sickle cell disease. Blood 1995;86:3676-3684. III

7. Vichinsky EP, Haberkern CM, Neumayr L, et al: A comparison of conservative and aggressive transfusion regimens in the perioperative management of sickle cell disease. N Engl J Med 1995;333:206-213. II

8. Amorosi EL, Ultmann JE: Thrombotic thrombocytopenic purpura: Report of 16 cases and review of the literature. Medicine (Baltimore) 1966;45:139-159. VI

9. Ridolfi RL, Bell WR: Thrombotic thrombocytopenic purpura. Report of 25 cases and review of the literature. Medicine (Baltimore) 1981;60:413-428. VI

10. Rock GA, Shumak KH, Buskard NA, et al: Comparison of plasma exchange with plasma infusion in the treatment of thrombotic thrombocytopenic purpura. Canadian Apheresis Group. N Engl J Med 1991;325:426-428. II

11. George JN: How I treat patients with thrombotic thrombocytopenic purpura–hemolytic uremic syndrome. Blood 2000;96:1223-1229. V

12. Rock GA: Thrombotic thrombocytopenic purpura: Outcome in 24 patients with impairment treated with plasma exchange. Canadian Apheresis Study Group. Transfusion 1992;32:710-714. VI

13. Vesely SK, Goerge JN, Adix L, et al: ADAMTS13 activity in thrombotic thrombocytopenic purpura-hemolytic uremic syndrome: Relation to presenting features and clinical outcomes in a prospective cohort of 142 patients. Blood. 2003;102:60-68. III

14. George JN: Thrombotic thrombocytopenic purpura: A syndrome that keeps evolving. J Clin Apher 2004;19:63-65. V

15. George JN: Thrombotic thrombocytopenic purpura. American College of Physicians Physician Information and Education Resource (PIER), April 7, 2005 http://pier.acponline.org/index.html. VI

16. Rizvi MA, et al: Complications of plasma exchange in 71 consecutive patients treated for clinically

suspected thrombotic thrombocytopenic purpura–hemolytic-uremic syndrome. Transfusion 2000;40:896-901. **VI**

17. Quintini G: Continuous intravenous infusion of dipyridamole as adjunctive therapy in the treatment of thrombotic thrombocytopenic purpura. Trans Apher Sci 2003;29:141-145. **VI**

18. Bobbio-Pallavinci E, Gugliotta L, Centurioni R, et al: Antiplatelet agents in thrombotic thrombocytopenic purpura (TTP). Results of a randomized multicenter trial by the Italian Cooperative Group for TTP. Haematologica 1997;82:429-435. **II**

19. Rock GA, Shumak KH, Sutton DM, et al: Cryosupernatant as replacement fluid for plasma exchange in thrombotic thrombocytopenic purpura. Members of the Canadian Apheresis Group. Br J Haematol 1996;94:383-386. **III**

20. Zeigler ZR, Shadduck RK, Gryn JF, et al: Cryoprecipitate poor plasma does not improve early response in primary adult thrombotic thrombocytopenic purpura (TTP). J Clin Apher 2001;16:19-22. **II**

21. Rock G, Anderson D, Clark W, et al: Does cryosupernatant plasma improve outcome in thrombotic thrombocytopenic purpura? No answer yet. Br J Haematol 2005;129: 79-86. **II**

22. Kappers-Klunne MC, Wijermans P, Fijnheer R, et al: Splenectomy for the treatment of thrombotic thrombocytopenic purpura. Br J Haematol 2005; 130:768-776. **III**

23. Tsai HM: Advances in the pathogenesis, diagnosis, and treatment of thrombotic thrombocytopenic purpura. J Am Soc Nephrol 2003;14:1072-1081. **V**

24. Tsai HM, Lian EC: Antibodies to von Willebrand factor cleaving protease in acute thrombotic thrombocytopenic purpura. N Engl J Med 1998;339:1585-1594. **III**

25. Fakhouri F, Vernant JP, Veyradier A, et al: Efficiency of curative and prophylactic treatment with rituximab in ADAMTS13-deficient thrombotic thrombocytopenic purpura: A study of 11 cases. Blood 2005;106: 1932-1937. **VI**

26. Bohm M, Betz C, Miesbach W, et al: The course of ADAMTS-13 activity and inhibitor titre in the treatment of thrombotic thrombocytopenic purpura with plasma exchange and vincristine. Br J Haematol 2005;129: 644-652. **VI**

27. Warkentin TE: New approaches to the diagnosis of heparin-induced thrombocytopenia. Chest 2005;127(Suppl):35S-45S. (V)

28. Warkentin TE, Greinacher A: Heparin-induced thrombocytopenia: Recognition, treatment, and prevention. The seventh ACCP Conference on Anthithrombotic and Thrombolytic Therapy. Chest 2004;126(Suppl):311S-337S. (VI)

29. Warkentin TE, Kelton JG: Temporal aspects of heparin-induced thrombocytopenia. N Engl J Med 2001;344: 1286-1292. (III)

30. Lubenow N, Kempf R, Eichner A, et al: Heparin-induced thrombocytopenia: Temporal pattern of thrombocytopenia in relation to initial use or reexposure to heparin. Chest 2002;122:37-42. (III)

31. Warkentin TE, Kelton JG: Delayed-onset heparin-induced thrombocytopenia and thrombosis. Ann Intern Med 2001;135:502-506. (VI)

32. Rice L, Attisha WK, Drexler A, Francis JL: Delayed-onset heparin-induced thrombocytopenia. Ann Intern Med 2002;136:210-215. (VI)

33. Warkentin TE, Bernstein RA: Delayed-onset heparin-induced thrombocytopenia and cerebral thrombosis after a single administration of unfractionated heparin. N Engl J Med 2003;348:1067-1069. (VI)

34. Warkentin TE, Sheppard JA, Moore JC, et al: Laboratory testing for the antibodies that cause heparin-induced thrombocytopenia: How much class do we need? J Lab Clin Med 2005;146:341-346. (III)

35. Rice L: Heparin-induced thrombocytopenia: Myths and misconceptions (that will cause trouble for you and your patient). Arch Intern Med 2004;164:1961-1964. (V)

36. Hirsh J, Heddle N, Kelton JG: Treatment of heparin-induced thrombocytopenia: A critical review. Arch Intern Med 2004;164:361-369. (I)

37. Calculations done by the author.

38. Lewis BE, Wallis DE, Berkowitz SD, et al: Argatroban anticoagulant therapy in patients with heparin-induced thrombocytopenia. Circulation 2001;103:1838-1843. (III)

39. Lewis BE, Wallis DE, Leya F, et al: Argatroban anticoagulation in patients with heparin-induced thrombocytopenia. Arch Intern Med 2003;163:1849-1856. (III)

40. Calculations by the author using data from references 38 and 39.

41. Lubenow N, Eichler P, Lietz T, et al: Lepirudin in patients with heparin-induced thrombocytopenia—Results of the third prospective study (HAT-3) and a combined analysis of HAT-1, HAT-2, and HAT-3. J Thromb Haemost 2005;3:2428-2436. **I**

42. Farner B, Eichler P, Kroll H, Greinacher A: A comparison of danaparoid and lepirudin in heparin-induced thrombocytopenia. Thromb Haemost 2001;85:950-957. **III**

43. Hassell K: The management of patients with heparin-induced thrombocytopenia who require anticoagulant therapy. Chest 2005;127(Suppl):1S-8S. **V**

44. Vincent JL, Baron JF, Reinhart K, et al: Anemia and blood transfusion in critically ill patients. JAMA 2002;288:1499-1507. **III**

45. Corwin HL, Parsonnet KC, Gettinger A: RBC transfusion in the ICU. Is there a reason? Chest 1995;108: 767-771. **III**

46. Corwin HL, Krantz SB: Anemia of the critically ill: "Acute" anemia of chronic disease. Crit Care Med 2000;28:3098-3099. **V**

47. Hebert PC, Tinmouth A, Corwin H: Anemia and red cell transfusion in critically ill patients. Crit Care Med 2003;31(Suppl):S672-S677. **V**

48. Leung JM, Weiskopf RB, Feiner J, et al: Electrocardiographic ST-segment changes during acute, severe, isovolemic hemodilution in humans. Anesthesiology 2000;93:1004-1010. **III**

49. Hebert PC, Wells G, Blajchman MA, et al: A multicenter, randomized, controlled clinical trial of transfusion requirements in critical care. N Engl J Med 1999;340: 409-417. **II**

50. Marik PE, Sibbald WJ: Effect of stored-blood transfusion on oxygen delivery in patients with sepsis. JAMA 1993;269:3024-3029. **III**

51. Rivers E, Nguyen B, Havstad S, et al: Early goal-directed therapy in the treatment of severe sepsis and septic shock. N Engl J Med 2001;345:1368-1377. **II**

52. Audet AM, Goodnough LT: Practice strategies for elective red blood cell transfusion. American College of Physicians. Ann Intern Med 1992;116:403-406. **IV**

Management of Diabetes Mellitus and Hyperglycemia in the Hospitalized Patient

Helen Azzam and C. Komal Jaipaul

1. In critically ill patients in the intensive care unit, what is the effect of strict glucose control versus less intensive glucose control on length of stay, morbidity, and mortality? In this population, what is the ideal blood glucose concentration?

Search Date: April 2006

Search Strategy: *PubMed, 1970 to 2006, search of "diabetes OR hyperglycemia" AND "critically ill OR intensive care" AND "glycemic control OR insulin." Limited to human and English language studies; 299 citations retrieved. Titles and abstracts scanned, with relevant citations selected. Bibliographies of all relevant citations reviewed. Search of the Cochrane Central Register of Controlled Trials, UpToDate, and the American Diabetes Association website yielded no additional studies.*

Hyperglycemia is common in critically ill patients and is associated with adverse outcomes. A review of the literature demonstrates a decrease in morbidity and mortality in diabetic and nondiabetic critically ill patients in the critical care unit (CCU), the surgical intensive care unit (ICU), and the mixed medical-surgical ICU when normoglycemia is maintained using intensive insulin therapy. Patients receiving intensive insulin therapy had reductions in ICU length of stay (but not in-hospital stay), septicemia, length of antibiosis, acute renal failure, need for red blood cell transfusions, and critical-illness polyneuropathy. A study in a strictly medical ICU population preliminarily confirms a decrease in morbidity when normoglycemia is maintained, but it shows only a decrease in mortality when length of stay exceeds 3 days. Although different target glucose ranges were used for each study, the largest in-hospital reduction in mortality was demonstrated when glucose levels were maintained between 80 and 99 mg/dL. Although glucose potassium insulin (GKI) infusions have been used in this country and abroad, particularly for cardiac critical care patients, the following studies address the use of insulin infusion alone.

MEDICAL ICUs

The earliest clinical trial showing deleterious effects of hyperglycemia was the DIGAMI study, in which 620 diabetic patients in the acute postmyocardial infarction period were randomized to strict glycemic control (126 to 196 mg/dL) with insulin infusion during the first 24 hours after infarction, followed by long-term subcutaneous insulin administration, versus standard glucose control.[1] There was a 25% relative reduction in mortality at 3.4 years in the strict control group, although it is not clear whether this reduction resulted from the insulin infusion peri-infarction or the long-term subcutaneous insulin.[1]

A study conducted strictly in medical ICU patients compared outcomes in 605 patients randomized to receive conventional treatment (i.e., insulin administered only when the blood glucose exceeded 215 mg/dL) and 595 patients who received intensive therapy (i.e., blood glucose maintained between 80 and 110 mg/dL by continuous insulin infusion).[2] Among all patients, regardless of length of stay, morbidity was reduced in the group receiving intensive insulin therapy compared with those receiving conventional treatment due to a decrease in development of renal injury (5.9% versus 8.9%, $P = .04$), reduction in weaning time from mechanical ventilation (HR = 1.21; 95% CI: 1.02 to 1.44; $P = .03$), and shorter length of stay in the ICU (HR = 1.15; 95% CI: 1.01 to 1.32; $P = .04$) and the hospital (HR = 1.16; 95% CI: 1.00 to 1.35; $P = .05$). In this population, there was no significant impact on mortality with aggressive insulin therapy. There was actually an increased mortality rate for patients who stayed in the ICU for less than 3 days when treated with aggressive insulin therapy compared with conventional therapy, although the study authors claim that the results differed when different analyses were used ($P = .05$ with the chi square test [HR = 1.09; 95% CI: 0.9 to 1.32]; $P = .35$ by uncorrected proportional-hazards analysis [HR = 1.09; 95% CI: 0.89 to 1.32]; $P = .41$ after correcting for baseline risk factors listed in the paper). In the patients who stayed at least 3 days in the ICU, aggressive insulin therapy led to a reduction in all-cause deaths while in the ICU (31.3% versus 38.1%, $P = .05$) and in-hospital deaths (43% versus 52.5%, $P = .009$). However, the study authors claim that their results are strictly preliminary and that a study with at least 5000 patients will be required to allow an adequate analysis.

SURGICAL AND MEDICAL-SURGICAL ICUs

Data on general surgical ICU patients come from a large, randomized, controlled trial by Van den Berghe and colleagues,[3] in which 1548 postoperative ventilated patients received strict glucose control by insulin infusion using a target range of 80 to 110 mg/dL or standard therapy with insulin administered only when the glucose level exceeded 200 mg/dL. Approximately 60% of these patients were postoperative from cardiac surgery, whereas the other 40% had had neurosurgery, cardiothoracic surgery, abdominal surgery, or vascular surgery or were trauma or burn patients. Patients in the strict control group had an adjusted relative reduction in in-ICU mortality of 32% (95% CI: 2% to 55%; $P < .04$) and a relative reduction in in-hospital mortality of 34% ($P = .01$). These results did not differ between different types of surgery. It is notable, however, that the 95% confidence interval for in-ICU mortality is extremely wide and approaches 1. There was also a relative reduction in septicemia by 46% ($P = .003$), in long-term antibiotic requirement by 35% ($P < .001$), in acute renal failure requiring hemodialysis or hemofiltration by 41% ($P = .007$), in the median number of red-cell transfusions by 50% ($P < .001$), and in critical-illness polyneuropathy by 44% ($P = .007$). For long-stay ICU patients (i.e., 5 days), there was a statistically significant relative reduction in the length of stay in the ICU from a mean of 15 days to a mean of 12 days ($P = .003$), although there was not a significant reduction in overall hospital length of stay (P value not provided). A follow-up study by the same investigators in 2003 showed that this benefit resulted from normoglycemia rather than the dose of insulin infused.[4]

A retrospective analysis expanded the study population by looking at 1826 patients in a medical-surgical ICU.[5] This study demonstrated an in-hospital mortality rate of 9.6% for patients with mean glucose levels between 80 and 99 mg/dL, 12.2% for patients with glucose levels between 100 and 199 mg/dL, and 42.5% for patients with a mean glucose level exceeding 300 mg/dL (P for all < .001).[5] In a follow-up retrospective study, the study authors studied the effect of implementation of an intensive insulin regimen in the same medical-surgical ICU and compared morbidity and mortality before and after the institution of a glucose management protocol.[6] Compared with the 800 preprotocol patients studied, the 800 postprotocol patients demonstrated a 29.3% relative reduction in mortality ($P = .002$), a 10.8% reduction in length of ICU stay ($P = .01$), 75% reduction in the development of acute renal failure ($P = .03$), and an 18.7% reduction in the number of patients necessitating red blood cell transfusions.

In a randomized, controlled trial looking specifically at nondiabetic patients in a surgical ICU, 61 patients were randomly assigned to receive strict insulin therapy (i.e., target glucose range of 80 to 120 mg/dL) or standard therapy (i.e., target glucose range of 180 to 220 mg/dL).[7] The investigators found statistically significant reductions in the incidence of nosocomial infections, including catheter-related infections and postoperative wound infections in the intensive control group ($P < .05$). The incidence of hypoglycemia, however, was higher in the strict insulin therapy group (32% versus 7.4% of patients, $P < .001$).

META-ANALYSES OF SURGICAL ICU PATIENTS

In a meta-analysis of 35 randomized, controlled trials, surgical ICU patients receiving strict insulin therapy had a 15% reduction in mortality (RR = 85%; 95% CI: 75% to 97%) compared with those receiving standard therapy.[7] The incidence of hypoglycemia, reported in 10 of these studies, was found to be approximately three times more likely in patients receiving intensive insulin therapy (RR = 3.4; 95% CI: 1.9 to 6.3). No adverse outcomes associated with hypoglycemia were observed in any of the 10 studies. The method of insulin administration affected outcomes, because the studies in which insulin therapy was administered as a GKI solution did not detect a significant decrease in mortality (RR = 0.90; 95% CI: 0.77 to 1.04). However, when the five trials in which insulin was administered by a method other than GKI were pooled, there was a 27% reduction in mortality (RR = 0.73; 95% CI: 0.56 to 0.95) with intravenous insulin therapy. The meta-analysis did not specify how insulin was administered in these latter five trials. This variation in insulin administration may explain why there was only a 15% reduction in mortality in this meta-analysis compared with larger decreases in the previously mentioned individual studies. Although meta-analyses have the benefit of larger numbers of patients, a clinician interested in the effects of insulin on a specific patient may be better served by looking at the data from a study addressing that population.

CONCLUSION

Based on this evidence, critically ill patients in an ICU setting with hyperglycemia should be placed on continuous insulin infusion, regardless of whether they are diabetic. The target fasting glucose range should probably be 80 to 110 mg/dL, although a slightly lower range (80 to 99 mg/dL) may be preferable if patients are monitored closely for hypoglycemia.

2. In patients admitted to the general floor, what is the effect of strict glucose control versus less intensive glucose control on length of stay, morbidity, and mortality? In this population, what is the ideal glucose concentration?

Search Date: April 2006

Search Strategy: *PubMed, 1970 to 2006, search of "diabetes OR hyperglycemia" AND "hospital OR inpatient" AND "glycemic OR glucose" AND "control OR management,"*

AND "morbidity OR mortality OR length of stay." Limited to human and English language studies; 414 citations retrieved. Titles and abstracts scanned, with relevant citations selected. Bibliographies of all relevant citations reviewed. The American Diabetes Association and the American College of Endocrinology websites were also searched for relevant position statements and references. Search of the Cochrane Central Register of Controlled Trials and UpToDate websites added no additional studies.

Hyperglycemia occurs in up to 38% of patients admitted to a general ward, with two thirds of this population carrying no history of diabetes before admission.[9] Although diabetes and hyperglycemia are associated with poor clinical outcomes,[9] there are no randomized, controlled trials that measure the effect of strict glycemic control on length of stay, morbidity, and mortality for general ward patients. Recommendations about target glucose range and the use of insulin on a general medical or surgical ward are therefore extrapolated from studies done in critically ill medical and surgical patients,[3,6,10] patients with acute myocardial infarctions,[1] and stroke patients.[11] The only available prospective trial in general medicine patients found a diabetes team to be effective in lowering mean finger-stick glucose values and improving outcomes such as length of stay and readmission rate.[12]

ASSOCIATION BETWEEN GLYCEMIC CONTROL AND CLINICAL OUTCOMES IN GENERAL INPATIENTS

The first study linking poor outcomes to hyperglycemia in patients on a general medical ward was published in 2002.[9] Medical records for 1886 patients admitted to a general hospital ward were reviewed. Compared with normoglycemic patients, patients with hyperglycemia had a higher in-hospital mortality rates (16% versus 1.7%, $P < .01$), a higher readmission rate to the ICU (29% versus 14%, $P < .01$), and increased likelihood of requiring skilled nursing or rehabilitation facilities at discharge (28% versus 14%, $P < .02$). Patients with newly diagnosed hyperglycemia had poorer outcomes than patients with a known history of diabetes with regard to length of stay (9 ± 0.7 days versus 5.5 ± 0.2 days,

$P < .001$), mortality (16% versus 3%, $P < .001$), and percentage discharged directly home (56% versus 74%, $P < .001$).[9]

The only prospective data on ward patients who are not critically ill come from a trial studying the effect of a diabetes team (i.e., diabetes nurse educator and an endocrinologist) on length of stay and rate of readmission.[12] In this study, 179 diabetic patients were randomized to the control group, in which they received care from physicians, nurses, nutritionists and social workers, or to the intervention group, in which a diabetes team also visited the patient daily. Patients in the control group had a longer length of stay than those in the intervention group (diabetes as primary diagnosis = 7.5 days [95% CI: 5 to 11 days] versus 5.5 days [95% CI: 4 to 8 days]; diabetes as secondary diagnosis = 10.5 days versus 10 days [95% CI: 8 to 13 days for both]). Seventy-five percent of patients in the intervention group maintained glucose levels between 80 and 180 mg/dL during the first month of the program compared with 46% in the control group ($P < .01$). The rate of readmission was higher for the control group than the intervention group (32% versus 15%, $P < .01$).[12] This study suggests that better glucose control in general ward patients is associated with decreased length of stay and rate of readmission, but effects of the diabetes team other than enhanced glycemic control may have influenced these outcomes.

CORTICOSTEROID INDUCED HYPERGLYCEMIA

There are no data examining treatment of hyperglycemia in inpatients requiring steroid treatment for exacerbations of asthma, chronic obstructive pulmonary disease (COPD), or autoimmune disorders. Two studies have shown that the incidence of hyperglycemia is higher among nondiabetic patients admitted for COPD exacerbation who are treated with steroids than among patients not treated with steroids. A systematic review found an odds ratio of 5.48 (95% CI: 1.58 to 18.96)[13] and a randomized, controlled trial showed that 15% of patients on steroids had hyperglycemic events compared with 4% of patients not on steroids ($P = .002$).[14] However, there are no randomized, controlled trials comparing outcomes for these patients.

SLIDING SCALE INSULIN IN HOSPITALIZED PATIENTS

Hyperglycemia in hospitalized patients is most commonly managed with sliding scale insulin (SSI), although there are few data supporting this reactive approach. A multicenter randomized, controlled trial enrolling hospitalized family medicine patients randomized to receive their routine outpatient diabetes medications or ISS plus their routine medications was unable to demonstrate any difference in the frequency of hyperglycemia (34.6% versus 33.6%, $P = .87$), hypoglycemia (9% versus 8%, $P = .83$), or mean length of stay (5.3 versus 5 days, $P = .86$).[15]

A prospective cohort study in 171 diabetic patients on medical inpatient services found no difference in hyperglycemic events in patients on an oral hypoglycemic or intermediate-acting subcutaneous insulin regimen alone compared with patients on one of these standing regimens plus ISS (95% CI crosses 1 for all RR comparisons). There was an increased rate of hyperglycemia in patients who received SSI without a standing dose of intermediate-acting insulin compared with patients who received no insulin at all (RR = 2.85 with a conservative ISS [95% CI: 1.07 to 7.59]; RR = 3.25 with an aggressive ISS [95% CI: 1.23 to 8.60]).[16] A retrospective study of 47 patients hospitalized with diabetic ketoacidosis suggested that proactive insulin therapy was better than a retroactive SSI approach or a combination of proactive and SSI therapy in terms of median glucose levels (199.9 versus 262.5 versus 221.2 mg/dL, respectively, $P < .05$) and length of stay (4.4 versus 6.3 versus 6.3 days, respectively, $P < .05$).[17]

OPTIMAL BLOOD GLUCOSE LEVEL IN GENERAL INPATIENT

Given the lack of randomized, controlled trials in general ward patients, the target blood glucose level is somewhat arbitrary. The American Diabetes Association, in a 2005 position statement, concludes that fasting glucose should be maintained under 126 mg/dL and that all random glucose levels should be less than 200 mg/dL based on the results of the Umpierrez study.[18] However, the American College of Endocrinology (ACE) 2004 position statement, citing the Van den Berghe study,[2] suggests that the target glucose range in general ward patients should be the range found to be most effective in decreasing morbidity and mortality in critically ill patients (i.e., fasting glucose level less than 110 mg/dL and random glucose level less than 180 mg/dL).[2,19]

Although there are no randomized, controlled trials looking specifically at general inpatients, it is reasonable to assume that hyperglycemia has a detrimental effect on morbidity, mortality, and length of stay and that the fasting and random glucose values should be maintained at less than 110 mg/dL and 180 mg/dL, respectively.[2,19,20] The ACE recommends using a continuous insulin infusion in selected patient populations (i.e., prolonged NPO, patients on TPN, perioperative patients, patients receiving glucocorticoids, or in patients requiring a dose-finding strategy before conversion to a subcutaneous insulin regimen). Although the ACE cites a number of references throughout the position statement that are also referenced in this paper, their recommendations regarding use of continuous insulin infusion in these specific populations appear to be based on expert opinion. In all other patients, it appears a proactive approach to glycemic control with long- or intermediate-acting subcutaneous insulin with or without oral agents should be used rather than SSI. Additional help from endocrinologists and diabetes nurses should be obtained as indicated.

3. In perioperative patients, what is the effect of strict glucose control versus less intensive glucose control on length of stay, morbidity, and mortality? In this population, what is the ideal blood glucose concentration?

Search Date: April 2006

Search Strategy: PubMed, 1970 to 2006, search of "perioperative OR preoperative OR intraoperative OR surgical" AND "diabetes OR hyperglycemia" AND "insulin OR glycemic control OR glucose control." Limited to human and English language studies; 427 citations retrieved. Titles and abstracts scanned, with relevant citations selected. Bibliographies of all relevant citations reviewed. The American Diabetes Association website was also used for position statements and consensus opinion. Search of the Cochrane Central Register of Controlled Trials and UpToDate yielded no additional studies.

Perioperative hyperglycemia in diabetic and nondiabetic patients has historically been difficult to manage[21] and is associated with increased perioperative morbidity and mortality.[22,23] A review of the literature demonstrates a decrease in morbidity and mortality in diabetic and nondiabetic patients with perioperative hyperglycemia when they received intensive perioperative insulin therapy. However, there are no randomized, controlled trials assessing the effect of tight glucose control in general surgery patients who do not require a postoperative ICU stay. In the populations studied, benefits were shown when perioperative glucose was maintained at less than 200 mg/dL in patients undergoing coronary artery bypass grafting (CABG), less than 110 mg/dL in post-CABG patients in a surgical ICU, and less than 120 mg/dL in patients in a general surgical ICU.

ASSOCIATION BETWEEN PERIOPERATIVE GLYCEMIC CONTROL AND CLINICAL OUTCOME

A prospective cohort study of diabetic patients undergoing CABG demonstrated that the incidence of postoperative deep sternal wound infection (DSWI) was reduced when the blood glucose level was maintained at less than 200 mg/dL.[24] This study compared two sequential groups of patients: 968 patients operated on between 1987 and 1991 who received SSI for perioperative glucose control and 1499 patients operated on between 1992 and 1997 who received continuous insulin infusion (CII). In both groups, perioperative glucose was maintained below 200 mg/dL from the day of surgery through the third postoperative day. Patients treated with the CII had a lower daily mean blood glucose level (176 ± 0.8 versus 206 ± 1.2 mg/dL on postoperative day 1, $P < .001$), tighter overall glycemic control (standard deviation of 36 mg/dL for SSI on postoperative day 1 versus 26 mg/dL for CII on postoperative day 1, $P < .001$), and a 34% relative risk reduction in DSWI (95% CI: 14% to 74%).[4]

A follow-up study on the same prospective data carried out to 2001 showed a 57% relative risk reduction in mortality in the CII group ($P < .001$).[10]

A randomized, controlled trial looking at postoperative cardiac patients who were mechanically ventilated in a surgical ICU showed decreased morbidity and mortality when blood glucose levels were maintained below 110 mg/dL.[2] A group of 1548 patients (diabetic and nondiabetic) were randomized to receive conventional therapy (i.e., insulin infusion only if the blood glucose level was > 200 mg/dL) or intensive therapy with insulin infusion (i.e., maintenance of blood glucose level between 80 and 110 mg/dL) until ICU discharge. Patients in the strict control group had an adjusted relative reduction in ICU mortality of 32% (95% CI: 2% to 55%) and a relative reduction of in-hospital mortality of 34% ($P = .005$). There was a relative reduction in septicemia of 46% ($P = .003$), long-term antibiotic requirement by 35% ($P < .001$), acute renal failure requiring hemodialysis or hemofiltration by 41% ($P = .007$), median number of red blood cell transfusions by 50% ($P < .001$), and critical-illness polyneuropathy by 44% ($P = .007$). In long-stay (≥ 5-day) surgical ICU patients, there was a statistically significant reduction in length of stay in the ICU from a mean of 15 days to a mean of 12 days ($P = .003$), although there was not a significant reduction in overall hospital length of stay (P value not given). A follow-up study showed that this benefit resulted from normoglycemia rather than the infused insulin dose.[2]

A randomized, controlled trial enrolling patients in a general surgical ICU demonstrated that strict glycemic control reduced the incidence of nosocomial infections in a predominately nondiabetic population.[6] Twenty-seven patients who received standard insulin therapy (i.e., target glucose level of 180 to 220 mg/dL) had a higher incidence of total nosocomial infections, including catheter-related, surgical wound, and bloodstream infections compared with 34 patients assigned to receive strict insulin therapy (i.e., target glucose level of 80 to 120 mg/dL) throughout their ICU stay ($P < .05$). In this study, the relative risk of hypoglycemia (glucose levels < 60 mg/dL) was increased by 25% ($P < .001$).[6] It is unclear whether these events were clinically significant.

COMPARISON OF INSULIN INFUSION WITH SUBCUTANEOUS INSULIN

Although tighter glucose control is associated with better outcomes in surgical patients, there is still debate over whether continuous insulin infusion is superior to subcutaneous insulin. Data in favor of insulin infusion come from the two studies of cardiac patients referenced earlier[10,24] and from two prospective trials looking at general surgical patients with diabetes. However, one is simply a feasibility study demonstrating that a postoperative insulin infusion algorithm effectively achieved and maintained glucose levels between 120 and 180 within 8 hours after surgery.[25] The second randomly divided 30 diabetic patients admitted for elective surgery into group A (i.e., intravenous insulin infusion and glucose-potassium infusion) and group B (i.e., subcutaneous insulin administration and glucose-potassium infusion), and the study found that intravenous insulin infusion achieved tighter glucose control intraoperatively ($P < .05$ at 1 hour, 2 hours, and 4 hours into surgery) but had no significant effect on glycemic control in the preoperative and postoperative periods ($P > .05$ at virtually all time points in the periods 24 hours before and 24 hours after surgery).[26] However, this observed intraoperative effect might have occurred because blood glucose levels were measured and acted on hourly during the surgery and only every 4 hours in the preoperative and postoperative periods. A randomized, controlled trial that attempted to determine the optimal method of glucose control was unable to show a significant difference in glycemic control between 19 diabetic patients randomized to receive strict glycemic control with subcutaneous insulin and 18 diabetic patients who received strict glycemic control with insulin infusion for 48 hours postoperatively ($P > .05$).[27]

TEMPORAL RELATIONSHIP BETWEEN GLYCEMIC CONTROL AND SURGERY AND THE ASSOCIATION WITH CLINICAL OUTCOMES

Several studies have looked specifically at the preoperative, intraoperative, and postoperative periods to determine when tight glucose control is most important.

A retrospective study evaluating diabetic patients undergoing CABG found that high preoperative mean glucose levels were the major risk factor for the development of postoperative infection.[28] In 400 study patients, insulin infusion was initiated 2 hours before surgery and serum blood glucose levels were maintained between 150 and 200 mg/dL and continued until the patient received oral nutrition. Despite similar postoperative glucose levels, diabetics who developed DSWI had higher preoperative serum glucose values (221 ± 10.5 mg/dL 2 days before surgery, 181 ± 9.45 mg/dL 1 day before surgery) compared with patients who did not develop DSWI (166 ± 36.38 mg/dL 2 days before surgery, 138 ± 30.53 mg/dL 1 day before surgery). However, because this is a retrospective trial, it is possible that the incidence of postoperative DSWI is related more to the preexisting severity of diabetes than to the glucose control in the 2 days immediately before surgery.

SUMMARY

The American Diabetes Association recommends maintaining fasting and preoperative glucose levels less than 126 mg/dL and random blood glucose levels less than 200 mg/dL.[18] It is reasonable to recommend, however, that all serum blood glucose levels in diabetic and nondiabetic patients, from 2 days before surgery to at least postoperative day 3 (or discharge from the ICU for critically ill patients), be maintained below 120 mg/dL in general surgical patients and in the range of 80 to 110 mg/dL in surgical ICU patients. This may be most easily and effectively accomplished with insulin infusion, although this requires a dedicated intravenous line, limits patient mobility, and may require additional nursing and house staff education and resources. The studies supporting a benefit of intravenous insulin infusion in general surgical patients are few, contain small numbers of patients, and are only observational in nature. Because neither method of insulin administration in perioperative non-ICU patients has been proved superior as long as blood glucose levels are maintained in the target range, the choice for each patient may remain guided by clinical situation and physician preference.

4.   In the hospitalized patient with diabetes mellitus, is there evidence to support the use of sliding scale insulin alone or in conjunction with a standing diabetic medication regimen?

Search Date: February 2006

Search Strategy: A search of Pub Med from the period 1966 to 2006 with the term "sliding scale insulin" with limits of English and humans yielded a total of 57 publications. Titles and abstracts were scanned, with relevant citations selected. Bibliographies of all relevant citations were reviewed. The American Diabetes Association 2005 position statement was also reviewed.

Despite a lack of data supporting the use of sliding scale insulin (SSI) regimens in the inpatient setting and the American Diabetes Association's position that "the traditional sliding scale insulin regimens, usually consisting of regular insulin without any intermediate or long-acting insulin, have been shown to be ineffective,"[29] these regimens continue to be commonly used.

Our review of the literature revealed five studies that have attempted to investigate the effects of SSI regimens. Two studies failed to demonstrate a benefit for the use of SSI regimens in conjunction with standing diabetic medications in patients with type 2 diabetes mellitus hospitalized with a comorbid illness.[15,16] A third study, likely consisting of type I diabetics, suggested that an SSI regimen alone resulted in poorer glucose control than did proactive or combination regimens.[17] A fourth study demonstrated that frequent adjustments of standing insulin regimens in lieu of SSI provided improved glycemic control compared with historical controls in whom SSI was used.[30] The final study demonstrated improved glycemic control in patients treated with twice-daily 70/30 insulin compared with patients receiving traditional SSI.[31]

RANDOMIZED CONTROLLED TRIALS EVALUATING THE USE OF SSI

The only randomized, controlled trial assessing the effects of an SSI regimen on glycemic control in patients with type 2 diabetes mellitus hospitalized for other conditions was performed by Dickerson and colleagues.[15]

This study failed to demonstrate a benefit from the addition of the SSI regimen to routine diabetes medications with respect to frequency of hyperglycemia, hypoglycemia, or length of hospitalization compared with routine diabetic medications alone.

In this study,[15] 153 type 2 diabetic patients admitted with a comorbid illness to 1 of 10 family medicine residency programs across the United States were randomized to one of two groups: SSI regimen in addition to routine diabetes medication (consisting of oral agents or standing insulin) during hospitalization (i.e., intervention group) or routine diabetes medications only during hospitalization (i.e., control group). Neither patients nor physicians were blinded, and in both groups, routine diabetes medications were adjusted, added, or discontinued as they would be during routine care. The primary outcome measures were the frequency of hyperglycemia (blood glucose level > 300 mg/dL), hypoglycemia (blood glucose level < 50 mg/dL), and glycemic events (combination of hyperglycemia and hypoglycemia). A secondary outcome measure was length of hospitalization.

There was no difference in the frequency of glycemic events or in the length of hospitalization between the two groups, as outlined in Table 9-1. The severity of hypoglycemia or hyperglycemia between the two groups was also not significantly different.

PROSPECTIVE COHORT STUDY EVALUATING THE USE OF SSI

An earlier study by Queale and associates[16] demonstrated that in patients not receiving a standing diabetic medication regimen, the SSI regimen was associated with a threefold increase in the risk of hyperglycemic events (Table 9-2). However, in patients receiving standing regimens consisting of oral agents or intermediate-acting insulin, the risk of hyperglycemia or hypoglycemia was not statistically significantly different with the addition of an SSI regimen.

The prospective cohort study by Queale and coworkers[16] was aimed at identifying predictors of hyperglycemic and hypoglycemic events in 171 diabetic patients (primarily type 2 diabetics) hospitalized with a comorbid illness to one of seven medical services at a single urban university hospital to determine whether

Table 9-1. Glycemic Control and Length of Stay for Patients Treated with Sliding Scale Insulin plus Routine Medications or with Routine Medications Alone

Measurement	SSI plus Routine Medications (Intervention, $n = 75$)	Routine Medications Only (Control, $n = 78$)	Significance
Patients with hyperglycemic events	33.3%	34.6%	$P = .87$
Patients with hypoglycemic events	8%	9%	$P = .83$
Mean number of glycemic events per patient	1.3 ± 2.9	1.3 ± 2.5	$P = .99$
Length of hospitalization in days	5.0 ± 4.2	5.3 ± 5.4	$P = .86$

SSI, sliding scale insulin.

Table 9-2. Hyperglycemic Episodes by Glycemic Control Regimen

Regimen	Adjusted RR (95% CI)		
	No SSI	Conservative SSI	Aggressive SSI
Standing regimen			
None	1.00 (reference)	2.85 (1.07-7.59)	3.25 (1.23-8.60)
Oral hypoglycemic agent	0.25 (0.05-1.33)	0.93 (0.29-2.98)	0.48 (0.10-2.36)
Intermediate acting insulin	1.38 (0.42-4.59)	1.82 (0.69-4.81)	0.60 (0.19-1.91)

RR, relative risk; SSI, sliding scale insulin.

SSI regimens were effective in improving glycemic control.

The standing glycemic control regimens in the hospital were categorized as follows: no standing regimen (37% of patients); oral hypoglycemic agent (25% of patients); or intermediate-acting insulin, with or without an oral hypoglycemic drug (37% of patients). Two types of SSI regimens were prescribed: an aggressive SSI regimen that started at a lower glucose level of less than 175 mg/dL (30% of patients) or a more conservative regimen that started at a higher glucose level of more than 175 mg/dL (46% of patients). Twenty-four percent of patients received no SSI regimen. Hyperglycemic and hypo-glycemic episodes were defined as blood glucose levels of 300 mg/dL or higher and as 60 mg/dL or less, respectively.

Of the 171 patients analyzed, 40% had at least one hyperglycemic event, and 23% had at least one hypo-glycemic event during the first 4 days of hospitalization. As shown in Table 9-2, patients treated with a conservative or aggressive SSI regimen in the absence of a standing regimen were three times more likely to develop hyper-glycemic events compared with their counterparts who did not receive glycemic control therapy (conservative regimen: adjusted RR = 2.85 [95% CI: 1.07 to 7.59]; aggressive regimen: adjusted RR = 3.25 [95% CI: 1.23 to 8.60]). Why patients who received SSI in the absence of a standing diabetic regimen should have poorer glycemic control that patients who received neither a standing regimen nor SSI is unclear. This finding raises the question of whether, in this nonrandomized study, patients who were more likely to be controlled by diet alone as an outpatient were assigned to the group that received neither a standing diabetic regimen nor SSI.

All other combinations of glycemic control regimens were statistically similar to one another. There was no significant interaction between the use of SSI regimens and hypoglycemic episodes.

The nonrandomized study by Queale and colleagues[16] may be subject to the potential bias that patients with more unstable diabetes were assigned to the SSI regimen and differed from those who were continued on their routine medications. The study conducted by Dickerson and coworkers[15] did not include a subgroup that was ran-domized to an SSI regimen only. Both studies, however, failed to demonstrate a benefit of SSI regimens when used in conjunction with a standing diabetic regimen, thereby casting doubt on the utility of SSI regimens as an adjunct to a standing diabetic regimen in hospitalized patients with type 2 diabetes.

RETROSPECTIVE STUDY COMPARING INSULIN REGIMENS IN TYPE I DIABETES

A third retrospective analysis by Gearhart and associates[17] compared the efficacy of a reactive SSI regimen, proactive insulin therapy, and a combination of the two methods in establishing glycemic control after the resolution of diabetic ketoacidosis in 47 diabetic patients hospitalized with a diagnosis of diabetic ketoacidosis. The treatment period began at the time that the intravenous insulin was discontinued and concluded at the time that there was a change in treatment protocol or the patient was discharged. Forty-seven patients were assigned to one of three treatment protocols: a reactive sliding scale regimen, in which patients received predetermined amounts of regular insulin based on the blood sugar levels measured at designated times (10 patients); a proactive regimen, in which patients were placed on a prospective regimen of any type of insulin subcutaneously in anticipation of glucose levels and no regular insulin was given retroactively in response to elevated blood sugar levels (14 patients); and a combination regimen, in which the patient was placed on scheduled intermediate- or short-acting insulin, or both, and received additional regular insulin for elevated blood sugar levels (23 patients).

Blood glucose control was assessed by evaluating the fluctuation of glucose values, median glucose values, degree of hyperglycemia and hypoglycemia, and the length of time necessary to achieve acceptable glucose values. The investigators developed four measures (i.e., deviation score, median score, high score, and low score) that allowed blood glucose control and degree of fluctuation to be assessed. The deviation score was calculated as the absolute difference between each measured glucose value from a baseline of 100 mg/dL divided by total number of glucose values. The median glucose value for all shifts was reported as the median score. A high score was defined as the number of shifts in which at least one glucose level of 250 mg/dL or higher was recorded divided by the number of shifts. A low score was defined as the number of shifts in which at least one glucose level of 80 mg/dL or lower was recorded divided by the number of shifts.

The deviation score was significantly higher for the reactive SSI group (167.4) than for the proactive (112.9) and combination (121.3) groups ($P < .01$). Median scores were also significantly higher for the reactive SSI group (262.5) than for the proactive (199.9) and combination (221.2) groups ($P < .05$). The reactive SSI group had a significantly higher number of shifts (0.70) in which a glucose level of 250 mg/dL or higher was recorded than in the proactive (0.37) and combination (0.40) groups ($P < .01$). Length of hospitalization was significantly shorter for the proactive group (4.4 days) than for the combination (6.3 days) and the reactive SSI groups (6.3 days) ($P < .01$). Proactive and combination groups did not differ significantly in high score, median score, or deviation score.

Patients who were treated with reactive SSI in the absence of a standing regimen had suboptimal blood sugar control compared with patients who received a standing insulin regimen alone or received an SSI regimen as an adjunct to a standing insulin regimen. Of even greater interest is the finding that blood sugar control in the group receiving a standing insulin regimen alone was not statistically different from that of the group receiving SSI in addition to a standing insulin regimen, suggesting that the addition of SSI to a standing diabetic regimen may not improve blood sugar control. Unlike the previous two studies, this retrospective study likely consisted of type I diabetics (given an initial presentation in diabetic ketoacidosis) who were lacking in endogenous basal insulin.

COMPARISON OF AGGRESSIVE ADJUSTMENT OF STANDING INSULIN WITH TREATMENT WITH SSI

Baldwin and colleagues[30] examined a program designed to re-educate medical house staff on the management of inpatient hyperglycemia without the use of SSI. Patients with a history of diabetes mellitus or a blood glucose level higher than 140 mg/dL admitted to two general medical house staff teams during an 8-week period were enrolled. Blood glucose was monitored preprandially and at bedtime. The outpatient diabetes regimen was continued for the initial 12 hours provided that the initial blood glucose level was less than 200 mg/dL. If the blood glucose concentration was higher than 200 mg/dL, oral agents were discontinued, and basal or bolus insulin was administered twice daily. Most insulin-treated patients received twice-daily doses of NPH and regular insulin; glargine and lispro/aspart were used only if they were preexisting therapy. Combination therapy with insulin and oral agents was not used, and standing orders were allowed for oral agents but not for insulin. SSI was not permitted. Doses were adjusted twice daily based on blood glucose values, with target fasting and preprandial glucose levels of 80 to 120 mg/dL and target bedtime glucose levels of 100 to 150 mg/dL. Glycemic control in the study group and in a group of historical control patients was compared. Results are outlined in Table 9-3.

This study[30] demonstrated that in inpatients, twice-daily adjustment of standing insulin regimens in lieu of an SSI regimen yielded improved glycemic control compared with historical controls in whom SSI was used. Although hypoglycemia occurred more frequently in the study group, the difference was not clinically relevant. The primary limitation of this study was the retrospective use of historical control patients.

In a small, nonrandomized, prospective, cohort study by Schoeffler and coworkers,[31] 20 type 2 diabetics admitted to two hospitals received twice-daily 70/30 insulin or SSI. Ten patients received 70/30 insulin adjusted twice daily based on glucose levels as indicated by a previously defined algorithm. The control group consisted of 10 patients who received SSI as prescribed by their physicians without concomitant standing insulin regimen. The study authors did not document how many patients received concomitant oral agents, other than to say that co-administration of oral agents was allowed. The mean daily glucose concentrations were significantly lower in the group receiving 70/30 insulin compared with the group receiving traditional SSI (151.3 versus 175.6 mg/dL, $P = .04$). Each subsequent day during the study period yielded a further improvement in glucose in the study group compared with the control (SSI) group. No hypoglycemic episodes (i.e., glucose level < 60 mg/dL) occurred in either group.

Table 9-3. Measurements of Glycemic Control

Measurement	Study Patients ($n = 88$)	Control Patients ($n = 99$)	Significance
Mean glucose ± SD (mg/dL)	150 ± 37	200 ± 51	$P < .01$
Glucose < 60 mg/dL (%)	3.60	1.40	$P = .01$
Hypoglycemia requiring D_{50} (%)	26	30	Not significant
Glucose > 250 mg/dL (%)	6.50	20.50	$P < .01$
Glucose 80-140 mg/dL (%)	43.80	22	$P < .01$
Glucose 80-180 mg/dL (%)	65.10	43.10	$P < .01$

Reprinted with permission from Baldwin D, Villanueva G, McNutt R, Bhatnagar S: Eliminating inpatient sliding-scale insulin: A Reeducation project with medical house staff. Diabetes Care 2005;28:1008-1011. Copyright © 2005, American Diabetes Association.

CONCLUSION

In summary, two studies of type 2 diabetics hospitalized with a comorbid condition failed to demonstrate a difference in glycemic control among patients who received SSI in addition to a standing diabetic regimen compared with patients who received a standing diabetic regimen alone.[15,16] A third study of type 1 diabetics suggests that use of SSI alone resulted in a greater degree of hyperglycemia compared with the use of a standing insulin regimen alone or the use of combination therapy consisting of the addition of SSI to a standing regimen.[17] This study of type 1 diabetics also failed to demonstrate a difference in glycemic control between patients receiving SSI in addition to a standing insulin regimen compared with patients receiving a standing insulin regimen alone. The two studies by Baldwin and colleagues[30] and Schoeffler and associates[31] suggest that replacing SSI with frequent (twice-daily) adjustment of insulin regimens based on blood sugars can result in improved glycemic control.

Additional randomized, controlled studies are needed to assess definitively whether SSI alone or in conjunction with a standing diabetic medication regimen improves glycemic control. The current data suggest that a proactive approach to blood sugar management in inpatients, rather than a reactive approach with SSI, is more likely to achieve improved glycemic control. However, this approach requires a greater time investment on the part of the physician, as evidenced by the study by Baldwin and associates.[30] It also requires changing a practice style that has become ingrained in the culture of medicine despite a lack of supporting evidence.

5. In hospitalized patients with diabetes mellitus receiving total parenteral nutrition, how is glycemic control most effectively achieved using insulin?

Search Date: February 2006

Search Strategy: *A search of Pub Med from the period 1966 to 2006 with the terms "enteral OR parenteral" AND "nutrition" AND "diabetes mellitus," with limits of English and human studies, yielded a total of 218 publications. Titles and abstracts were scanned, with relevant* *citations selected. Bibliographies of all relevant citations as well as the American Diabetes Association position statement regarding the inpatient management of diabetes and hyperglycemia[18] were reviewed.*

Achieving adequate blood sugar control in hospitalized patients with type 2 diabetes mellitus who are receiving total parenteral nutrition (TPN) can be challenging. Park and coworkers[32] reported that 77% of patients with type 2 diabetes who were not previously receiving insulin subsequently required insulin to achieve glycemic control while receiving TPN. Of the patients with type 1 diabetes mellitus, 67% required an increase in their insulin dose while receiving TPN.

There are no randomized, controlled trials examining the most effective method by which to achieve glycemic control in diabetic patients receiving TPN. The traditional method of achieving glycemic control involves adding incremental doses of insulin to the TPN bag until control is achieved, a process that may take several days. Although the American Diabetes Association recommends that regular insulin be added to the TPN bag directly, they also suggest that the practitioner consider using a separate intravenous insulin infusion for 24 hours to determine the daily insulin requirement.[18] They recommend adding two thirds of this calculated daily insulin requirement (as regular insulin) to subsequent TPN bags or adding two thirds of the total units of insulin administered subcutaneously the previous day (if an intravenous insulin infusion is not used) to the next day's TPN bag (as regular insulin) until a daily dose is determined.

EFFICACY AND SAFETY OF IV INSULIN IN PATIENTS RECEIVING TPN

The American Diabetes Association's suggestion to consider a separate intravenous insulin infusion is based on two studies that investigated the efficacy and safety of the use of a separate intravenous infusion of insulin in patients receiving TPN. Wolfson and colleagues[33] conducted an observational study in which patients received an intravenous infusion of insulin, with the rate and concentration of insulin infusion adjusted based on blood glucose levels instead of SSI based on regularly scheduled glucose measurements. Thirty-nine patients in medical and surgical ICUs received intravenous insulin at the initiation of TPN. Blood glucose was measured hourly, and the infusion rate of insulin was adjusted based on predetermined blood glucose levels until the concentration was stable (i.e., between 125 and 200 mg/dL for 3 consecutive hours).

In this study,[33] the median time to stabilization of blood glucose was 9 hours, with time to stabilization for individual patients ranging from 5 to 32 hours. No episodes of symptomatic hypoglycemia occurred; however, it was not uncommon for concentrations to fall to 45 to 70 mg/dL after returning to the normal range. Results of this study suggest that the use of a separate insulin infusion safely facilitates glycemic control in patients receiving TPN.

A study by Sajbel and coworkers[34] evaluated the efficacy, safety, and cost-effectiveness of a separate continuous insulin infusion in the treatment of TPN-induced hyperglycemia. Sixteen patients between the ages of 17 and 80 years were enrolled based on a blood glucose level of more than 100 mg/dL at a TPN infusion rate of less than 75% of their calculated caloric requirement. Five of the 16 patients were known to have diabetes, and 8 of the patients were treated in an ICU. The patients were started on a continuous insulin infusion, which was titrated to keep the blood glucose concentration between 130 and 230 mg/dL with no glycosuria. When the blood glucose level was stable within this range for 24 hours and the TPN had been advanced to the target, the amount of insulin per unit time of each TPN bottle was calculated and added to the subsequent bottles of TPN.

The average time on an insulin infusion was 3.5 days (range, 1.0 to 22 days), with 73% of the glucose measurements in the range of 100 to 250 mg/dL. It was estimated that compared with the amount used when incremental doses of insulin were added to the TPN bag, the insulin infusion saved an average of 7.3 liters of TPN solution per patient, corresponding to a cost savings of $395 at the study institution after accounting for the costs of the insulin infusion setup and pump. With regard to safety, no blood sugar level below 50 mg/dL was recorded; however, one patient did experience two hypoglycemic reactions, both as a result of preventable errors related to incorrect insulin infusion.

CONCLUSION

These studies suggest that it may be prudent to consider using a separate insulin infusion as an efficacious and safe alternative to achieving glycemic control in patients receiving TPN. However, randomized, controlled trials comparing separate insulin infusion with traditional methods of insulin replacement in patients receiving TPN are needed before definitive recommendations can be made. The higher resource use associated with separate insulin infusion suggests that this approach may be better suited to settings in which there is adequate nursing support to allow for more intensive monitoring (e.g., unit settings or floors with higher nurse to patient ratios). We, therefore, recommend that until additional data, including randomized, controlled trials, become available, clinicians should tailor their practice to individual patients.

6. In patients with acute stroke, is blood glucose concentration associated with clinical outcomes?

Search Date: February 2006

Search Strategy: A search of Pub Med from the period 1966 to 2005 with the term "acute stroke" AND "hyperglycemia," with limits of English and humans, yielded a total of 165 publications. Titles and abstracts were scanned, with relevant citations selected. Repeating the search by replacing the term "acute stroke" with "acute cerebrovascular accident" did not yield additional relevant citations. Bibliographies of all relevant citations as well as the American Diabetes Association position statement regarding the inpatient management of diabetes and hyperglycemia[18] were reviewed.

Although several observational studies have suggested associations among blood glucose levels, morbidity, mortality, and outcomes for patients presenting with acute stroke, no randomized, controlled trials have assessed the impact of intensive glucose control on outcomes of patients with acute stroke.

The Glucose Insulin in Stroke Trial (GIST) was a randomized, controlled trial that examined the safety of a glucose potassium insulin (GKI) infusion to achieve a target glucose concentration of 72 to 126 mg/dL in patients presenting with acute stroke.[35] Fifty-three acute stroke patients presenting within 24 hours of onset of symptoms and having mild to moderate hyperglycemia (i.e., glucose levels between 126 and 306 g/dL) were randomized to receive a 24-hour infusion of normal saline or a GKI infusion (i.e., 16 units of insulin and 20 mmol of potassium chloride in 500 mg of 10% glucose) at a rate of 100 mL/hour. Of the 25 patients who received GKI, one required intravenous glucose for symptomatic hypoglycemia. Plasma glucose levels were not significantly lower in the GKI group during the infusion period. The 4-week mortality rate was not significantly different for the two groups. This study confirmed the safety of a GKI infusion in acute stroke patients with mild to moderate hyperglycemia but was not powered to detect differences in outcomes at 4 weeks.

ASSOCIATION BETWEEN ADMISSION GLUCOSE LEVEL AND CLINICAL OUTCOMES IN PATIENTS WITH ACUTE STROKE

Capes and colleagues[11] performed a systematic review and meta-analysis of 31 articles describing 32 cohort studies evaluating the relationship between glucose levels after acute stroke and outcomes. The investigators found that in nondiabetic patients, an admission glucose level of 110 to 126 mg/dL after acute ischemic stroke was associated with an increased risk of in-hospital or 30-day mortality (RR = 3.28; 95% CI: 2.32 to 4.64). Admission hyperglycemia after hemorrhagic stroke, however, was not associated with higher mortality rates for diabetic or nondiabetic patients.

Williams and coworkers[36] studied 656 patients hospitalized with acute ischemic stroke. Hyperglycemia, defined as an admission glucose level of 130 mg/dL or higher, was associated with a longer length of stay (7.2 versus 6.0 days, $P = .015$) and increased the risk of death at 30 days (HR = 1.87; 95% CI: 1.05 to 3.32), 1 year (HR= 1.75; 95% CI: 1.14 to 2.67), and 6 years (HR = 1.41; 95% CI: 1.02 to 1.94) after stroke. Hyperglycemia was not associated with an increased risk of in-hospital mortality.

Pulsinelli and associates[37] retrospectively evaluated stroke outcome in diabetics compared with nondiabetics and prospectively assessed stroke outcome based on the admission blood glucose levels of nondiabetics. The neurologic status at discharge of 72 nondiabetic and 35 diabetic patients admitted with a diagnosis of ischemic stroke was used to grade the severity of stroke as good, fair, or poor based on functional status. The neurologic outcome for diabetic patients with stroke was significantly worse than for nondiabetic patients ($P < .05$). Stroke-related deaths were also more common in the diabetic group ($P < .05$). In the prospective study, among nondiabetics, neurologic outcome was worse for patients who had a blood glucose level on admission above 120 mg/dL. This difference, however, was not statistically significant ($P = .061$).

Parson and colleagues[38] prospectively evaluated 63 acute stroke patients. Multiple regression analysis demonstrated that doubling of the blood glucose concentration from 90 to 180 mg/dL was associated with a 60% decrease in penumbral salvage and a 56 cm^3 increase in infarct size.

Demchuk and coworkers[39] investigated whether blood glucose concentration was an independent predictor of intracranial hemorrhage associated with recombinant tissue plasminogen activator (rt-PA) in 138 consecutive patients presenting with ischemic stroke. Baseline serum glucose concentration (99 mg/dL increments) was an independent predictor of symptomatic hemorrhage (OR = 2.26; 95% CI: 1.05 to 4.83; $P = .03$) and all hemorrhage (OR = 2.26; 95% CI: 1.07 to 4.69; $P = .04$). When excluding glucose level, a history of diabetes mellitus was also a significant predictor of all hemorrhage (OR = 3.61; 95% CI: 1.43 to 9.14; $P = .007$) and symptomatic hemorrhage (OR = 7.46; 95% CI: 2.68 to 96.4; $P = .002$).

A post hoc analysis of the National Institute of Neurologic Disorders and Stroke (NINDS) rt-PA Stroke Trial investigated the relationship between admission blood glucose levels and clinical outcomes for 624 patients presenting with acute ischemic stroke.[40] The mean admission glucose concentration was 150g/dL, and 21% of patients had a history of diabetes mellitus. In multivariate analysis, an increase in the admission glucose level was associated with a decrease in the odds for neurologic improvement (OR = 0.76 per 100 mg/dL increase in admission glucose; 95% CI: 0.61 to 0.95; P = .01). As the admission glucose level increased, the odds for symptomatic intracranial hemorrhage also increased (OR = 1.75 per 100 mg/dL increase in admission glucose; 95% CI: 1.11 to 2.78; P = .02). However, the relationship between admission glucose concentrations and favorable outcomes depended in part on the admission mean blood pressure, with hyperglycemia during acute ischemic stroke appearing to be more detrimental when associated with a higher admission mean blood pressure.

ASSOCIATION BETWEEN PERSISTENT HYPERGLYCEMIA AND OUTCOMES IN PATIENTS PRESENTING WITH ACUTE STROKE

Although most studies have assessed the association between admission blood glucose levels and outcomes after stroke, Baird and associates[41] looked at whether persistent hyperglycemia after stroke affected radiographic or clinical outcomes, as defined by the National Institutes of Health Stroke Scale (NIHSS) and modified Rankin Scale (mRS) scores. Twenty-five patients presenting within 24 hours of anterior circulation ischemic symptoms were enrolled, five of whom were subsequently excluded. All patients received HbA_{1C} and admission blood glucose testing, followed by 4-hour capillary glucose readings. Hyperglycemia was defined as an admission blood glucose level of 144 g/dL or higher, mean capillary glucose level of 126 g/dL or higher over the 72-hour monitoring period, and admission HbA_{1C} level of 6.2% or higher. All patients had magnetic resonance imaging (MRI) within 24 hours of symptom onset (acute), between 3 and 6 days after presentation (subacute), and at 3 months (outcome). Unlike previous studies, neither admission glucose nor admission HbA_{1C} concentrations showed a statistically significant association with radiographic or clinical outcomes. However, mean capillary glucose levels over the 72-hour monitoring period did show significant positive correlations with infarct volume change between acute and subacute MRIs (r = .60; P < .01), acute and outcome MRIs (r = .56; P = .01), outcome NIHSS (r = .53; P < .02), and outcome mRS (r = .53; P < .02). Acute and final infarct volume change and clinical outcomes were significantly worse for patients with mean blood glucose levels of 126 g/dL or higher.

SUMMARY

In summary, some observational data suggest an association between improved glycemic control and improved morbidity and mortality rates for patients presenting with acute stroke. However, randomized trials comparing strict control with less aggressive glucose control in patients with acute stroke are needed to definitively answer this question.

REFERENCES

1. Malmberg K, Ryden L, Efendic S, et al: Randomized trial of insulin-glucose infusion followed by subcutaneous insulin treatment in diabetic patients with acute myocardial infarction (DIGAMI study): Effects on mortality at 1 year. J Am Coll Cardiol 1995;26:57-65. II

2. Van den Berghe G, Wilmer A, Milants I, et al: Intensive insulin therapy in the medical ICU. N Engl J Med 2006;354:449-461. II

3. Van den Berghe G, Wouters P, Weekers F, et al: Intensive insulin therapy in critically ill patients. N Engl J Med 2001;345:1359-1367. II

4. Van den Berghe G, Wouters P, Bouillon R, et al: Outcome benefit of intensive insulin therapy in the critically ill: Insulin dose versus glycemic control. Crit Care Med 2003;31:359-366. II

5. Krinsley JS: Association between hyperglycemia and increased hospital mortality in a heterogeneous population of critically ill patients. Mayo Clin Proc 2003; 78:1471-1478. III

6. Krinsley JS: Effect of an intensive glucose management protocol on the mortality of critically ill adult patients. Mayo Clin Proc 2004;79:992-1000. III

7. Grey NJ, Perdrizet GA: Reduction of nosocomial infections in the surgical intensive-care unit by strict glycemic control. Endocr Pract 2004;10:46-52. II

8. Pittas AG, Siegel RD, Lau J: Insulin therapy for critically ill hospitalized patients: A meta-analysis of randomized controlled trials. Arch Intern Med 2004;164: 2005-2011. I

9. Umpierrez GE, Isaacs SD, Bazargan N, et al: Hyperglycemia: An independent marker of in-hospital

mortality in patients with undiagnosed diabetes. J Clin Endocr Metab 2002;87:978-982. **III**

10. Furnary AP, Gao G, Grunkemeier GL, et al: Continuous insulin infusion reduces mortality in patients with diabetes undergoing coronary artery bypass grafting. J Thorac Cardiovasc Surg 2003;125:1007-1021. **III**

11. Capes S, Hunt D, Malmberg K, et al: Stress hyperglycemia and prognosis of stroke in nondiabetic and diabetic patients: a systematic overview. Stroke 2001;32:2426-2432. **I**

12. Koproski J, Pretto Z, Poretsky L: Effects of an Intervention by a diabetes team in hospitalized patients with diabetes. Diabetes Care 1997;20:1553-1555. **II**

13. Wood-Baker RR, Gibson PG, Hannay M, et al: Systemic corticosteroids for acute exacerbations of COPD. Cochrane Database Syst Rev 2005;(1):CD001288. **III**

14. Niewoehner DE, Erbland ML, Deupree RH, et al: Effect of systemic glucocorticoids on exacerbations of COPD. N Engl J Med 1999;340:1941-1947. **III**

15. Dickerson LM, Ye X, Sack JL, Hueston WJ. Glycemic control in medical inpatients with type 2 diabetes mellitus receiving sliding scale insulin regimens versus routine diabetes medications: A multicenter randomized controlled trial. Ann Fam Med 2003;1:29-35. **II**

16. Queale WS, Seidler AJ, Brancati FL: Glycemic control and sliding scale insulin use in medical inpatients with diabetes mellitus. Arch Intern Med 1997;157:545-552. **III**

17. Gearhart JG, Duncan JL, Replogle WH, et al: Efficacy of sliding-scale insulin therapy: a comparison with prospective regimens. Fam Pract Res J 1994:14:313-322. **III**

18. Clement S, Braithwaite SS, Magee MF, et al: American Diabetes Association reviews/commentaries/position statements technical review: Management of diabetes and hyperglycemia in hospitals. Diabetes Care 2004; 27:553-591. **IV**

19. American College of Endocrinology: Position statement on inpatient diabetes and metabolic control. Endocr Pract 2004;10:77-82. **IV**

20. Moghissi ES, Hirsch IB: Hospital management of diabetes. Endocr Metab Clin 2005;34:1-16. **V**

21. McAlister FA, Man J, Bistritz L, et al: Diabetes and coronary artery bypass surgery: An examination of perioperative glycemic control and outcomes. Diabetes Care 2003;26:1518-1524. **III**

22. Schade DS: Surgery and diabetes. Med Clin North Am 1988;72:1531-1543. **V**

23. Alberti KG, Gill GV, Elliott MJ: Insulin delivery during surgery in the diabetic patient. Diabetes Care 1982;5:65-77. **V**

24. Furnary AP, Zerr KJ, Grunkemeier GL, Starr A: Continuous intravenous insulin infusion reduces the incidence of deep sternal wound infection in diabetic patients after cardiac surgical procedures. Ann Thor Surg 1999;67:352-360. **III**

25. Watts NB, Gebhart SS, Clark RV, Phillips LS: Postoperative management of diabetes mellitus: Steady-state glucose control with bedside algorithm for insulin adjustment. Diabetes Care 1987;10:722-728. **III**

26. Pezzarossa A, Taddei F, Cimicchi MC, et al: Perioperative management of diabetic subjects. Subcutaneous versus intravenous insulin administration during glucose-potassium infusion. Diabetes Care 1988; 11:52-58. **III**

27. Gonzalez-Michaca L, Ahumada M, Ponce-de-Leon S: Insulin subcutaneous applications vs. continuous infusion for postoperative blood glucose control in patients with non-insulin-dependent diabetes mellitus. Arch Med Res 2002;33:48-52. **II**

28. Guvener M, Pasaoglu I, Demircin M, Mehmet OC: Perioperative hyperglycemia is a strong correlate of postoperative infection in type II diabetic patients after coronary artery bypass grafting. Endocr J 2002;49:531-537. **III**

29. Standards of medical care in diabetes. Diabetes Care 2005;28:S4-S36. **IV**

30. Baldwin D, Villanueva G, McNutt R, Bhatnagar S: Eliminating inpatient sliding-scale insulin: A reeducation project with medical house staff. Diabetes Care 2005;28:1008-1011. **III**

31. Schoeffler JM, Rice DAK, Gresham DG: 70/30 Insulin algorithm versus sliding scale insulin. Ann Pharmacother 2005;39:1606-1610. **III**

32. Park RH, Hansell DT, Davidson LE, et al: Management of diabetic patients requiring nutritional support. Nutrition 1992;8:316-320. **III**

33. Woolfson AMJ: An improved method for blood glucose control during nutritional support. J Parenter Enteral Nutr 1980;5:436-440. **III**

34. Sajbel TA, Dutro MP, Radway PR: Use of separate insulin infusions with total parenteral nutrition. J Parenter Enteral Nutr 1986;11:97-99. **III**

35. Scott JF, Robinson GM, French JM, et al: Glucose potassium insulin infusions in the treatment of acute stroke patients with mild to moderate hyperglycemia: The Glucose Insulin in Stroke Trial (GIST). Stroke 1999;30:793-799. **II**

36. Williams LS, Rotich J, Qi R, et al: Effects of admission hyperglycemia on mortality and costs in acute ischemic stroke. Neurology 2002;59:67-71. **III**

37. Pulsinelli WA, Levy DE, Sigsbee B, et al: Increased damage after ischemic stroke in patients with hyperglycemia with or without established diabetes mellitus. Am J Med 1983;74:540-544. **III**

38. Parsons MW, Barber A, Desmond PM, et al: Acute hyperglycemia adversely affects stroke outcome: A magnetic resonance imaging and spectroscopy study. Ann Neurol 2002;52:20-28. **III**

39. Demchuk AM, Morgenstern LB, Krieger DW, et al: Serum glucose level and diabetes predict tissue plasminogen activator-related intracerebral hemorrhage in acute ischemic stroke. Stroke 1999;30:34-39. **III**

40. Bruno A, Levine SR, Frankel MR, et al: Admission glucose level and clinical outcomes in the NINDS rt-PA stroke trial. Neurology 2002;59:669-674. **III**

41. Baird TA, Parsons MW, Phanh T, et al: Persistent poststroke hyperglycemia is independently associated with infarct expansion and worse clinical outcome. Stroke 2003;34:2208-2214. **III**

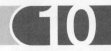

Endocrine Issues During Acute Illness, Sepsis, and the Perioperative Period

Kathryn E. Ackerman
and Jennifer S. Myers

1. Do supplemental steroids need to be given to all patients undergoing surgery who are on chronic or intermittent corticosteroid therapy?

Search Date: October 2005

Search Strategy: Pub Med, 1980 to 2005, search of "corticosteroids" AND "surgery OR perioperative." Limited to human and English language studies. Titles and abstracts scanned with relevant citations selected. Bibliographies from relevant citations and UpToDate also scanned. Cochrane Collaboration also searched.

The need for supplemental or "stress-dose" steroids before a surgical procedure is a common question in medical consultation. The practice of routinely prescribing supplemental steroids to patients on chronic steroid therapy became commonplace after a case report in 1952 that described a patient who developed perioperative circulatory shock as a result of preoperative withdrawal from glucocorticoid therapy.[1] Since that time, there has been a paucity of evidence to support the practice of routine steroid supplementation in supraphysiologic doses for all patients undergoing surgery. However, there is a small body of literature that can guide the clinician in making more evidence-based choices for the individual patient.

There are some generally accepted indications for providing supplemental steroids during periods of physiologic stress such as surgery or critical illness. These include administering steroids to those with impaired responsiveness to a test of adrenocortical reserve (e.g., the adrenocorticotropin-releasing hormone [ACTH] stimulation test) and to those with clinical findings of Cushing's syndrome or otherwise unexplained signs of adrenal insufficiency (e.g., hyponatremia, hypokalemia). Providing coverage to those at risk for adrenal insufficiency based on historical accounts of prior steroid therapy is more controversial. There is a wide variability in the hypothalamic-pituitary-adrenal (HPA) axis that cannot be predicted with certainty based on age, sex, dose, or duration of steroid therapy. An observational study of 279 patients receiving 5 to 30 mg of prednisone daily (or its equivalent) for 1 to 15 years showed a poor correlation between the plasma cortisol response to a test of adrenocortical reserve and the dose or duration of steroid therapy.[2]

DOSING SUPPLEMENTAL STEROIDS BASED UPON STEROID HISTORY

In many clinical scenarios, taking a careful steroid history may prevent the overtreatment of all patients on chronic glucocorticoids with supplemental steroids. It is generally accepted that patients taking small (≤ 5 mg/day of prednisone or its equivalent) or alternate-day doses of steroids do not require steroid supplementation. In a retrospective study of rheumatology patients, current steroid dose was the only significant predictor of HPA axis function.[3] In this study, all patients receiving daily doses of 5 mg of prednisone or less had normal responses to the ACTH stimulation test. Doses greater than 5 mg produced variable results. Similarly, two older studies suggested that alternate-day corticosteroid regimens also do not suppress the HPA axis.[4,5] In contrast, patients taking more than 20 mg of prednisone or its equivalent per day for more than 3 weeks and patients who have a cushingoid appearance are generally considered to have some degree of biochemical HPA axis suppression.[6] Patients on intermediate regimens have more variable rates of suppression.

DURATION OF HPA AXIS SUPPRESSION AFTER STEROID CESSATION

The duration of functional HPA axis suppression after the cessation of glucocorticoid therapy is also uncertain.

Recovery from steroid-induced HPA suppression is time dependant, spontaneous, and a function of the doses administered before tapering began. It is also sometimes difficult to determine the date of steroid cessation when steroid use has been erratic or purposely intermittent.[6] The HPA axis is considered to respond normally to stress 1 year after the cessation of prolonged steroid therapy. The time course of recovery for the pituitary and adrenal glands is illustrated in a study of 14 patients with Cushing's syndrome resulting from an adrenal tumor or exposure to exogenous glucocorticoids for 1 to 10 years.[7] In this study, after the tumor was removed or exogenous steroids were discontinued, plasma ACTH and cortisol levels were measured periodically at 6 AM for up to 1 year. Although pituitary function had returned to normal by the second to fifth month after steroid withdrawal, adrenocortical function remained impaired for up to 9 months after withdrawal. In a separate study, adrenocortical function, as measured by the plasma cortisol response to insulin-induced hypoglycemia, returned to normal after 1 year.[8]

Recovery from short bursts of steroids may be more rapid. In patients receiving a short course of 25 mg of prednisone daily for 5 days, peak cortisol responses to hypoglycemia and ACTH were suppressed at 2 days into therapy but returned to normal 5 days after the conclusion of therapy.[9] Similarly, HPA function recovered 1 week after a short course of prednisone (40 mg three times daily, then tapered over 4 days).[10]

EVIDENCE FOR LACK OF UTILITY OF SUPPLEMENTAL STEROIDS IN CERTAIN POPULATIONS

Lack of utility of supplemental steroids has been documented in a variety of patient populations. In the general surgical population, 18 patients with documented secondary adrenal insufficiency (determined by the ACTH stimulation test) were randomized in a double-blind fashion to receive an intravenous cortisol infusion followed by cortisol injections for 3 days postoperatively or identical injection amounts of saline.[11] Subjects underwent major operations such as joint replacements and abdominal surgery. Pulse and blood pressure rates were similar throughout surgery in both groups.

One patient from each group experienced hypotension, but both improved their blood pressures with volume replacement alone. The small sample size in this study, however, limits the generalizability of these findings. In the renal transplant population, 52 renal allograft recipients received their usual immunosuppressive doses of prednisone (5 to 10 mg/day) during 58 operations.[12] No clinical or laboratory (as measured by cortisol levels and 24-hour urinary free cortisol levels in the non-stressed and perioperative period) evidence for adrenal insufficiency was seen. In the orthopedic population, 28 patients who were receiving chronic corticosteroid replacement and undergoing 35 major orthopedic operations had no clinical or laboratory evidence of adrenal insufficiency as measured by 24-hour urinary free-cortisol levels before and during the operative procedure.[13] Previous literature has suggested that supplemental steroids may be unnecessary in glucocorticoid-dependant patients in the perioperative setting, but these studies were largely limited by the fact that biochemical testing of adrenal function was not performed.

Evidence of adrenal suppression on a laboratory test of the HPA axis does not predict clinical events; it only identifies those at greater risk for perioperative adrenal insufficiency. Some patients on glucocorticoids with abnormal responses on tests of adrenal function have tolerated anesthesia and surgery without additional steroids.[14] The reasons for this are uncertain. It is possible that there is adrenocortical reserve in stressful clinical scenarios that cannot be measured with a biochemical test. There may also be individual variability in the circulating level of cortisol required to maintain vascular tone in various settings.[6]

2. What dose of supplemental steroids should be given to patients at risk for secondary adrenal insufficiency in the perioperative period?

Search Date: October 2005

Search Strategy: *Pub Med, 1980 to 2005, search of "corticosteroids" AND "surgery OR perioperative." Limited to human and English language studies. Titles and* *abstracts scanned with relevant citations selected. Bibliographies from relevant citations and UpToDate also scanned. Cochrane Collaboration also searched.*

The normal cortisol secretion rate in response to major surgery and general anesthesia is estimated to be 75 to 150 mg/day (50 mg/day for minor operations).[14] Larger doses of supplemental steroids are not necessary or advised, because cortisol rates rarely exceed 200 mg/day in the perioperative period.[14] These estimates are based on older studies that documented the cortisol secretion rate after major surgery in very small numbers of patients (n = 2 to 10). Recommendations for supplemental steroids therefore should be in amounts comparable to the normal cortisol response to surgical stress. There is no evidence that prolonged regimens or tapering regimens are necessary in the postoperative period unless an additional stressor (e.g., infection, myocardial infarction) exists. When postoperative stressors are present, continuation of supplemental glucocorticoids is advised until the clinical scenario improves. Circulating cortisol levels have been shown to return to normal in most patients by 24 to 48 hours after surgery.[15]

There is evidence that adrenocortical secretion during surgical stress is proportional to the severity of surgery. Chernow and colleagues[15] demonstrated this by measuring serum cortisol levels 1 hour after the onset of surgery in patients undergoing a variety of surgical procedures. Serum cortisol levels ranged from 18 to 23 μg/dL (roughly equivalent to 5 to 10 mg of prednisone or 25 to 50 mg of hydrocortisone) for minor procedures such as laparoscopy to 32 μg/dL (roughly equivalent to 12 to 20 mg of prednisone or 50 to 75 mg of hydrocortisone) for more stressful procedures such as appendectomy or hysterectomy to 52 μg/dL (roughly equivalent to 25 to 50 mg of prednisone or 100 to 150 mg of hydrocortisone) for the most stressful procedures such as aortofemoral bypass or colectomy. A prospective cohort study of 30 non–steroid-dependant patients undergoing elective knee arthroscopy or total knee arthroplasty revealed a significant difference (P < .001) between the two groups with respect to change in baseline cortisol values in response to the procedure. The cortisol levels in the less invasive arthroscopy group did not change significantly in response to the procedure.[16] Depending on the patient's current steroid dose, it is often possible to continue the daily maintenance dose throughout the perioperative period because therapeutic steroid doses often approach or exceed the amount of cortisol secreted during surgical stress. For example, if a patient takes 20 mg of prednisone daily for sarcoidosis and is undergoing a laparoscopic cholecystectomy (i.e., minor surgical stress), the physician can recommend continuing the current steroid dose without additional supplementation throughout the perioperative period.

Based on the available literature and knowledge of the physiology of the HPA axis, a multidisciplinary group has made recommendations regarding perioperative glucocorticoid therapy for patients deemed to require supplemental steroids based on the duration and severity of the surgical procedure[14] (Table 10-1). These recommendations are not based on controlled clinical trials, because no such trials exist to answer this question. It is possible that even the doses recommended are excessive. When using perioperative supplemental steroids, most experts agree that coverage should begin on call to the operating room and continue for 24 to 48 hours after the operation.

3. Do patients receiving inhaled corticosteroids need to be considered for supplemental steroids in the perioperative period?

Search Date: October 2005

Search Strategy: *Pub Med, 1980 to 2005, search of "inhaled corticosteroids" AND "adrenal insufficiency." Limited to human and English language studies. Titles and abstracts scanned with relevant citations selected. Bibliographies from relevant citations and UpToDate also scanned. Cochrane Collaboration also searched.*

Inhaled corticosteroids (ICs) have become the first-line anti-inflammatory treatment for asthma. Consequently, the number of patients receiving these agents is large. Although ICs have significantly fewer systemic side effects than oral steroids, biochemical evidence of

Table 10-1. Recommendations for Perioperative Steroids in Glucocorticoid Dependant Patients

Degree of Surgical Stress	Examples of Surgery	Steroid Dose per Day	Duration of Steroid
Minor	Inguinal hernia repair, other short operative procedures	Hydrocortisone (25 mg) or prednisone (5 mg)	1 day
Moderate	Joint replacements, lower extremity revascularization, hysterectomy	Hydrocortisone (50-75 mg) or prednisone (12-20 mg)	1-2 days
Major	Cardiac surgery involving cardiopulmonary bypass, pancreatoduodenectomy	Hydrocortisone (100-150 mg) or prednisone (25-40 mg)	2-3 days

Data from Salem M, Tainsh RE, Bromberg J, et al: Perioperative glucocorticoid coverage: A reassessment 42 years after emergence of a problem. Ann Surg 1994;219:416-425.

adrenal suppression has been proved to occur with these agents. The degree of adrenal suppression is a function of the dose and drug type. A meta-analysis of 21 studies of urinary cortisol levels and 13 studies of suppression of 8 AM plasma cortisol levels showed significant adrenal suppression at higher doses (> 750 µg/day for fluticasone; > 1500 µg/day for all other ICs) of inhaled corticosteroids.[17] Most studies included in this meta-analysis were randomized trials in adults; four trials enrolled children. For urinary cortisol values, fluticasone had significantly greater dose-related suppression than beclomethasone ($P < .05$; CI: 1.0 to 60.6), budesonide ($P < .001$; CI: 20.9 to 76.1), or triamcinolone ($P < .05$; CI: 3.7 to 88.1). Similar results were seen for 8 AM plasma cortisol suppression. Because therapeutically equivalent doses were compared, these differences cannot be accounted for by increased drug potency alone.

Fluticasone has been shown to have a higher lipophilicity than the other ICs.[18] This presumably leads to a longer plasma half-life, increased tissue distribution, and prolonged glucocorticoid receptor occupancy. In clinical practice, there is a widely accepted 2:1 ratio between fluticasone and the other ICs in terms of drug potency. The risk of secondary adrenal insufficiency in patients receiving fluticasone has been well described in numerous case reports and case series of adults and children.[19,20] These descriptions illustrate that subclinical adrenal insufficiency can be unmasked during the tapering of an IC or during the switch from a more potent IC to a less potent IC (e.g., switching from fluticasone to budesonide).[21] The other ICs have been known to cause adrenal insufficiency, albeit less commonly. A combination of topical bioactivity and systemic bioactivity is likely with all ICs when they are given in high doses. The decision to increase the dose of an IC for an individual patient should be performed carefully, taking into account the risk-benefit ratio of these agents at their higher doses. In an observational study, doubling the dose of fluticasone from 1 to 2 mg/dL did not result in any improvement in asthma severity but resulted in a highly significant increase in adrenal suppression.[22]

ICs have been compared with oral corticosteroids in a few studies. For example, fluticasone (440 to 1750 µg) produced suppression of 8 AM plasma cortisol levels that was comparable to adrenal suppression seen with prednisolone (5 to 20 mg).[23] This is supported by the fact that there is a persistent degree of adrenal suppression in asthmatics who are being weaned from prednisolone therapy with high-dose fluticasone (2000 µg).[24]

Although clinical and subclinical forms of adrenal insufficiency have been demonstrated in patients using ICs, clinically important perioperative adrenal crises seem rare. This may be related to the ability of the HPA axis to tolerate lesser degrees of surgical stress when the adrenal glands are only partially suppressed. It is reasonable to withhold supplemental glucocorticoids in patients taking ICs unless they have signs or symptoms of adrenal insufficiency. In these cases, a test of adrenal function should be performed preoperatively. Unexplained perioperative hemodynamic instability in this population should alert the clinician to the possibility of secondary adrenal insufficiency. In a broader outpatient general medicine and pediatric population, unexplained hypoglycemia, growth retardation, weight loss, fatigue, and other nonspecific systemic symptoms in patients receiving ICs should prompt a test of adrenal function. Potent topical steroid preparations have been associated with HPA axis suppression as well and should be considered similarly.[25,26]

4. How can glucocorticoid insufficiency be diagnosed during an acute illness?

Search Date: October 2005

Search Strategy: *PubMed, 1990 to 2005, search of "adrenal insufficiency OR corticosteroid insufficiency" AND "sepsis OR illness" AND "diagnosis." Limited to humans and English language studies; 226 citations retrieved. Titles and abstracts scanned, with relative citations selected. Bibliographies of all relevant citations reviewed. Search of practice guidelines from the American College of Chest Physicians and the Society of Critical Care Medicine was also conducted.*

During stresses such as acute illness, trauma, anesthesia, and surgery, the HPA axis is activated, resulting in increased cortisol levels. However, in some instances, the activation is not adequate (i.e., relative adrenal insufficiency), conferring an increased risk of mortality to the patient. This suppression during stress may be a result of the systemic inflammatory response that results in the release of interleukin-1α (IL-1α), IL-6, and tumor necrosis factor-α (TNF-α). In vitro, these cytokines have been shown to suppress the adrenal response to ACTH and the pituitary response to corticotropin-releasing hormone.[27,28] Because many critically ill patients are not able to mount an appropriate cortisol response to stress, it is often important to determine whether the HPA axis is truly suppressed.

CLINICAL FEATURES OF ADRENAL INSUFFICIENCY

Although corticosteroid insufficiency during acute illness can be difficult to detect, there are some clinical features that are suggestive. In patients with pre-existing adrenal insufficiency, fatigue, anorexia, nausea, myalgias, postural hypotension, and depression may be experienced. Increased skin pigmentation may be seen in patients with increased corticotropin levels, and those with Addison's disease may display vitiligo. Hypopituitarism may present as amenorrhea or cold intolerance. Unfortunately, many of the clinical findings in corticosteroid insufficiency are seen in many acutely ill patients, independent of their steroid response to stress. Hemodynamic instability, tachycardia, fever, hypoglycemia, and multiple organ failure are seen in corticosteroid insufficiency but are certainly not specific. Laboratory findings may include hyponatremia, hyperkalemia, hypoglycemia, eosinophilia, and elevated thyrotropin levels, but in isolation, these findings are not sensitive or specific for the diagnosis of adrenal insufficiency.[29] Although many of these findings are detected in a variety of clinical scenarios in the critical care setting, findings of hypoglycemia and eosinophilia should lower the threshold for testing for adrenal insufficiency.[30]

CORTISOL VALUES IN THE CRITICALLY ILL

There is no consensus on what is considered the lower limit of normal for cortisol values in critically ill patients. Cortisol levels in such patients have been shown to vary from normal to as high as 3350 nmd (121 µg/dL).[31,32] Despite these levels, many intensive care unit (ICU) patients with have experienced improvements in hemodynamic status after receiving low-dose hydrocortisone.

There is diurnal variation in cortisol secretion, with peak levels of cortisol usually occurring between 8 and 9 AM. A morning cortisol level is commonly used to assess adrenal insufficiency in the unstressed patient. However, during critical illness and stress, the diurnal variation is disrupted, making the interpretation of such levels more difficult.[33]

DIAGNOSTIC TESTS FOR ADRENAL INSUFFICIENCY

Several tests can assist clinicians in the evaluation of adrenal insufficiency. The most clinically relevant are discussed here and summarized in Table 10-2. The gold standard for assessing adrenal insufficiency is the use of the insulin tolerance test (ITT). This involves the intravenous injection of 0.1 to 0.15 units of regular insulin per kilogram of body weight to stimulate the entire HPA axis and induce severe hypoglycemia (i.e., plasma glucose concentration < 40 mg/dL). Plasma glucose and cortisol (and sometimes cosyntropin) are measured before injection and again at 15, 30, 45, 60, 75, and 90 minutes after the insulin injection. In normal subjects, the plasma cortisol concentration increases to at least 18 to 20 µg/dL. In critically ill patients, however, this test is typically not performed because of cost and matters of practicality. It is also unpleasant for the patient, considered unsafe in unstable or unconscious patients, and contraindicated in patients with coronary heart disease or seizures.[33,34]

PROGNOSTIC VALUE OF THE COSYNTROPIN STIMULATION TEST IN THE CRITICALLY ILL

Cosyntropin is a synthetic peptide made of the first 24 amino acids of ACTH. The cosyntropin stimulation test is more commonly used to assess relative adrenal insufficiency in the critically ill patient. Tests using two separate doses have most frequently been used and studied. The first involves measuring a baseline cortisol level, administering 250 µg of cosyntropin intravenously or intramuscularly, and then measuring the plasma cortisol level again 30 or 60 minutes after injection. Unfortunately, there

Table 10-2. Diagnostic Options to Assess Adrenal Function in the Acutely Ill Patient

Diagnostic test	Pros	Cons	Most Common Test Interpretation in Critical Illness
Insulin tolerance test	Gold standard	Expensive; difficult to perform; contraindicated in unconscious or clinically unstable patients and those with coronary heart disease or seizures	Increase in plasma cortisol concentration to at least 18-20 µg/dL considered normal
Morning serum cortisol (between 8 and 9 AM)	Only one laboratory draw	Unless result very high or very low, need further testing; possible delay in treatment if waiting until next day for morning cortisol; diurnal variation of cortisol frequently disrupted during stress	No upper-limit standard in acute illness established. Outside of critical illness, values can be interpreted as follows: cortisol ≤ 3 µg/dL, adrenally insufficient; if cortisol ≥ 19 µg/dL, adrenal insufficiency ruled out
Random serum cortisol	Can be performed quickly	Interpretation of results depends on level of illness; no consensus on cutoff values; often requires further assessment with ACTH level, renin level, or follow-up cosyntropin stimulation test	Minimum levels of appropriate baseline random cortisol range of 10-34 µg/dL
Cosyntropin stimulation test: 250 µg IV	Good specificity compared with 1-µg test	Poorer sensitivity compared with 1-µg test; supraphysiologic dose; no consensus on interpretation	Basal cortisol level = 18 µg/dL and/or those whose cortisol level rises by > 9 µg/dL considered normal
Cosyntropin stimulation test: 1 µg	Good sensitivity compared with 250-µg test	Poorer specificity compared with 250-µg test; no consensus on interpretation	Basal cortisol level = 18 µg/dL and/or those whose cortisol level rises by > 9 µg/dL considered normal

are many proposed threshold levels for random cortisol and post-stimulation cortisol that may rule out adrenal insufficiency, with no consensus on which to use. Minimum levels of appropriate baseline random cortisol range from 10 to 34 µg/dL in critically ill patients.[29]

Annane and coworkers[35] investigated the prognostic value of different basal levels of cortisol and cosyntropin response in patients who met specific clinical criteria for septic shock. Three groups based on patients' prognoses were identified: good (i.e., basal cortisol level ≤ 34 µg/dL and an increase of > 9 µg/dL after 250 µg of intravenous cosyntropin; 28-day mortality rate of 26%), intermediate (i.e., basal cortisol level of 34 µg/dL and an increase of ≤ 9 µg/dL after 250 µg of intravenous cosyntropin or basal cortisol level > 34 µg/dL and an increase of > 9 µg/dL after 250 µg of intravenous cosyntropin; 28-day mortality rate of 67%), and poor (basal cortisol level > 34 µg/dL and an increase ≤ 9 µg/dL after 250 µg of intravenous cosyntropin; 28-day mortality rate of 82%). These results suggest that basal plasma cortisol levels were higher in patients who had the highest risk of mortality, with 34 µg/dL as the most appropriate cut-off point to discriminate between survivors and nonsurvivors from septic shock in this population. This study also demonstrated that patients with a weaker cortisol response had a higher risk of death, with a difference of 9 µg/dL between basal cortisol levels and post-cosyntropin stimulation being the best value to discriminate between survivors and nonsurvivors.[35]

LOW DOSES VERSUS HIGH DOSE COSYNTROPIN STIMULATION TESTS IN THE CRITICALLY ILL

Because the 250-µg intravenous cosyntropin stimulation test involves a dose that is 100 times greater than the maximum physiologic ACTH stress dose, there is concern that those who mount a cortisol response to 250 µg of intravenous cosyntropin may not respond to a normal, physiologic dose of ACTH. Thus, these patients would have false-negative cosyntropin stimulation tests.[34]

A second type of cosyntropin ACTH test involves using only 1 µg of intravenous cosyntropin for stimulation of the adrenal gland. Although mixed results have been seen in noncritically ill patients given the 1-µg versus 250-µg intravenous cosyntropin stimulation tests compared with the gold-standard ITT, there have only been three studies comparing low-dose and high-dose cosyntropin tests in critically ill patients.[34] The first trial examined 28 patients positive for human immunodeficiency virus (HIV) treated in medical ICUs. This study highlighted the fact that various cut-offs for defining adrenal insufficiency as well as various doses of cosyntropin stimulation could highly affect which patients were considered adrenally insufficient. The patients received 1 µg of intravenous cosyntropin (i.e., low-dose test), followed 60 minutes later by 60 µg of intravenous cosyntropin (i.e., high-dose test). The subjects had serum cortisol levels measured at baseline and then 30 and 60 minutes after each of the intravenous doses of cosyntropin. When adrenal insufficiency was defined as a baseline cortisol level less than 25 µg/dL, 75% (21 of 28) patients were considered adrenally insufficient. When adrenal insufficiency was defined as a baseline cortisol level less than 25 µg/dL and a post-test low-dose stimulation cortisol level less than 25 µg/dL, 46% (13 of 28) patients were considered adrenally insufficient. When adrenal insufficiency was defined as a baseline cortisol level less than 25 µg/dL and a post-test high-dose stimulation cortisol level less than 25 µg/dL, 21% (6 of 28) patients were considered adrenally insufficient. As a higher dose of cosyntropin was given, fewer patients were considered adrenally insufficient. These numbers followed a similar trend when a lower cut-off was used. When adrenal insufficiency was defined as a baseline cortisol level less than 18 µg/dL, 50% (14 of 28) of patients were considered adrenally insufficient. When adrenal insufficiency was defined as a baseline cortisol level less than 18 µg/dL and a post-test low-dose stimulation cortisol level less than 18 µg/dL, 21% (6 of 28) of patients were considered adrenally insufficient. When adrenal insufficiency was defined as a baseline cortisol level less than 18 µg/dL and a post-test high-dose stimulation cortisol level less than 18 µg/dL, only 7% (2 of 28) of patients were considered adrenally insufficient. This study found that there is a high incidence of adrenal insufficiency in critically ill HIV-infected patients that varies with the criteria used to diagnose adrenal insufficiency. The low-dose stimulation test was more sensitive than the high-dose test for diagnosing adrenal insufficiency in this population.[36]

A second trial looked at 59 ICU patients with septic shock. The patients had baseline cortisol measured and then received 1 µg of intravenous cosyntropin, followed 60 minutes later by 249 µg of intravenous cosyntropin. All patients were administered hydrocortisone (100 mg IV every 8 hours) for the first 24 hours while awaiting results of the cosyntropin tests. Steroid responsiveness was defined as the cessation of the need for norepinephrine to maintain a mean arterial pressure of more than 65 mm Hg within 24 hours of the first dose of hydrocortisone. In this study, 47% of patients died. The mean baseline cortisol level was 20.9 ± 12.1 µg/dL in the survivors and 31.9 ± 20.5 µg/dL in the nonsurvivors ($P = .01$) Thirty-six patients (61%) had adrenal insufficiency when defined as a baseline cortisol concentration of less than 25 µg/dL. When the standard diagnostic threshold of post–cosyntropin-stimulated cortisol of less than 18 µg/dL was used, 13 (22%) patients had adrenal insufficiency by the low-dose test and 5 (8%) patients by the high-dose test. Ninety-five percent of steroid-responsive patients had a baseline cortisol concentration less than 25 µg/dL. When a baseline cortisol of 25 µg/dL was used as the reference method, the low-dose test had a sensitivity of 62%, whereas the high-dose test had a sensitivity of 24%. Fifty-four percent of steroid responders had a diagnostic low-dose test result, and 22% had a diagnostic high-dose test result. This study found the 1-µg intravenous cosyntropin stimulation test to be more sensitive than the 250-µg test.[37]

The third study addressing the issue of the low-dose versus high-dose cosyntropin test has been published only in abstract form, and methodologic details are limited. Fifty ICU patients with clinically suspected adrenal insufficiency or pressor support for more than 24 hours were studied. Each received 1 µg of cosyntropin, followed by an additional 250 µg 5 hours later. Normal response was defined as a peak cortisol that doubled from baseline to reach a value greater than an unstated reference range maximum. Sixty-one percent of patients were diagnosed with adrenal insufficiency after the 1-µg cosyntropin stimulation versus 35% after the 250-µg cosyntropin test. Although details were limited, the investigators also concluded that the 1-μg stimulation test might be more sensitive than the 250-μg test.[38]

CORTISOL-BINDING PROTEINS IN THE CRITICALLY ILL

A study by Hamrahian and coworkers[39] brought to light the relevance of cortisol-binding proteins in cosyntropin testing. They found that many critically ill patients have decreased cortisol-binding proteins (55% in their study), and by measuring total serum cortisol rather than free cortisol levels after a cosyntropin stimulation test, an inaccurate assessment of available cortisol may be obtained. Critically ill patients with decreased cortisol-binding proteins had lower baseline and cosyntropin-stimulated serum total cortisol concentrations compared with critically ill patients with normal binding protein levels ($P < .001$). However, the mean baseline serum free cortisol levels were similar in the two groups of ill patients and were significantly higher than the values in normal patients who were not ill ($P < .001$ for both comparisons).[38] More studies are needed to elucidate the importance of routine measurement of cortisol-binding proteins in addition to cortisol levels to assess adrenal insufficiency.[39]

SUMMARY

There are no universal guidelines that recommend the most appropriate cosyntropin dose or the most appropriate baseline or post-stimulation cortisol level when evaluating acutely ill patients for adrenal insufficiency. Most large clinical trials looking at outcomes of various steroid treatments in septic patients used the 250-μg cosyntropin test. However, the three studies mentioned previously all showed a higher sensitivity for detecting adrenal insufficiency using the 1-μg cosyntropin test. Use of the 1-μg cosyntropin test, however, may lead to overtreatment of patients with steroids. Conversely, use of the 250-μg cosyntropin test may result in overstimulation of the adrenal glands, thereby missing some patients who have true adrenal insufficiency and would benefit from the use of steroids during periods of critical illness and beyond. This dilemma may not be resolved until a safe method of comparing the two tests against a gold standard (e.g., ITT) can be performed in large clinical trials and the outcomes of steroid treatment in patients with various cosyntropin stimulation test results are studied.

With few studies using the same definitions of adrenal insufficiency or cosyntropin response, a conservative approach to detecting relative adrenal insufficiency in critically ill patients may consist of measuring a baseline cortisol level followed by administration of 1 µg of cosyntropin and measurement of the serum cortisol level 60 minutes later. Individuals with a basal cortisol level below 18 µg/dL or those whose cortisol level rose by 9 µg/dL or less can be considered to have relative adrenal insufficiency.

5. Should glucocorticoids be used routinely in patients with septic shock and other critical illnesses? If so, at what dose and for what duration?

Search Date: October 2005

Search Strategy: PubMed, 1990 to 2005, search of "glucocorticoids OR steroids" AND "septic shock OR critical illness." Limited to human and English language studies; 502 citations retrieved. Titles and abstracts scanned, with relative citations selected. Bibliographies of all relevant citations reviewed. Search of practice guidelines from the American College of Chest Physicians and the Society of Critical Care Medicine was also conducted.

The use of steroids to treat septic shock became routine practice in the late 1970s and early 1980s based on animal data and a 1976 clinical trial.[40-43] During the mid-1980s, randomized trials explored the use of high-dose steroids to treat sepsis. Two of the largest and best-designed trials were the Veterans Administration Trial and a study by Bone and colleagues.[45]

TRIALS OF HIGH DOSE STEROIDS IN THE CRITICALLY ILL

The Veterans Administration Trial randomized 233 patients with clinical signs of systemic sepsis and a normal sensorium to methylprednisolone (30 mg/kg followed by 5 mg/kg/hr for 9 hours) or placebo. No reduction in clinical complications or in 14-day mortality was demonstrated. However, patients treated with placebo had a statistically significant improvement in resolution of infection at 14 days (12 of 23) compared with patients who received glucocorticoid treatment (3 of 16) ($P = .03$).[44]

Bone and coworkers[45] randomized 381 patients with clinically suspected severe sepsis or septic shock to methylprednisolone (30 mg/kg given in four infusions beginning within 2 hours of diagnosis) or placebo. No significant differences were found in the prevention or reversal of shock or in overall mortality. In a subgroup of patients with elevated serum creatinine levels (> 2 mg/dL) at enrollment, the mortality rate at 14 days was significantly increased among those receiving methylprednisolone (46 of 78 [59%] versus 17 of 58 [29%] among those receiving placebo, $P < .01$).[45] Results of these two studies argue against the use of high-dose steroids in the treatment of severe sepsis and septic shock.

Two meta-analyses of randomized, controlled trials primarily using high-dose steroids in sepsis were published in 1995. The first looked at nine trials involving 1232 patients with sepsis or septic shock who received steroids (various doses between 1 and 30 mg/kg/day of methylprednisolone, dexamethasone, betamethasone, or hydrocortisone) or placebo. Although corticosteroids appeared to increase mortality among patients with severe infection, the confidence interval crossed 1 (RR = 1.13; 95% CI: 0.99 to 1.29). No beneficial effect was demonstrated in the subgroup of patients with septic shock (RR = 1.07; 95% CI: 0.91 to 1.26). Studies with the highest methodologic quality scores also found a trend toward increased mortality overall (RR = 1.10; 95% CI: 0.94 to 1.29), but the confidence interval crossed 1.[46] The second meta-analysis examined 10 prospective, randomized, controlled trials, assessing the mortality difference between treatment with predominantly high-dose steroids versus placebo in patients with sepsis or septic shock. In this analysis, there was only a −0.2% difference in mortality favoring steroids (95% CI: −9.2% to 8.8%), and the confidence interval crossed 1.[47] There is agreement among clinicians and researchers that high-dose, short-course therapy with methylprednisolone or dexamethasone in septic shock does not reduce mortality or improving outcomes and that it instead may be harmful.[42,48]

TRIALS OF LOWER DOSE STEROIDS IN THE CRITICALLY ILL

Subsequent studies have evaluated the appropriateness of lower-dose supplemental steroids in critically ill patients. Three notable randomized, controlled trials of lower doses of hydrocortisone replacement in septic shock have demonstrated improved hemodynamics and decreased need for vasopressor therapy. A 1998 study by Bollaert and associates[49] randomized 41 intensive care patients (from two clinical centers) with persistent septic shock to hydrocortisone (100 mg IV three times daily for 5 days with subsequent reductions by one half every 3 days) or placebo. Sixty-eight percent of the patients receiving hydrocortisone achieved shock reversal, defined as a stable systolic arterial pressure of more than 90 mm Hg for 24 hours or longer without volume expansion or catecholamine use (except for a < 5 µg/kg/min infusion of dopamine used for renal therapy) and a blood lactate concentration of less than 2 mmol/L, compared with 21% of patients receiving placebo (P = .007). However, mortality rates at 28 days were not significantly different between the two groups (32% in the hydrocortisone group versus 63% in the placebo group, P = .091). The two groups were not well matched, with higher baseline cortisol levels and a greater proportion of nonresponders to cortisol stimulation before enrollment in the placebo group.[49]

Briegel and colleagues[50] randomized 40 septic shock patients in a single clinical center to receive hydrocortisone (100 mg IV, followed by 0.18 mg/kg/hr IV for ≥ 6 days, followed by a taper over 6 days after shock reversal) or to placebo. Most patients in both groups achieved shock reversal, but it was achieved more quickly in the steroid group (median time of 2 days on vasopressor support in the hydrocortisone group versus 7 days in the placebo group, P = .005). There were no significant differences in mortality or in the number of patients who experienced resolution of septic shock between the two groups. Side effects seen in the treatment group included increases in serum sodium concentration to the upper normal range as well as increases in blood glucose, blood urea nitrogen, and liver enzymes.[50]

Annane and colleagues performed a placebo-controlled, randomized, double-blind, parallel-group trial in 19 ICUs in France, where 300 patients with septic shock were randomized to receive hydrocortisone (50 mg IV every 6 hours) and fludrocortisone (50 μg orally once daily) or placebo for 7 days. A comparable proportion of patients in each group (114 of 150 patients in the steroid group and 115 of 149 patients in the placebo group) were nonresponsive to a cortisol stimulation test (i.e., cortisol level increase of < 9 μg/dL) before treatment. Vasopressor therapy was able to be withdrawn within 28 days in 57% of nonresponders in the steroid group and 40% of nonresponders in the placebo group (P = .001). There was no significant difference in resolution of septic shock between those who responded to cortisol stimulation in both groups.[51] Although this study was large, well designed, and well executed, there has been debate about the definition of *relative adrenal insufficiency* used by the investigators to describe the nonresponders. Unlike this study, many prior studies did not include patients whose peak cortisol levels were above 18 μg. Because the mean peak cortisol levels were higher in the placebo group, this may have skewed the results such that patients with higher cortisol levels at baseline may have been sicker before treatment.

A later trial also supported the use of hydrocortisone in ICU patients with severe community-acquired pneumonia (defined as meeting two minor or one major 1993 American Thoracic Society criterion for severe pneumonia). Hydrocortisone treatment (200 mg IV loading bolus, followed by an infusion of 10 mg/hr for 7 days) compared with placebo was associated with a significant reduction in length of hospital stay (P = .03) and in-hospital mortality (P = .009). No increase in complications was seen in the treatment group.[54]

META-ANALYSES ON STEROIDS IN THE CRITICALLY ILL

In a 2004 systemic review and meta-analysis, 23 studies of corticosteroid use in septic patients were identified. Seven studies were excluded based on lack of information, study design, or lack of heterogeneity of patient population. Sixteen were included, and a unique distinction was observed. Sorting all relevant clinical trials by year of publication showed that before 1992, almost all trials demonstrated a relative risk of death of more than 1.0 for septic patients receiving steroids compared with those who did not, whereas all trials published after 1992 demonstrated a relative risk of death of less than 1.0 in similar patient populations. In 1992, a consensus was reached regarding the definition of sepsis, and information was published discussing the observation that septic shock is often associated with relative adrenal insufficiency. Later trials in this meta-analysis had more homogenous subjects, used stricter definitions, and more often used longer courses of low-dose steroids. Subgroup analysis of patients receiving long courses (≥ 5 days) of low-dose corticosteroids (≤ 300 mg of hydrocortisone daily or equivalent) found a relative risk for mortality of 0.80 at 28 days (five trials, $N = 465$; 95% CI: 0.67 to 0.95) and 0.83 at hospital discharge (five trials, $N = 465$; 95% CI: 0.71 to 0.97) in patients treated with supplemental corticosteroids. Use of corticosteroids decreased mortality in ICUs (four trials, $N = 425$; RR = 0.83; 95% CI: 0.70 to 0.97) and increased likelihood of shock reversal at 7 days (four trials, $N = 425$; relative benefit = 1.60; 95% CI: 1.27 to 2.03) and 28 days (four trials, $N = 425$; relative benefit = 1.26; 95% CI: 1.04 to 1.52) without inducing side effects.[52]

Another meta-analysis from 2004 compared the same five trials mentioned previously to trials performed before 1989 and concurred with the results described earlier. The study authors also found a linear relationship between the dose of steroids and their effect on survival, characterized by benefit at low doses and increasing harm at higher doses ($P = .02$). The lower dose effect may be beneficial through augmentation of adrenal function in the stressed state or limited anti-inflammatory properties that do not cause harmful immunosuppression.[53]

CLINICAL PRACTICE GUIDELINES ON STEROIDS IN THE CRITICALLY ILL

Based on the previously described work and other trials assessing specific physiologic parameters affected by corticosteroids, the Surviving Sepsis Campaign,[48] developed by 11 international professional societies in various specialties, recommends the following:

1. Use of moderate doses of steroids (200 to 300 mg/day of hydrocortisone administered in divided

doses or by continuous infusion) in septic patients after adequate fluid resuscitation

2. Consideration of fludrocortisone (50 µg/day), even though hydrocortisone has intrinsic mineralocorticoid activity

3. Use of steroid supplementation in patients with shock (not sepsis alone) and preexisting adrenal insufficiency

4. Consideration of tapering dosage of steroids after resolution of septic shock (there are no comparative studies between a fixed duration of steroids and a clinically guided protocol)[32]

The use of the ACTH stimulation test was deemed optional, resulting from the conflicting expert opinions regarding appropriate ACTH dosage and adequate physiologic baseline cortisol and response to stimulation. The task force commented that if the ACTH stimulation test were to be performed, dexamethasone could be initiated before the injection of cosyntropin pending results of the ACTH stimulation test. Unlike hydrocortisone or methylprednisolone, dexamethasone does not have cortisol-like metabolites, which interfere with the cortisol assay.[48] The American College of Critical Care Medicine Task Force, in contrast, recommends use of steroids only in patients with hypotension refractory to catecholamine vasopressors or in patients known to be adrenally insufficient.[55]

One review[56] described a reasonable approach to steroid use in critical illness. The study authors suggest that in patients presenting with septic shock, a 250-µg corticotropin test should be performed immediately, followed by administration of 200 to 300 mg/day of hydrocortisone. If adrenal insufficiency is confirmed (≤ 9-µg/dL increase in serum cortisol after corticotropin testing), hydrocortisone is continued for 7 days. If results do not suggest adrenal insufficiency, hydrocortisone treatment is stopped.

More research is needed to specify appropriate doses in different clinical settings and the timing of initial treatment, ideal choice of glucocorticoid, and duration of therapy. This is particularly true regarding the potential addition of fludrocortisone.

6. How should thyroid function tests be interpreted in the asymptomatic perioperative or critically ill patient?

Search Date: February 2006

Search Strategy: PubMed, 1990 to 2006, search of "sick euthyroid OR critical illness" AND "thyroid OR critically ill" AND "thyroid OR perioperative AND thyroid." Limited to human and English language studies; 444 citations retrieved. Titles and abstracts scanned, with relative citations selected. Bibliographies of all relevant citations reviewed. Search of practice guidelines from the American College of Chest Physicians, American Endocrine Society, and the Society of Critical Care Medicine was also conducted.

Thyroid function testing in perioperative and critically ill patients has long posed a challenge for clinicians. Many factors affect the results of typical thyroid tests, making interpretation of such values quite difficult. To better understand the utility of various thyroid function tests, we first review the physiology of the thyroid during various stressful states.

Under typical conditions, the hypothalamus secretes thyrotropin-releasing hormone (TRH), which stimulates the pituitary to produce thyrotropin (thyroid-stimulating homrone [TSH]), subsequently stimulating the thyroid to produce thyroid hormones. The thyroid gland produces thyroxine (T_4) and triiodothyronine (T_3). This is the only source of T_4. However, most of T_3 (75% to 80%) is produced peripherally from 5'-deiodination of T_4 to T_3, which is catalyzed by 5'-monodeiodinase in different organs, including the kidneys and liver. Various deiodinases are responsible for conversion of T_4 to the biologically active T_3, which exerts most of the thyroid's effects. There are also deiodinases that convert T_4 to the inactive reverse T_3 (rT_3). Both T_3 and rT_3 are further converted to diiodothyronine (T_2) by other deiodinases. Thyroid hormones exert feedback on TRH and TSH secretion[57,58] (Fig. 10-1).

Euthyroid sick syndrome (ESS) or *nonthyroidal illness syndrome* (NTIS) are terms that have been used to describe various thyroid test abnormalities in perioperative patients, fasting patients, and those with systemic

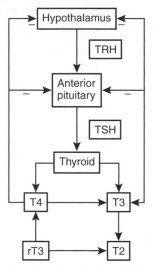

Figure 10-1. Hypothalamic-pituitary-thyroidal axis. rT_3, reverse triiodothyronine; T_2, diiodothyronine; T_4, thyroxine; TRH, thyroid-releasing hormone; TSH, thyroid-stimulating hormone.

nonthyroid illnesses (NTIs), such as critically ill ICU patients. NTIS is replacing ESS as proper nomenclature because many patients with thyroid abnormalities in such settings may not truly be euthyroid.[59]

The abnormalities in NTIS have been classified as low T_3 syndrome, low T_3-low T_4 syndrome, high T_4 syndrome, and other thyroid abnormalities.[59,60] The classic presentation is a low serum level of total T_3, normal to low level of total T_4, and normal level of TSH.[61]

CHANGES IN THYROID AXIS DURING ILLNESS

The hypothalamic-pituitary-thyroid (HPT) axis undergoes modifications during severe stress and illness. Even during caloric restriction and mild illnesses, 5′-monodeiodinase is decreased. In the acute phase of critical illness, TSH and T_4 levels are elevated briefly. Less T_4 is converted to T_3, but similar amounts of rT_3 are formed as during the healthy state. However, less rT_3 is converted to T_2, leading to a subsequent increase in rT_3. With more chronic stress and illness, TRH, TSH, and therefore T_4 levels fall, and even a greater ratio of rT_3 to T_3 is formed from T_4. The rT_3 to T_2 conversion is further diminished, with a more pronounced rT_3/T_3 ratio[57,62] (Fig. 10-2).

Other factors have been implicated in various NTIS changes. The presence of certain drugs (e.g., dopamine, corticosteroids, anticonvulsants), increased cortisol levels, and catecholamines can decrease serum TSH levels. Changes in glycosylation and abnormal regulation during NTIS affect TSH levels. There is a transient increase in serum TSH in the early and recovery phases of NTIS.[57,59]

Low serum levels of T_4 may be caused by decreased serum binding. This may be a direct result of decreased or abnormal thyroid-binding globulin (TBG); binding inhibitors such as heparin, furosemide, and some non-steroidal anti-inflammatory drugs (NSAIDs); or increased

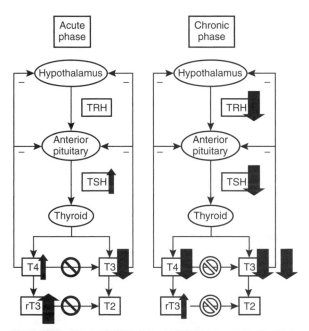

Figure 10-2. Changes in the thyroid axis during acute and chronic critical illness. (Adapted from Van den Berghe G: Novel insights into the neuro-endocrinology of critical illness. Eur J Endocrinol 2000;143:1-13.)

T_4 clearance. T_4 levels can also be lowered as a direct effect of decreased TSH concentration. High serum levels of T_4 can be the result of increased TBG concentration, decreased tissue uptake, or decreased T_4 clearance.

The decreased 5'-monodeiodinase activity leading to decreased T_3 production may be influenced by decreased nutrition, free radicals, increased cortisol or exogenous steroids, other drugs, decreased tissue uptake of T_4, decreased selenium levels, circulating inhibitors, cytokines, and increased levels of rT_3. Serum T_3 may also be diminished in response to decreased serum binding and decreased TSH levels. Serum rT_3 levels are elevated because of decreased clearance, which may be from decreased conversion to T_2 or from decreased tissue uptake.[57,63]

There is debate regarding whether decreases in circulating thyroid hormones are beneficial or detrimental to the critically ill or perioperative patient. Some clinicians and investigators argue that hypothyroxinemia may be a beneficial adaptive response to critical illness and stress and that giving T_3 or T_4 to ICU or perioperative patients may inhibit an important TSH response during recovery.[64,65]

Abnormal thyroid function test results are found at least as frequently in NTIS as in pure thyroid illnesses.[59] Lower levels of TSH, T_4, and T_3 and higher levels of rT_3 have correlated with a poor prognosis for critically ill patients.[66-69] For example, in one study by Slag and associates[67] of 86 ICU patients, an initial T_4 value less than 3 mg/dL correlated with an 84% mortality rate ($P < .01$). However, there is no substantial evidence to suggest that supplemental thyroid hormone therapy in NTIS improves outcomes.

HORMONE SUPPLEMENTATION IN NONTHYROIDAL ILLNESS SYNDROME

In a randomized, prospective study by Brent and coworkers[65], patients admitted to a medical ICU who had a total serum T_4 concentration less than 5 µg/dL were randomly assigned to T_4 treatment (1.5 µg/kg IV for 2 weeks; $n = 11$) or a control group ($n = 12$). In the treatment group, serum total T_4 and free T_4 concentrations significantly increased by day 3 and were normal on day 5; TSH levels decreased significantly, as did the

TSH response to TRH. A significant rise in serum T_3 occurred in the control group on day 7 but did not occur until day 10 in the treatment group. Mortality rates were equivalent in the two groups (73% treatment group versus 75% control group). Regardless of group assignment, survivors and nonsurvivors were distinguishable completely based on baseline T_3/T_4 ratios (17.0 ± 1.8 ng/µg in survivors versus 7.0 ± 0.7 in nonsurvivors, $P < .001$). T_4 therapy was not beneficial and might have slowed the T_3 increase in the treatment group.[65] Studies of T_3 therapy in NTIS have also demonstrated no benefit or minimal improvement in rat studies and in small human cohorts.[70-72]

During and after cardiopulmonary bypass surgery, changes occur in thyroid hormone laboratory values similar to those described previously as common in NTIS: depression of T_3 and free T_3 concentrations with a concomitant increase in rT_3 levels.[73] In one randomized, double-blind study by Mullis-Jansson and colleagues,[74] the effects of supplemental T_3 in patients undergoing elective coronary artery bypass grafting were examined. On removal of the aortic cross-clamp after coronary bypass, 170 patients were randomized to receive intravenous T_3 (0.4-µg/kg bolus plus 0.1-µg/kg/hr infusion administered over a 6-hour period, $n = 81$) or placebo ($n = 89$). The patients randomized to T_3 had higher cardiac indices and lower inotropic requirements after the operation. They also had a significantly lower incidence of postoperative myocardial ischemia (4% versus 18%, $P = .007$) and pacemaker dependence (14% versus 25%, $P = .013$). Seven patients in the placebo group required postoperative mechanical assistance (intra-aortic balloon pump, $n = 4$; left ventricular assist device, $n = 3$), compared with none in the T_3 group ($P = .01$). There were no deaths in the treatment group but two in the placebo group, a difference that was not statistically significant. Although a history of thyroid disease or history of thyroid replacement therapy were exclusion criteria, baseline and follow-up thyroid function tests were not reported for group.[74]

In a similar randomized, placebo-controlled study by Klemperer and coworkers,[75] T_3 (intravenous bolus of 0.8 µg/kg plus a 0.113-µg/kg/hr infusion over 6 hours) or placebo was given to 142 patients with coronary artery disease and depressed left ventricular function after the aortic cross-clamp was removed following coronary bypass surgery. In the treatment and control groups, the mean serum T_3 concentration was in the low-normal range before the start of surgery and had decreased by approximately 40% 30 minutes after the initiation of cardiopulmonary bypass. Similar to the previously described study, the mean postoperative cardiac index was higher in the T_3 group (2.97 ± 0.72 versus 2.67 ± 0.61 L/min/m², P = .007), and systemic vascular resistance was lower (1073 ± 314 versus 1235 ± 387 dyn·sec·cm⁻⁵, P = .003). However the two groups did not differ significantly in the incidence of arrhythmia or the requirement of inotropic and vasodilator drugs during the 24 hours after surgery or in perioperative mortality and morbidity rates.[75] Both studies demonstrated some changes in hemodynamics with T_3 but found no statistically significant mortality benefit.

Even less favorable results occurred in a randomized, double-blind, placebo-controlled trial by Bennett-Guerrero and colleagues.[76] At release of the aortic cross-clamp, 211 patients undergoing coronary artery surgery at high risk for requiring inotropic drug support were given intravenous infusion of T_3 (intravenous bolus of 0.8 µg/kg plus a 0.12-µg/kg/hr infusion over 6 hours), dopamine (5-µg/kg/min infusion for 6 hours), or placebo. The T_3 level did not change hemodynamic variables or inotropic drug requirements, heart rate increased (P < .001), and a trend toward decreased use of inotropic agents was found in the dopamine group only.[76]

Van den Berghe and colleagues[77] looked at combined supplementation of growth hormone–releasing peptide-2 (GHRP-2), TRH, and gonadotropin-releasing hormone (GnRH) in 33 critically ill men who had baseline decreased percentages of pulsatile TSH and decreased total T_3 and T_4 concentrations compared with healthy controls. Patients were randomly assigned to 5 days of placebo (n = 7), GHRP-2 (1 µg/kg/hr, n = 9), GHRP-2 plus TRH infusion (1 µg/kg/hr + 1 µg/kg/hr, n = 9), or pulsatile GnRH (0.1 µg/kg every 90 minutes) with GHRP-2 plus TRH infusion (n = 8). Multiple endocrine parameters were measured and demonstrated that co-administration of GHRP-2, TRH, and GnRH reactivated the growth hormone, TSH, and luteinizing hormone axes in these critically ill men and evoked beneficial metabolic effects that were absent with GHRP-2 infusion alone and only partially present with GHRP-2 plus TRH. Serum lactate levels and white blood cell count were increased by GHRP-2 infused alone and in combination with TRH but not by GHRP-2 plus TRH plus GnRH. These results suggest that attempts to improve metabolism through an endocrine pathway in prolonged critical illness should possibly involve a combined strategy designed to normalize pituitary function as a whole and may be more effective and safer than single-hormone interventions. However, these results need to be repeated in larger, more diverse cohort and randomized, controlled trials and should include additional treatment and mortality end points.[77]

Although no standard recommendations exist for treatment of NTIS alone, missing overt hypothyroid or hyperthyroid disorders being masked by an NTIS presentation can be worrisome. If any true thyroid disorder is suspected in an NTIS patient, the clinician should begin with a good history and physical examination. Although this is often challenging in an ICU setting, obtaining historical and physical clues helps to differentiate NTIS from another underlying thyroid disorder. Special attention should be paid to the medication list for possible interactions. Laboratory work should begin with TSH, free T_4, and free T_3 levels. Because decreases in TBG levels and thyroid binding affinity are common in critically ill patients, laboratory assays that estimate free circulating T_3 and T_4 concentrations are more helpful than total T_3 and T_4 levels.

NONTHYROIDAL ILLNESS SYNDROME AND LOW THYROID-STIMULATING HORMONE LEVELS

In an NTIS patient with primary hyperthyroidism, the serum TSH concentration should be undetectable (< 0.01 mU/L), with high-normal or elevated levels of free T_3 and T_4.[78] The serum TSH concentration is undetectable in less than 7% of nonhyperthyroid NTIS patients, and it is most common in those who have been treated with dopamine or corticosteroids.[79] If laboratory values suggest hyperthyroidism, treatment (usually with propylthiouracil or methimazole) should be considered in the appropriate clinical context (i.e., multiple hyperthyroidism signs, including tachycardia, moist skin, trembling, or proptosis)[78] However, no controlled studies have assessed the optimal therapeutic regimen for such patients.

NONTHYROIDAL ILLNESS SYNDROME AND HIGH THYROID-STIMULATING HORMONE OR LOW TRIIODOTHYRONINE AND THYROXINE LEVELS

In NTIS patients with TSH levels higher than 10 mU/L and the appropriate clinical signs (e.g., dry skin, goiter, decreased deep tendon reflexes, cardiac arrhythmias, pericardial effusions, hypothermia), hypothyroidism should be considered. The TSH concentration is elevated in only about 12% of NTIS patients.[80] A low free T_4 concentration in NTIS patients not receiving TSH-suppressive drugs also suggests hypothyroidism. In patients with TSH levels higher than 10 mU/L, it may be reasonable to treat with levothyroxine at 50 to 100 μg/day, depending on level of suspicion and the overall medical condition of the patient. With TSH levels between 5 and 10 mU/L, the clinician may consider repeating the thyroid function tests over the course of a few days for confirmation before treating.[59] The rT_3 level is not a useful test when the TSH concentration is less than 10 mU/L, because rT_3 levels have been shown to be low, normal, and high in this TSH range. However, the rT_3 level is not usually elevated in hypothyroid NTIS patients with TSH levels above 10 mU/L, and in that context, a non-elevated rT_3 level may aid in the diagnosis.[81] Hashimoto's thyroiditis, is characterized by goiter and positive antithyroid antibodies. Secondary or tertiary hypothyroidism may require additional tests to assess the secretion of other hormones from the pituitary or hypothalamus.[59, 78]

NONTHYROIDAL ILLNESS SYNDROME AND NORMAL THYROID-STIMULATING HORMONE LEVELS

The multiple interactions and changes in hormonal regulation that occur during NTIS produce complicated clinical scenarios. Extremely low or high TSH levels lead the clinician to suspect and possibly treat hyperthyroidism and hypothyroidism, respectively. However, there is no good evidence to suggest treating NTIS abnormalities when the TSH concentration is within a normal range. If the free T_4 concentration is extremely low and the TSH level is in the normal range, levothyroxine therapy can be considered. However, if thyroid illness is suspected, and the TSH level is not overtly abnormal, without further large-scale prospective studies, the most prudent approach would be to repeat thyroid function tests in a few days for confirmation (Box 10-1).

Box 10-1. Approach to Thyroid Testing and Treatment in the Asymptomatic Perioperative or Critically Ill Patient

NTIS and Undetectable TSH Levels

- Values may be consistent with hyperthyroidism in the setting of high-normal or elevated free T_3 and T_4.

- Consider treating the patient with propylthiouracil or methimazole.

- This profile can be seen in patients treated with dopamine and corticosteroids.

NTIS and High TSH and/or Low T_3 and/or Low T_4 Levels

- If TSH > 10 mU/L, free T_4 is low, and appropriate clinical signs (e.g., dry skin, goiter, decreased deep tendon reflexes, cardiac arrhythmias, pericardial effusions, hypothermia) are present, hypothyroidism should be considered. The rT_3 value may be useful for diagnosis.

- If the TSH value is between 5 and 10 mU/L, consider repeating the thyroid function tests over the course of a few days for confirmation before treating the patient.

- If Hashimoto's thyroiditis is suspected, evaluate for goiter and antithyroid antibodies.

- Clinical clues, multiple thyroid function tests, and possibly cortisol, prolactin, and/or gonadotropin levels may be necessary in complicated presentations of mildly elevated TSH levels.

NTIS and Normal TSH Levels

- Evidence does not support treating NTIS abnormalities when the TSH value is within the normal range.

- If clinical signs suggest thyroidal illness, consider additional thyroid function tests.

NTIS, nonthyroidal illness syndrome; rT_3, inactive reverse T_3; T_3, triiodothyronine; T_4, thyroxine; TSH, thyroid-stimulating hormone.

REFERENCES

1. Fraser CG, Preuss FS, Bigford WD: Adrenal atrophy and irreversible shock associated with cortisone therapy. JAMA 1952;149:1542-1543. **VI**

2. Schlaghecke R, Kornely E, Santen RT, et al: The effect of long-term glucocorticoid therapy on pituitary-adrenal responses to exogenous corticotropin-releasing hormone. N Engl J Med 1992;236:226-230. **III**

3. LaRochelle GE, LaRochelle AG, Ratner RE, et al: Recovery of the hypothalamic-pituitary-adrenal (HPA) axis in patients with rheumatic diseases receiving low-dose prednisone. Am J Med 1993;95:258-264. **III**

4. Ackerman GL, Nolsn CM: Adrenocortical responsiveness after alternate-day corticosteroid therapy. N Engl J Med 1968;278:405-409. **III**

5. Fauci AS: Alternate-day corticosteroid therapy. Am J Med 1978;64:729-731. **V**

6. Axelrod L: Perioperative management of patients treated with glucocorticoids. Endocrinol Metab Clin North Am 2003;32:367-383. **V**

7. Graber AL, Ney RL, Nicholson WE, et al: Natural history of pituitary-adrenal recovery following long-term suppression with corticosteroids. J Clin Endocrinol Metab 1965;25:11-16. **III**

8. Livanou T, Ferriman D, James VHT: Recovery of hypo-thalamo-pituitary-adrenal function after corticosteroid therapy. Lancet 1967;2:856-859. **III**

9. Streck WF, Lockwood DH: Pituitary adrenal recovery following short-term suppression with corticosteroids. Am J Med 1979;66:910-914. **III**

10. Carella MJ, Srivastava LS, Gossain VV, Rovner DR: Hypothalamic-pituitary-adrenal function one week after a short burst of steroid therapy. J Clin Endocrinol Metab 1993;76:1188-1191. **III**

11. Glowniak JV, Loriaux DL: A double-blind study of perioperative steroid requirements in secondary adrenal insufficiency. Surgery 1997;121:123-129. **II**

12. Bromberg JS, Baliga P, Cofer JB, et al: Stress steroids are not required for patients receiving a renal allograft and undergoing operation. J Am Coll Surg 1995;180:532-536. **III**

13. Friedman RJ, Schiff CF, Bromberg JS: Use of supplemental steroids in patients having orthopaedic operations. J Bone Joint Surg Am 1995;77:1801-1806. **III**

14. Salem M, Tainsh RE, Bromberg J, et al: Perioperative glucocorticoid coverage: A reassessment 42 years after emergence of a problem. Ann Surg 1994;219: 416-425. V

15. Chernow B, Alexander HR, Thompson WR, et al: Hormonal responses to graded surgical stress. Arch Intern Med 1987;147:1273-1278. III

16. Leopold SS, Casnellie MT, Warme WJ, et al: Endogenous cortisol production in response to knee arthroscopy and total knee arthroplasty. J Bone Joint Surg Am 2003;85:2163-2167. III

17. Lipworth BJ: Systemic adverse effects of inhaled corticosteroid therapy. A systematic review and meta-analysis. Arch Intern Med 1999;159:941-955. I

18. Pederson S, O'Byrne P: A comparison of the efficacy and safety of inhaled corticosteroids in asthma. Allergy 1997;52(Suppl):1-34. V

19. Todd G, Buck J, Ross-Russel R, et al: Acute adrenal crisis in asthmatics treated with high-dose fluticasone propionate [abstract]. Chest 2001;120:139S. VI

20. Patel L, Wales JK, Kibirige MS, et al: Symptomatic adrenal insufficiency during inhaled corticosteroid treatment. Arch Dis Child 2001;85:330-334. VI

21. Todd GR, Wright D, Ryan M: Acute adrenal insufficiency in a patient with asthma after changing from fluticasone propionate to budesonide. J Allergy Clin Immunol 1999;103:956-957. VI

22. Ayres JG, Bateman ED, Lundback B, Harris TAJ: High dose fluticasone propionate, 1 mg daily, versus fluticasone propionate, 2 mg daily, or budesonide, 1.6 mg daily, in patient with chronic severe asthma. Eur Respir J 1995:8:579-586. III

23. Wilson AM, Lipworth BJ: Systemic dose-response relationships with oral and inhaled corticosteroids in asthmatics. Thorax 1997;52(Suppl 6):A57. III

24. Noonan M, Chervinsky P, Busse WW, et al: Fluticasone propionate reduces oral prednisolone use while it improves asthma control and quality of life. Am J Respir Crit Care Med 1995;152:1467-1473. II

25. Walsh P, Aeling JI, Huff L, Weston WL: Hypothalamus-pituitary-adrenal axis suppression by superpotent topical steroid. J Am Acad Dermatol 1993;29:501. II

26. Katz HI, Hien NT, Prawer SE, et al: Superpotent topical steroid treatment of psoriasis vulgaris: Clinical efficacy

and adrenal function. J Am Acad Dermatol 1987; 16:804. II

27. Marik PE, Zaloga GP: Adrenal insufficiency in the critically ill: A new look at an old problem. Chest 2002;122:1784-1796. V

28. Dorin RI, Qualls CR, Crapo LM: Diagnosis of adrenal insufficiency. Ann Intern Med 2003;139:194-204. I

29. Cooper MS, Stewart PM: Corticosteroid insufficiency in acutely ill patients. N Engl J Med 2003;348:727-734. V

30. Beishuizen A, Vermes I, Hylkema BS, Haanen C: Relative eosinophilia and functional adrenal insufficiency in critically ill patients. Lancet 1999;353:1675-1676. V

31. Ligtenberg JJ, Zijlstra JG: The relative adrenal insufficiency syndrome revisited: Which patients will benefit from low-dose steroids? Curr Opin Crit Care 2004;10:456-460. V

32. Keh D, Boehnke T, Weber-Cartens S, et al: Immunologic and hemodynamic effects of "low-dose" hydrocortisone in septic shock: A double-blind, randomized, placebo-controlled, crossover study. Am J Respir Crit Care Med 2003;167:512-520. II

33. Oelkers W: Adrenal insufficiency. N Engl J Med 1996;335:1206-1212. V

34. Kozyra EF, Wax RS, Burry LD: Can 1 microg of cosyntropin be used to evaluate adrenal insufficiency in critically ill patients? Ann Pharmacother 2005; 39:691-698. I

35. Annane D, Sebille V, Troche G, et al: A 3-level prognostic classification in septic shock based on cortisol levels and cortisol response to corticotropin. JAMA 2000; 283:1038-1045. II

36. Marik PE, Kiminyo K, Zaloga GP: Adrenal insufficiency in critically ill patients with human immunodeficiency virus. Crit Care Med 2002;30:1267-1273. II

37. Marik PE, Zaloga GP: Adrenal insufficiency during septic shock. Crit Care Med 2003;31:141-145. II

38. Yamashita S, Drynan J, Guest C: Comparison of low-dose 1 μg with conventional dose cosyntropin 250 μg for adrenal insufficiency testing in critical illness [abstract]. Crit Care Med 2001;29:A164. II

39. Hamrahian AH, Oseni TS, Arafah BM: Measurements of serum free cortisol in critically ill patients. N Engl J Med 2004;350:1629-1638. II

40. Shapiro NI, Howell M, Talmor D: A blueprint for a sepsis protocol. Acad Emerg Med 2005;12:352-359. V

41. Balk RA: Steroids for septic shock: back from the dead? (Pro). Chest 2003;123:490S-499S. V

42. Sessler CN: Steroids for septic shock: back from the dead? (Con). Chest 2003;123:482S-489S. V

43. Schumer W: Steroids in the treatment of clinical septic shock. Ann Surg 1976;184:333-341. II

44. The Veterans Administration Systemic Sepsis Cooperative Study Group: Effect of high-dose glucocorticoid therapy on mortality in patients with clinical signs of systemic sepsis. N Engl J Med 1987;317:659-665. II

45. Bone RC, Fisher CJ Jr, Clemmer TP, et al: A controlled clinical trial of high-dose methylprednisolone in the treatment of severe sepsis and septic shock. N Engl J Med 1987;317:653-658. II

46. Cronin L, Cook DJ, Carlet J, et al: Corticosteroid treatment for sepsis: A critical appraisal and meta-analysis of the literature. Crit Care Med 1995;23:1430-1439. I

47. Lefering R, Neugebauer EA: Steroid controversy in sepsis and septic shock: A meta-analysis. Crit Care Med 1995;23:1294-1303. I

48. Dellinger RP, Carlet JM, Masur H, et al: Surviving Sepsis Campaign guidelines for management of severe sepsis and septic shock. Crit Care Med 2004;32:858-873. IV

49. Bollaert PE, Charpentier C, Levy B, et al: Reversal of late septic shock with supraphysiologic doses of hydrocortisone. Crit Care Med 1998;26:645-650. II

50. Briegel J, Forst H, Haller M, et al: Stress doses of hydrocortisone reverse hyperdynamic septic shock: A prospective, randomized, double-blind, single-center study. Crit Care Med 1999;27:723-732. II

51. Annane D, Sebille V, Charpentier C, et al: Effect of treatment with low doses of hydrocortisone and fludrocortisone on mortality in patients with septic shock. JAMA 2002;288:862-871. II

52. Annane D, Bellissant E, Bollaert PE, et al: Corticosteroids for severe sepsis and septic shock: A systematic review and meta-analysis. BMJ 2004;329:480. I

53. Minneci PC, Deans KJ, Banks SM, et al: Meta-analysis: The effect of steroids on survival and shock during sepsis depends on the dose. Ann Intern Med 2004;141:47-56. I

54. Confalonieri M, Urbino R, Potena A, et al: Hydrocortisone infusion for severe community-acquired pneumonia: A preliminary randomized study. Am J Respir Crit Care Med 2005;171:242-248. II

55. Hollenberg SM, Ahrens TS, Annane D, et al: Practice parameters for hemodynamic support of sepsis in adult patients: 2004 update. Crit Care Med 2004; 32:1928-1948. IV

56. Annane D: Glucocorticoids in the treatment of severe sepsis and septic shock. Curr Opin Crit Care 2005;11:449-453. V

57. Vanhorebeek I, Van den Berghe G: The neuroendocrine response to critical illness is a dynamic process. Crit Care Clin 2006;22:1-15. V

58. Utiger RD: Altered thyroid function in nonthyroidal illness and surgery. To treat or not to treat? N Engl J Med 1995;333:1562-1563. V

59. Chopra IJ: Clinical review 86: Euthyroid sick syndrome: Is it a misnomer? J Clin Endocrinol Metab 1997; 82:329-334. V

60. Chopra IJ, Hershman JM, Pardridge WM, Nicoloff JT: Thyroid function in nonthyroidal illnesses. Ann Intern Med 1983;98:946-957. V

61. Stathatos N, Levetan C, Burman KD, Wartofsky L: The controversy of the treatment of critically ill patients with thyroid hormone. Best Pract Res Clin Endocrinol Metab 2001;15:465-478. V

62. Van den Berghe G: Novel insights into the neuroendocrinology of critical illness. Eur J Endocrinol 2000;143:1-13. V

63. Peeters RP, van der Geyten S, Wouters PJ, et al: Tissue thyroid hormone levels in critical illness. J Clin Endocrinol Metab 2005;90:6498-6507. II

64. Brierre S, Kumari R, Deboisblanc BP: The endocrine system during sepsis. Am J Med Sci 2004; 328:238-247. V

65. Brent GA, Hershman JM: Thyroxine therapy in patients with severe nonthyroidal illnesses and low serum thyroxine concentration. J Clin Endocrinol Metab 1986;63:1-8. II

66. Peeters RP, Wouters PJ, can Toor H, et al: Serum 3,3', 5'-triiodothyronine (rT3) and 3,5,3'-triiodothyronine/rT3 are prognostic markers in critically ill patients and are associated with postmortem tissue deiodinase activities. J Clin Endocrinol Metab 2005;90:4559-4565. II

67. Slag MF, Morley JE, Elson MK, et al: Hypothyroxinemia in critically ill patients as a predictor of high mortality. JAMA 1981;245:43-45. III

68. Kaptein EM, MacIntyre SS, Weiner JM, et al: Free thyroxine estimates in nonthyroidal illness: Comparison of eight methods. J Clin Endocrinol Metab 1981;52: 1073-1077. **III**

69. Chinga-Alayo E, Villena J, Evans AT, Zimic M: Thyroid hormone levels improve the prediction of mortality among patients admitted to the intensive care unit. Intensive Care Med 2005;31:1356-1361. **III**

70. Hesch RD, Husch M, Kodding R, et al: Treatment of dopamine-dependent shock with triiodothyronine. Endocr Res Commun 1981;8:229-237. **III**

71. Dulchavsky SA, Kennedy PR, Geller ER, et al: T3 preserves respiratory function in sepsis. J Trauma 1991;31:753-758. **III**

72. Dulchavsky SA, Hendrick SR, Dutta S: Pulmonary biophysical effects of triiodothyronine augmentation during sepsis-induced hypothyroidism. J Trauma 1993;35:104-108. **III**

73. Holland FW 2nd, Brown PS Jr, Weintraub BD, Clark RE: Cardiopulmonary bypass and thyroid function: A "euthyroid sick syndrome." Ann Thorac Surg 1991;52:46-50. **III**

74. Mullis-Jansson SL, Argenziano M, Corwin S, et al: A randomized double-blind study of the effect of triiodothyronine on cardiac function and morbidity after coronary bypass surgery. J Thorac Cardiovasc Surg 1999;117:1128-1134. **II**

75. Klemperer JD, Klein I, Gomez M, et al: Thyroid hormone treatment after coronary-artery bypass surgery. N Engl J Med 1995;333:1522-1527. **II**

76. Bennett-Guerrero E, Jiminez JL, White WD, et al: Cardiovascular effects of intravenous triiodothyronine in patients undergoing coronary artery bypass graft surgery. A randomized, double-blind, placebo-controlled trial. Duke T3 study group. JAMA 1996;275:687-692. **II**

77. Van den Berghe G, Baxter RC, Weekers F, et al: The combined administration of GH-releasing peptide-2 (GHRP-2), TRH and GnRH to men with prolonged critical illness evokes superior endocrine and metabolic effects compared to treatment with GHRP-2 alone. Clin Endocrinol (Oxf) 2002;56:655-669. **II**

78. Nylen ES, Muller B: Endocrine changes in critical illness. J Intensive Care Med 2004;19:67-82. **V**

79. Spencer C, Eigen A, Shen D, et al: Specificity of sensitive assays of thyrotropin (TSH) used to screen for thyroid

disease in hospitalized patients. Clin Chem 1987;33:1391-1396. III

80. Spencer CA: Clinical utility and cost-effectiveness of sensitive thyrotropin assays in ambulatory and hospitalized patients. Mayo Clin Proc 1988; 63:1214-1222. V

81. Burmeister LA: Reverse T3 does not reliably differentiate hypothyroid sick syndrome from euthyroid sick syndrome. Thyroid 1995;5:435-441. III

11

Infectious Disease Issues in Medical Consultation

*Sean Pierre Pickering and
Daniel C. R. Chen*

1. What are the indications for a urinary catheter?

Search Date: April 2005

Search Strategy: *PubMed, 1978 to April 2005, search for "infection AND catheter AND urinary," limited to English and human studies.*

The indications for urethral catheterization include surgery, urine output measurement, urine retention, and urinary incontinence. A study in 1995 showed unjustified urinary catheterization in 21% of patients and unjustified continued use in 47%.[1] More than one third of catheter days were potentially avoidable in another study.[2] After 30 days of catheterization, most patients have bacteriuria.[3]

2. How can catheter-associated urinary tract infections be prevented?

Search Date: April 2005

Search Strategy: *PubMed, 1978 to April 2005, search for "infection AND catheter AND urinary," limited to English and human studies.*

The most consistent forms of prevention involve avoiding the use of urinary catheters,[1,4] shortening the duration of use,[1] and minimizing manipulation of the catheter itself.[5-8] Several alternatives to indwelling catheters have been investigated. Condom catheters have been investigated as an alternative means of catheterization for men. Urine within and around these condoms can develop high concentrations of bacteria. No well-designed studies have shown benefit to the use of condom catheters over indwelling catheters in the short term, but most studies have shown a trend favoring condom catheters in the short term and clearer benefit in chronic cases. In parallel studies done at the same institution, indwelling catheters resulted in 106 symptomatic infections in 514 patient-months at risk (0.21 per patient-month at risk),[9] compared with 0.08 per patient-month at risk in 497 patients with external catheters.[10] Intermittent catheterization has shown reduced rates of bacteriuria compared with indwelling catheters and is the standard of care for spinal injury patients.[11] Suprapubic catheters have also been associated with fewer catheter-associated urinary tract infections (CAUTIs).[12] They are an option for patients requiring long-term catheterization.

Silver is a bactericidal agent that prevents the formation of biofilms and has been studied in the prevention of CAUTIs.[13-18] In a prospective, 2-year surveillance study in 10 patient units using historical control data, the introduction of silver alloy and silver hydrogel-coated catheters resulted in a decrease in urinary tract infections (UTIs) and cost savings.[13] In another study using hydrogel-coated catheters and comparing UTI rates with historical UTI rates, there was a nonsignificant reduction in infections with a moderate cost savings.[17] In a randomized study comparing catheters coated with hydrogel and silver salts with traditional noncoated catheters, the incidence of infections among 199 patients was 11.9% for the control group and 10% for the coated-catheter group.[14] These results were not significant.

Reminders to practitioners about urinary catheter indications and discontinuation best practices is another CAUTI prevention strategy.[19] One study showed that prompting physicians to remove unnecessary catheters resulted in decreased catheter duration and reduction of CAUTIs.[20]

GUIDELINES FOR THE TREATMENT OF CAUTIs

Guidelines for prevention of CAUTIs by the Centers for Disease Control and Prevention (CDC) have been available for the past 20 years without significant revision.[21] Later guidelines with weighted recommendations from the U.S. Department of Health have been developed. Most of the recommendations pertain to nursing care, but for the consultant, a few important points can be summarized[6]:

- Only use indwelling urethral catheters after considering alternative methods of management.
- Review regularly the patient's clinical need for continuing urinary catheterization, and remove the catheter as soon as possible.
- Document catheter insertion and care.
- Catheterization is an aseptic procedure.
- Clean the urethral meatus before insertion of the catheter (studies on proper meatal care, such as iodine solutions, soap and water, or silver sulfadiazine cream, have shown widely varying results so expert opinion is often used).
- Use an appropriate lubricant from a single-use container to minimize urethral trauma and infection.
- Do not change catheters unnecessarily or as part of routine practice.
- Routine personal hygiene is all that is needed to maintain meatal hygiene.

3. How are the complications of catheter-associated urinary tract infections managed?

Search Date: April 2005

Search Strategy: PubMed, 1978 to April 2005, search for "infection AND catheter AND urinary," limited to English and human studies.

In immunocompetent hosts, the treatment of asymptomatic bacteriuria in short-term–catheterized patients is not usually indicated.[3,22] Patients undergoing urologic procedures are an exception. Removal of the catheter (considering the possibility of a biofilm being present) should be performed in patients with symptomatic bacteriuria[3]. Two thirds of bacteriuria cases in these patients clear within a week.[23] In patients with signs of bacteremia, other sources should be considered, and blood and urine cultures should be drawn. Asymptomatic candiduria is usually a long-term complication of urinary catheterization and can usually be treated by simply removing the catheter.

4. What are the strategies for the prevention of surgical site infections?

Search Date: April 2005

Search Strategy: *PubMed, 1971 to April 2005, search for "surgical AND wound" OR "site AND infection NOT dental." Both limited to English and human studies; search run limited to guidelines, then to reviews, then to randomized, controlled trials, and then to clinical trials, all done by PubMed Date search order.*

The risk factors and organisms associated with surgical site infections (SSIs) are important for understanding the strategies used for prevention of these infections. Tables 11-1 and 11-2 are adapted from the CDC guidelines for SSI prevention.[24]

Table 11-1. **Patient and Operative Characteristics that may Influence the Risk of Surgical Site Infection**

Source	Characteristics
Patient	Age Nutritional status Diabetes Smoking Obesity Coexistent infections Colonization with microorganisms Altered immune response Length of preoperative stay
Operation	Duration of surgical scrub Skin antisepsis Preoperative shaving Preoperative skin preparation Duration of operation

Continued

Table 11-1. Patient and Operative Characteristics that may Influence the Risk of Surgical Site Infection—cont'd

Source	Characteristics
	Antimicrobial prophylaxis
	Operating room ventilation
	Inadequate sterilization of instruments
	Foreign material in the surgical site
	Surgical drains
	Surgical technique
	Poor hemostasis
	Failure to obliterate dead space
	Tissue trauma

Adapted from Mangram AJ, Horan TC, Pearson ML, et al: Guideline for prevention of surgical site infection, 1999. Hospital Infection Control Practices Advisory Committee. Infect Control Hosp Epidemiol 1999;20:250-278.

Table 11-2. Likely Pathogens in Surgical Site Infections

Surgical Procedures	Likely Pathogens
Placement of all grafts, prostheses, or implants	*Staphylococcus aureus*, coagulase-negative staphylococci
Cardiac operations	*S. aureus*, coagulase-negative staphylococci
Neurosurgery	*S. aureus*, coagulase-negative staphylococci
Breast surgery	*S. aureus*, coagulase-negative staphylococci
Ophthalmic surgery (limited data, but common in procedures such as anterior segment resection, vitrectomy, and scleral buckles)	*S. aureus*, coagulase-negative staphylococci, streptococci, gram-negative bacilli
Orthopedic surgery (total joint replacement; closed fractures; use of nails, bone plates, and other internal fixation devices; functional repair without an implant or device; trauma)	*S. aureus*, coagulase-negative staphylococci, gram-negative bacilli

Table 11-2. Likely Pathogens in Surgical Site Infections—cont'd

Surgical Procedures	Likely Pathogens
Noncardiac thoracic surgery (lobectomy, pneumonectomy, wedge resection, other noncardiac mediastinal procedures, closed tube thoracostomy)	S. aureus, coagulase-negative staphylococci, Streptococcus pneumoniae, gram-negative bacilli
Vascular surgery	S. aureus, coagulase-negative staphylococci
Appendectomy	Gram-negative bacilli, anaerobes
Biliary tract surgery	Gram-negative bacilli, anaerobes
Colorectal surgery	Gram-negative bacilli, anaerobes
Gastroduodenal	Gram-negative bacilli, streptococci, oropharyngeal anaerobes (e.g., peptostreptococci)
Head and neck surgery (major procedures with incision through the oropharyngeal mucosa)	S. aureus, streptococci, oropharyngeal anaerobes (e.g., peptostreptocococci)
Obstetric and gynecologic surgery	Gram-negative bacilli, enterococci, group B streptococci, anaerobes
Urologic surgery (tests may not be beneficial if urine is sterile)	Gram-negative bacilli

Adapted from Mangram AJ, Horan TC, Pearson ML, et al: Guideline for prevention of surgical site infection, 1999. Hospital Infection Control Practices Advisory Committee. Infect Control Hosp Epidemiol 1999;20:250-278.

Pharmacologic and nonpharmacologic prevention strategies have been described for the prevention of SSIs. Nonpharmacologic interventions include maintaining normothermia, supplemental oxygen, avoiding shaving surgical sites, and careful regulation of blood glucose.[25]

Hypothermia significantly increases the risk of SSI and prolongs hospital stays.[26] Hypothermia results in tissue vasoconstriction, decreased oxygen-dependent superoxide radical killing by neutrophils, and decreased collagen deposition (i.e., scar formation).[25]

Theoretically, supplemental oxygen is effective in reducing infection because it improves phagocytosis and oxidative killing by macrophages. A 100% FIO_2 compared with 30% FIO_2 has been shown to diminish the decrease in macrophage function.[27] Until recently, few studies provided evidence supporting the use of supplemental oxygen, and consequently, the practice of routinely administering oxygen in the postoperative setting varied widely. In one randomized, controlled trial, the use of supplemental FIO_2 of 0.80 rather than 0.30 in 500 subjects reduced the risk of infection from 11% to 5%.[28]

For hair removal before surgery, studies and practice guidelines recommend the use of clippers rather than skin shaving (if hair removal is necessary).[24,29] Shaving increases the rate of SSIs.[30] The increased risk of infection is believed to result from microscopic cuts in the skin that later serve as foci for bacterial entry.

Glucose control was studied in 1548 intubated surgical intensive care unit patients in a randomized, controlled trial.[31] Those receiving tight glucose control (serum glucose level < 110 mg/dL) compared with less tight control (serum glucose level < 215 mg/dL) had significant improvements in mortality (4.6% compared with 8%).[31] The greatest effect was seen among those with multiorgan failure with a proven septic focus. Sternal wound infections have also been significantly reduced by tight glucose control with intravenous insulin infusion.[32]

PHARMACOLOGIC PREVENTION OF SURGICAL SITE INFECTIONS

The National Surgical Infection Prevention Project (NSIPP) was formed in 2004 to minimize the morbidity and mortality associated with SSIs. Three performance measures were determined to have importance in the development of SSIs.[33]

1. The proportion of patients who have parenteral antimicrobial prophylaxis initiated within 1 hour before surgical incision
2. The proportion of patients who are provided an antimicrobial agent that is consistent with published guidelines
3. The proportion of patients whose prophylactic antimicrobial therapy is discontinued within 24 hours after surgery

These three points were the focus of a large, retrospective, cohort study looking at ways in which we can improve the use of antimicrobial prophylaxis. Although appropriate antimicrobials were used in more than 90% cases, the recommended timing of initiation of antibiotics and termination of antibiotics was reached in only one half of cases.[34] The NSIPP advisory statement is summarized in Table 11-3.[33] The American Society of Health-System Pharmacists recommends continued antimicrobial

Table 11-3. Surgical Infection Prevention Guidelines: Writers Workgroup Consensus Positions	
Antibiotic Selection	**Consensus Position**
Selection by Principle	
Antibiotic timing	Infusion of the first antimicrobial dose should begin within 60 minutes before the surgical incision.*
Duration of prophylaxis	Prophylactic antimicrobials should be discontinued within 24 hours after the end of surgery.
Screening for β-lactam allergy	For operations for which cephalosporins represent the most appropriate antimicrobials for prophylaxis, the medical history should be adequate to determine whether the patient has a history of allergy or serious adverse antibiotic reaction. Alternative testing strategies (e.g., skin testing) may be useful for patients with reported allergies.
Antimicrobial dosing	The initial antimicrobial dose should be adequate based on the patient's body weight, adjusted dosing weight, or body mass index. An additional antimicrobial dose should be provided intraoperatively if the operation is still continuing two half-lives after the initial dose.
Selection by Procedure	
Abdominal or vaginal hysterectomy	Cefotetan therapy is preferred; cefazolin or cefoxitin are alternatives. Metronidazole monotherapy also is used.† If the patient has a β-lactam allergy, use clindamycin combined with gentamicin or ciprofloxacin‡

Continued

Table 11-3. Surgical Infection Prevention Guidelines: Writers Workgroup Consensus Positions—cont'd

Antibiotic Selection	Consensus Position
	or aztreonam; metronidazole with gentamicin or ciprofloxacin[‡]; or clindamycin monotherapy.
Hip or knee arthroplasty	Use cefazolin or cefuroxime. If the patient has a β-lactam allergy, use vancomycin or clindamycin.
Cardiothoracic and vascular surgery	Use cefazolin or cefuroxime. If the patient has a β-lactam allergy, use vancomycin or clindamycin.
Colon surgery	For oral antimicrobial prophylaxis, use neomycin plus erythromycin base or neomycin plus metronidazole. For parenteral antimicrobial prophylaxis, use cefotetan, cefoxitin, or cefazolin plus metronidazole. If the patient has a β-lactam allergy, use clindamycin combined with gentamicin, ciprofloxacin, or aztreonam, or use metronidazole combined with gentamicin or ciprofloxacin.[‡]

*When fluoroquinolone or vancomycin are indicated, infusion of the first antimicrobial dose should begin within 120 minutes before the incision.
[†]Metronidazole monotherapy is included in the Practice Bulletin of the American College of Obstetricians and Gynecologist as an alternative to β-lactams for patients undergoing hysterectomy, although it may be less effective as a single agent for prophylaxis.
[‡]A single 750-mg dose of levofloxacin may be substituted for ciprofloxacin.
Adapted from Bratzler D, Houck PM, for the Surgical Infection Prevention Guidelines Writers Workgroup: Antimicrobial prophylaxis for surgery: An advisory statement from the National Surgical Infection Prevention Project. Clin Infect Dis 2004;38:1706-1715.

prophylaxis for up to 72 hours after wound closure. These are the only guidelines that support extension of antimicrobial prophylaxis after surgical wound closure.[35]

Although newer antimicrobials are available, many antimicrobials from even a decade ago are still efficacious and considered standard prophylaxis. Recommended antimicrobial agents are summarized in Table 11-4.[36] There are decisions regarding SSI prevention that will be made by the primary surgery or anesthesiology team before the consultant's involvement in the case. These areas include operating room characteristics, preparation techniques, surgical techniques, instrument and gown

Table 11-4. Antimicrobial Prophylaxis for Surgical Wounds

Operations	Bacteria	Intravenous Administration of Antimicrobial	Dose*
Cardiac: all with sternotomy, cardiopulmonary bypass	*Staphylococcus aureus, Staphylococcus epidermidis,* diphtheroids, gram-negative enterics	Cefazolin (vancomycir)	1 to 2 g (1g slowly) preinduction, 1-2 g every 8 hr for 48 hr
Noncardiac vascular: aortic resection and prosthetic bypass	*S. aureus, S. epidermidis,* diphtheroids, gram-negative enterics	Cefazolin (vancomycin)	1g (1g slowly) preinduction, 2 postoperative doses
Orthopedic: insertion of prosthetic joints, open operations	S aureus, *S. epidermidis*	Cefazolin (vancomycin)	1g (1g slowly) preinduction
Neurosurgery	S. aureus, S. epidermidis	Cefazolin (vancomyc n)	1g (1g slowly) preinduction
Head and neck: operations involving the mucous membranes and deep tissue	Oral aerobes and anaerobes, S. aureus, streptococci	Cefazolin	2 g preinduction

Continued

Table 11-4. Antimicrobial Prophylaxis for Surgical Wounds—cont'd

Operations	Bacteria	Intravenous Administration of Antimicrobial	Dose*
General thoracic: pulmonary and esophageal	Oral anaerobes, S. aureus, streptococci, gram-negative enterics	Cefazolin	1 to 2 g preinduction
Gastroduodenal: bariatric, ulcer patients treated with H$_2$-blockers, bleeding duodenal ulcer, genitourinary or gastric cancer	Oropharyngeal flora and gram-negative enterics, S. aureus	Cefazolin	1 to 2 g preinduction
Biliary: all open and laparoscopic procedures (chronically intubated biliary tract)	Gram-negative enterics, S. aureus, Enterococcus fecalis, clostridia (plus Pseudomonas species)	Cefazolin (culture-based selection)	1 to 2 g preinduction (preinduction dose and repeat interval based on drug kinetics)
Colorectal: operations that open the colon or rectum	Enteric aerobes and anaerobes	Oral neomycin or erythromycin (cefoxitin or cefotetan or cefmetazole)	Operating room day 1:1 g at 1, 2, and 11 PM (1 g preinduction)

Appendectomy; simple appendicitis (antibiotics are empirical or definitive for complicated appendicitis)	Enteric aerobes and anaerobes	Cefoxitin or cefotetan or cefmetazole	1 g preinduction
Cesarean section	Enteric aerobes and anaerobes, E. fecalis, group B streptococci	Cefazolin	1 g after umbilical cord is clamped
Hysterectomy	Enteric aerobes and anaerobes, E. fecalis, group B streptococci	Cefazolin	1 g preinduction
Abdominal trauma	Enteric aerobes and anaerobes	Cefoxitin	2 g preinduction

*Parenthetic text refers to alternate antibiotic or situation. Current data suggest repeat dosing for operations lasting longer than the serum half-life. Preinduction indicates dosing in the operating room before initiating anesthesia.

Adapted from Page CP, Bohnen JM, Fletcher JR, et al: Antimicrobial prophylaxis for surgical wounds: Guidelines for clinical care. Arch Surg 1993;128:79-88.

sterilization, and even skin antisepsis and antimicrobial prophylaxis.

5. Is mupirocin effective in eradicating *Staphylococcus aureus* nasal carriage?

Search Date: April 2005

Search Strategy: PubMed, January 1980 to April 2005, for "staphylococcus aureus," "surgery," "antibiotic," "antimicrobial," "infection, nasal." Limit: English language, meta-analysis, randomized, controlled trial, clinical, practice guideline, review.

Mupirocin calcium ointment (pseudomonic acid) is a topical antimicrobial agent with broad-spectrum activity effective against many gram-positive bacteria, including *Staphylococcus aureus*, methicillin-resistant *S. aureus* (MRSA), and vancomycin-resistant *S. aureus*. The side effects of this drug are mild and can include headache, rhinitis, and taste changes.

EPIDEMIOLOGY OF STAPHYLOCOCCUS AUREUS NASAL CARRIAGE

S. aureus is a common cause of SSIs. The source of *S. aureus* infections is thought to be the patient's endogenous flora, and the ecologic niche is the anterior nares. At any time, 25% to 30% of the whole population is colonized.[37] *S. aureus* nasal carriers are two to nine times more likely to acquire a SSI.[37]

MUPIROCIN ERADICATION OF STAPHYLOCOCCUS AUREUS

Mupirocin is effective in eliminating carriage of *S. aureus* in the nares. The efficacy of mupirocin in the eradication of *S. aureus* nasal carriage has been proved in a double-blind, placebo-controlled study of 68 health care workers with *S. aureus* nasal carriage. When applied twice daily for 5 days, mupirocin decreased *S. aureus* nasal carriage and hand carriage within 72 hours of completion of treatment. At 3 months, 71% of subjects who received mupirocin remained free of nasal *S. aureus* compared with 18% of controls.[38] In a group of 143 volunteers with stable nasal carriage of *S. aureus*, 91% of those receiving mupirocin treatment for 5 days had a clearance of colonization within 48 to 96 hours after completing treatment, compared with 6% in the control group of volunteers. Moreover, 74% of volunteers who cleared the nasal carriage of *S. aureus* by 4 days remained clear of colonization at the end of 4 weeks.[39] In one clinical trial,[37] 83% of nasal carriage of *S. aureus* was eliminated in general, gynecologic, neurologic, and cardiothoracic surgery patients receiving three to five doses of mupirocin. Carriage was eliminated in 93% of patients receiving six or more doses of mupirocin.

6. What is the role of mupirocin in reducing surgical site infections with *S. aureus*?

The role of mupirocin in reducing *S. aureus* SSIs has been studied. The Mupirocin and the Risk of *Staphylococcus aureus* (MARS) study was a randomized, placebo-controlled trial looking at prophylactic intranasal application of mupirocin and its effect on SSIs with *S. aureus* in patients undergoing elective and nonemergent cardiothoracic, general, oncologic, gynecologic, or neurologic procedures. The intervention group of patients received mupirocin twice daily to the nares for up to 5 days before the operation. Patients were monitored for 1 month after the surgery to determine whether they had acquired an *S. aureus* infection. The study treated 1933 patients with mupirocin and had 1931 patients as controls. *S. aureus* SSIs were found in 2.3% of patients receiving mupirocin and 2.4% of patients receiving placebo. This difference was not statistically significant, but in patients who had known nasal carriage of *S. aureus*, there was a statistical difference in SSIs in patients receiving mupirocin versus placebo (4.0% versus 7.7%; OR for infection = 0.49; 95% CI: 0.25 to 0.92; P = .02).[37]

CARDIOTHORACIC SURGERY SITE INFECTIONS

The effects of mupirocin on sternal wound infections after cardiothoracic surgery have been assessed in several studies. In a case-control study, Kluytmans and colleagues[40] assessed 752 consecutive cardiothoracic surgery patients receiving intranasal mupirocin and compared them with 928 historical and 116 concurrent controls undergoing cardiothoracic surgery. In the treatment group, mupirocin calcium ointment was applied twice daily for 5 consecutive days, and the first dose was administered on postoperative day 1. The intervention and control groups had comparable rates of *S. aureus* nasal carriage (16% and 15%, respectively) before surgery. Overall, there was a statistically significant reduction in SSIs (2.8% versus 7.8%) with *S. aureus* and other organisms in the treatment arm. The investigators observed that the reduction of deep SSIs was greater than the reduction of incisional SSIs in the treated groups.[40] Cimochowski and associates[41] compared 992 consecutive historical controls with 854 prospectively followed patients undergoing cardiothoracic surgery. All intervention patients, regardless of *S. aureus* nasal carriage status, received mupirocin intranasally 1 day before surgery and for 5 days postoperatively. The rate of sternal wound infections was 2.7% in the control group and 0.9% in the treatment group. A subgroup analysis looking at *diabetics* found that there was a statistical difference in the rate of infection in the untreated and treated groups (5.1% versus 1.9%). In the nondiabetic population, the differences were less (1.8% and 0.5%, respectively).[41] In a study of 3800 cardiothoracic surgery patients at a community hospital, intranasal mupirocin ointment significantly decreased overall sternal wound infections from 2.62% to 1.24% ($P = .007$). In subgroup analyses, the incidence of deep ($P = .025$) as opposed to superficial ($P = .14$) wound infections was significantly decreased. In this study, patients were not screened for *S. aureus* nasal carriage.[42]

MUPIROCIN ERADICATION IN ORTHOPEDIC AND NEUROSURGERY POPULATIONS

Mupirocin has been studied in other surgical populations as well. A case-control study of orthopedic surgery patients treated with mupirocin showed a decrease in the incidence of SSIs. The general surgical wound infection rates were 1.3% in the intervention group and 2.7% in the untreated group ($P = .02$). However, when specifically looking at surgical wound infections caused by *S. aureus*, results were not significant (treatment group had 0.7% infections compared with 1.1% in control group; $P = .3$).[43] In the MARS study, there was no statistical difference in patients carrying nasal *S. aureus* and receiving mupirocin or placebo and undergoing orthopedic surgery or neurosurgery, but there were relatively small numbers in these subgroups.[37]

MUPIROCIN ERADICATION IN ABDOMINAL SURGERY PATIENTS

A randomized trial by Suzuki and colleagues[44] studied 395 patients undergoing abdominal surgery. Subjects were randomly assigned to receive preoperative intranasal mupirocin (193 patients) or usual care (202 patients). Most postoperative SSIs in this study were caused by gram-negative bacteria. For the 21 gram-positive SSIs, no difference was found between the groups. Although this study suggests that intranasal mupirocin treatment had no significant impact on SSIs after abdominal surgery, the baseline incidence of nasal *S. aureus* carriage was not ascertained.[44]

7. Aside from mupirocin, what other strategies have been studied to eradicate *S. aureus* colonization?

Other strategies, such as systemic administration of antimicrobials and bacterial interference with a modified *S. aureus* strain, have been attempted to eliminate nasal carriage of *S. aureus.* These have failed because of development of antimicrobial resistance or recolonization of the nares with the original bacteria or a resistant strain. A combinations of intranasal bacitracin and rifampin was shown to eradicate *S. aureus* colonization from the anterior nares of patients undergoing hemodialysis, but this strategy needs further investigation with regard to its efficacy in reducing subsequent infections.[45]

8. What is the incidence of bacteremia after diagnostic medical procedures?

Search Dates: April 2005

Search Strategy: *PubMed, January 1980 to April 2005, search for "murmur," "antibiotic," "prophylaxis," "valve," "endocarditis." Limited to English language, meta-analysis, randomized, controlled trial, clinical, practice guideline, review.*

Endocarditis often follows occult bacteremia. Certain health care procedures can introduce bacteria into the bloodstream. Although it is not always possible to prove that a particular procedure caused an individual case of endocarditis, a causal relationship is often inferred based on the temporal nature of the procedure to the occurrence of disease.

The frequency of bacteremia after health care procedures has been studied. The incidence of bacteremia usually is highest after dental and oral procedures. The relative frequency of endocarditis after diagnostic procedures is shown in Table 11-5. Bacteremias associated with procedures are short lived, and the frequency of positive blood cultures after dental procedures is highest 30 seconds after a tooth extraction and usually lasts less than 10 minutes.[46] Bacteria associated with common diagnostic and therapeutic procedures are usually sensitive to antibiotics. Strategies that incorporate preprocedural

Table 11-5. **Rates of Bacteremia after Dental, Diagnostic, and Therapeutic Procedures**

Procedure and Site	Incidence (Range) %
None (spontaneous bacteremia)	< 1 (0-3)
Oral cavity	
Tooth extraction	60 (18-85)
Periodontal surgery	88 (60-90)
Brushing teeth or irrigation	40 (7-50)
Tonsillectomy	35 (33-38)
Respiratory tract	
Tracheal intubation	10 (0-16)
Nasotracheal suctioning	16
Bronchoscopy	
Rigid bronchoscope	15
Flexible bronchoscope	0
Genitourinary tract	
Catheter insertion or removal	13 (0-26)
Prostatectomy	
Sterile urine	12 (11-13)
Infected urine	60 (58-82)
Dilation of strictures	28 (19-86)
Normal delivery	3 (1-5)
Insertion or removal of an intrauterine device	0

Table 11-5. Rates of Bacteremia after Dental, Diagnostic, and Therapeutic Procedures—cont'd

Procedure and Site	Incidence (Range) %
Gastrointestinal tract	
Upper gastrointestinal endoscopy	4 (0-8)
Transesophageal echocardiography	1 (0-17)
Endoscopic retrograde	5 (0-6)
cholangiopancreatography	10 (5-11)
Barium enema	5 (0-5)
Colonoscopy	
Sigmoidoscopy	5
Rigid sigmoidoscope	0
Flexible sigmoidoscope	2
Proctoscopy	8
Hemorrhoidectomy	45
Esophageal dilation	
Vascular system	
Cardiac catheterization	2 (0-5)

Adapted from Durack DT: Prevention of infective endocarditis. N Engl J Med 1995;332;38-43.

and periprocedural empirical antibiotic have been adopted to decrease the incidence of endocarditis for specific patient populations.

9. In what circumstances should prophylaxis for bacterial endocarditis be recommended?

Although bacteremia occurs after various procedures, most endocarditis is not procedure related. Only 4% to 19% of cases can be attributed to such procedures. Van der Meer and colleagues[47] assessed the efficacy of antibiotic prophylaxis for the prevention of endocarditis in a case-control study in the Netherlands. They observed that most patients with endocarditis with a known, preexisting cardiac lesion did not get endocarditis when a dental or medical procedure was performed. The study authors concluded that if total compliance with prophylaxis were adhered to, endocarditis could have been prevented in only 6% of patients with native-valve endocarditis.[47] Although this is a small percentage, the prevention of endocarditis is highly desirable because this disease carries significant morbidity and mortality.

The guidelines from the American Heart Association (AHA) have been adopted as principles for initiating antibiotic prophylaxis for the prevention of endocarditis after medical procedures (Tables 11-6, 11-7, and 11-8). The AHA recommendations are based on a combination of experimental animal models of efficacy of prophylaxis, in vitro data about pathogens known to cause endocarditis, analysis of procedure-related endocarditis literature, and retrospective analysis of cases of human endocarditis and associated prophylactic use. There have been no randomized trials to definitively establish the efficacy of antibiotic prophylaxis in the prevention of endocarditis for specific patient populations.

10. How is a true penicillin allergy identified?

Search Strategy: PubMed, search for "penicillin AND cephalosporin AND allergy," "penicillin AND desensitization AND allergy," "hypersensitivity AND skin testing." Limited to English and human studies. Search run limited to guidelines, then to randomized, controlled trials, then to clinical trials, all done by PubMed date search order.

There continues to be much debate on the management of patients who report penicillin allergies. About 10% of the population reports a penicillin allergy, but more than 90% of these patients lack penicillin-specific IgE antibodies and could therefore receive β-lactam antibiotics safely.[50,51] Many of these patients were told to avoid penicillins by their parents or pediatricians since childhood. Others recall reactions to penicillins that probably do not represent true allergies.[52]

For patients who report penicillin allergies, several options exist when deciding on the safety of future β-lactam use. Skin testing is often recommended to determine the existence of a true allergy.[52,53] If skin test results are negative, β-lactams are considered safe to administer. If an alternative drug is not available and skin testing is not an option due to time constraints or patient or physician preference, the patient can be desensitized

Table 11-6. Cardiac Lesions for Which Bacterial Endocarditis Prophylaxis Is or Is Not Recommended

Endocarditis Prophylaxis Is Recommended

High-risk category
    Prosthetic cardiac valves, including bioprosthetic and homograft valves
    Previous bacterial endocarditis, even in the absence of heart disease
    Complex cyanotic congenital heart disease (e.g., single-ventricle states,
        transposition of the great arteries, tetralogy of Fallot)
    Surgically constructed systemic pulmonary shunts or conduits
    Moderate-risk category
    Most congenital cardiac malformations (other than those listed above
        and below)
    Rheumatic and other acquired valvular dysfunction even after valvular
        surgery
    Hypertrophic cardiomyopathy
    Mitral valve prolapse with valvular regurgitation
        Mitral regurgitation determined by the presence of a murmur or by
            echo Doppler
        Men older than 45 years without a consistent murmur may warrant
            prophylaxis, even in the absence of resting regurgitation.

Endocarditis Prophylaxis Is Not Recommended

Negligible risk category (no greater than in the general population)
    Isolated secundum septal defect
    Surgical repair of atrial septal defect, ventricular septal defect or patent
        ductus arteriosus (without residua beyond 6 months)
    Previous coronary artery bypass graft surgery
    Mitral valve prolapse without valvular regurgitation (individuals with
        mitral valve prolapse associated with thickening or redundancy of
        the valve leaflets may be at increased risk for bacterial endocarditis)
Physiologic, functional, or innocent heart murmurs
Previous Kawasaki disease without valvular dysfunction
Previous rheumatic fever without valvular dysfunction
Cardiac pacemakers (intravascular and epicardial) and implanted
    defibrillators

*Adapted with permission from Dajani AS, Taubert KA, Wilson W, et al: Prevention of
bacterial endocarditis. Recommendations by the American Heart Association. JAMA
1997;277:1794-1801.*

Table 11-7. Procedures for Which Bacterial Endocarditis Prophylaxis Is or Is Not Recommended

Procedure	Prophylaxis Recommended	Prophylaxis Not Recommended
Dental	Dental extractions Periodontal procedures Dental implant placement, reimplantation of avulsed teeth Endodontic (root canal) instrumentation or surgery Subgingival placement of antibiotic fibers or strips Initial placement of orthodontic bands Intraligamentary local anesthetic injections Prophylactic cleaning of teeth or implants	Restorative dentistry (e.g., filling cavities, replacement of missing teeth) Local anesthetic injections Intracanal endodontic treatment Placement of rubber dams Postoperative suture removal Placement of removable prosthodontic or orthodontic appliances and adjustment of appliances Taking of oral impressions Fluoride treatments Taking of oral radiographs Shedding of primary teeth
Respiratory tract	Tonsillectomy and/or adenoidectomy Surgical operations involving respiratory mucosa Bronchoscopy with a rigid bronchoscope	Endotracheal intubation Bronchoscopy with a flexible bronchoscope with or without biopsy Tympanostomy tube insertion

Gastrointestinal tract	Sclerotherapy for esophageal varices (not banding) Esophageal stricture dilation ERCP with suspected biliary obstruction Biliary tract surgery Surgical operations involving intestinal mucosa	Transesophageal echocardiography Endoscopy with or without gastrointestinal biopsy
Genitourinary tract	Prostatic surgery Cystoscopy Urethral dilation	Vaginal hysterectomy Vaginal delivery Cesarean section In uninfected tissue: urethral catheterization, uterine dilatation/curettage, therapeutic abortion, sterilization procedures, insertion/removal of IUDs
Other		Cardiac catheterization, including balloon angioplasty or stents Implanted cardiac pacemakers or defibrillators Incision or biopsy or surgically scrubbed skin Circumcision

ERCP, endoscopic retrograde cholangiopencreatography; IUD, intrauterine device.
Adapted from Dajani AS, Taubert KA, Wilson W, et al: Prevention of bacterial endocarditis. Recommendations by the American Heart Association. JAMA 1997;277:1794-1801.

Table 11-8. **Antimicrobial Therapy**

Procedures and Patient Groups	Therapy
Dental/Oral Or Upper Respiratory Tract	
Standard	Amoxicillin (2 g) orally 1 hour before procedure
If penicillin allergic	Clindamycin (600 mg), cephalexin (2 g), or azithromycin (500 mg) 1 hour before procedure
If unable to use oral therapy	Ampicillin (2 g IV or IM) 30 minutes before procedure or clindamycin (600 mg IV) or cefazolin (1 g IV) 30 minutes before procedure if penicillin allergic
Gastrointestinal or Genitourinary Tract	
If high-risk patient	Ampicillin (2 g IV) plus gentamycin (1.5 mg/kg IV) 30 minutes before procedure, followed by amoxicillin (1 g PO/IV/IM) 8 hours later
If penicillin allergic	Gentamycin (1.5 mg/kg IV) and van comycin (1 g IV) 30 minutes before procedure
If moderate-risk patient	Amoxicillin (2 g PO) or ampicillin (2 g IV or IM) 30 minutes before procedure
If penicillin allergic	Vancomycin (IV) if penicillin allergic
Special Cases	
Pregnancy	Prophylaxis should be given if otherwise indicated.
Antibiotics for other indications	For patients taking antibiotics for other indications at the time of dental or invasive procedures, another antibiotic of a different class should be taken.
At high or moderate risk for endocarditis	Patients at high or moderate risk for endocarditis undergoing procedures involving infected tissue should receive an antimicrobial expected to cover the causative organism.

Adapted from Dajani AS, Taubert KA, Wilson W, Bolger AF, et al: Prevention of bacterial endocarditis. Recommendations by the American Heart Association. JAMA 1997;277:1794-1801.

to penicillin (discussed later).[52,54] Another approach is to avoid β-lactam antibiotics altogether without skin testing. Survey studies among physicians have shown significant variation in the prescribing patterns of β-lactam antibiotics and the use of skin testing in patients who report a penicillin allergy.[55,56]. In clinical practice, many variables, such as good history taking, urgency of the final decision, type of infection, and suitable antibiotic alternatives, contribute to the decision-making process. Given the cost of broad-spectrum antibiotics and the increased prevalence of multidrug-resistant organisms, the need for more penicillin allergy education is clear.

11. What is the difference between an adverse reaction to penicillin and a true penicillin allergy?

An adverse reaction is an unwanted or unintended response to a drug. A true allergy (i.e., anaphylaxis) has four varieties (Table 11-9). Penicillin has been associated with several of these allergy types, but only one is immediately life threatening, a type I allergy. A type I allergy is IgE mediated and can be determined by skin testing. Knowing the difference between adverse reactions and the various types of allergies can assist in directing the history in patients who report a prior penicillin allergy. Examples of useful, directed questions to use in the patient who reports a penicillin allergy are shown in Box 11-1.

12. How accurate is the penicillin skin test in identifying patients who are not allergic to penicillin?

The penicillin skin test is useful in patients with a concerning or questionable history of a type I allergic reaction to penicillin and when no suitable alterative antimicrobial agents are available. Skin testing typically takes about 40 minutes and is therefore less useful in urgent situations. Certain medications, such as antihistamines, tricyclic antidepressants, and adrenergic drugs, can inhibit the skin test and require discontinuation at least 48 hours before testing. Skin testing involves an epidermal prick followed by an intradermal injection. It can reliably predict only IgE-mediated drug reactions.[52,58]

Table 11-9. Immunologic Classification of Allergic Reactions to Drugs

Immunologic Class	Antibody Class	Typical Onset	Common Clinical Manifestations	Examples
Type I (anaphylactic, immediate hypersensitivity)	IgE	≤ 60 min	Ranges from urticaria to bronchoconstriction, laryngeal edema, hypotension, and circulatory collapse	Penicillin, blood products, vaccines, dextran
Type II (cytotoxic)	IgG, IgM	5-12 hr	Hemolytic anemia, granulocytopenia, thrombocytopenia	Penicillin, sulfonamides
Type III (immune complex)	IgG, IgM	3-8 hr	Serum sickness symptoms, drug fever, glomerulonephritis	Penicillin, sulfonamides
Type IV (cell mediated)	None known	24-48 hr	Contact dermatitis, graft rejection	Preservatives
Type V (idiopathic)	Unknown	Varies, usually > 72 hr	Maculopapular rash, Stevens-Johnson syndrome, eosinophilia	Penicillin, sulfonamides

Adapted from Golembiewski JA: Allergic reactions to drugs: Implications for perioperative care. J Perianesth Nurs 2002;17:393-398.

Box 11-1. Questions to Ask during the Penicillin Allergy History

- What was the patient's age at the time of the reaction?

- Does the patient recall the reaction? If not, who informed them of it?

- How long after beginning penicillin did the reaction begin?

- What were the characteristics of the reaction?

- What was the route of administration?

- Why was the patient taking penicillin?

- What other medications was the patient taking? Why and when were they prescribed?

- What happened when the penicillin was discontinued?

- Has the patient taken antibiotics similar to penicillin (for example, amoxicillin, ampicillin, cephalosporins) before or after the reaction? If yes, what was the result?

Adapted from Salkind AR, Cuddy PG, Foxworth JW: The rational clinical examination. Is this patient allergic to penicillin? An evidence-based analysis of the likelihood of penicillin allergy. JAMA 2001;285:2498-505.

Systemic reactions occur in about 1% of those skin tested and are usually mild. However, when systemic reactions do occur, they can be serious, and skin testing therefore should be done only under the supervision of physicians familiar with the test.

For patients with negative skin test results and a history of penicillin allergy, IgE-mediated reactions occur in 2% to 15% of patients who are treated subsequently with penicillins, depending on the clinical history. These reactions, however, are mild and self-limited. Anaphylaxis in the setting of a negative result for a penicillin skin test has not been documented in the United States. The positive predictive value of skin testing is unable to be determined because skin test–positive patients are not subsequently treated with penicillins.[59]

Ideally, all major determinants (e.g., β-lactam ring, benzyl penicilloyl) and as many minor determinants (e.g., side chains, penicillin G) of β-lactams as possible should be included in the skin test. Using major determinants alone can detect 75% to 95% of potential allergies. Using major and minor determinants can detect up to 99% cases.[60,61] A negative penicillin test result rules out the potential for an allergy with a 97% to 99% success rate.[50,51] Aside from the time required for testing, there are few limitations to the procedure. Reliable estimates of the sensitivity and specificity for penicillin skin testing compared with a reference standard such as an oral challenge have never been generated, mostly because few studies have compared the two.[52] There are no formal contraindications to performing the test. Figures 11-1, 11-2, and 11-3 provide more information about the appropriate scenarios for penicillin skin testing.

13. In patients who report antibiotic allergies, when is drug desensitization required?

Desensitization is indicated when a patient has a clear history of a type I allergy and there are no alternative antibiotic substitutions. It is indicated each time the patient is re-exposed to a course of the antibiotic. Desensitization is a procedure in which small incremental doses of the drug are given at 15- or 20-minute intervals (as tolerated), based on established protocols for oral and parenteral treatment, respectively, until therapeutic doses are achieved. Typically, about 14 to 18 incremental doses are administered in total. The antibiotic may then safely be given at therapeutic doses, with care to avoid lapses in therapy. It is hypothesized that IgE is neutralized or mast cells are slowly degranulated during the course of the desensitization procedure.[58,64] If desensitization is halted for 48 hours, the process must be restarted. Mild skin reactions occur in up to a third of patients, but severe reactions have not been documented.[64]

14. What is the cross-reactivity between cephalosporin and penicillin antibiotics?

Previous studies have shown inconsistent results regarding cross-reactivity between penicillins and

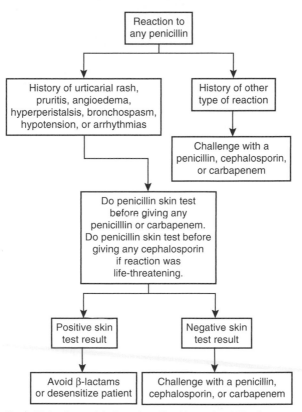

Figure 11-1. Approach to the patient with a history of penicillin allergy. (Adapted from Robinson J, Hameed T, Carr S: Practical aspects of choosing an antibiotic for patients with a reported allergy to an antibiotic. Clin Infect Dis. 2002;35:26-31.)

cephalosporins.[53,62] Early studies showed that patients allergic to penicillin had a fourfold increased risk for developing a reaction when treated with cephalosporins, with a higher risk correlating with first-generation cephalosproins.[62] Few studies with large numbers of subjects have challenged patients who had positive penicillin skin test results with cephalosporins. One review[63] tallied data from seven studies and found that among

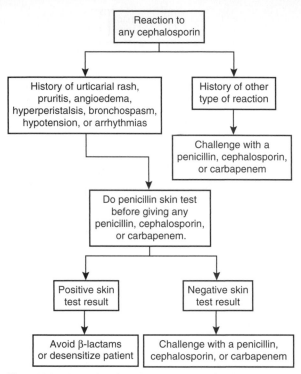

Figure 11-2. Approach to the patient with a history of cephalosporin allergy. (Adapted from Robinson J, Hameed T, Carr S: Practical aspects of choosing an antibiotic for patients with a reported allergy to an antibiotic. Clin Infect Dis 2002;35:26-31.)

135 patients, 6 had reactions. This indicates a 4.4% cross-reactivity rate for cephalosporins in patients with type I allergies to penicillin.[63]

The importance of the side chain of the β-lactam antibiotic rather than the β-lactam ring itself (considered the main antigenic determinant) has been highlighted. The side chain is an antigenic determinant. Older cephalosporins have a side chain similar to the side chain of penicillin, and this may have resulted in the initial reports of anaphylactic reactions to cephalosporins. Older cephalosporins may also have contained trace amounts of penicillin.

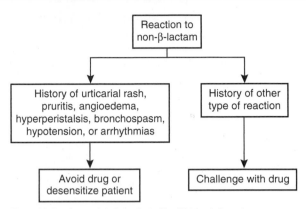

Figure 11-3. Approach to the patient with a history of allergy to a non-β-lactam drug. (Adapted from Robinson J, Hamood T, Carr S: Practical aspects of choosing an antibiotic for patients with a reported allergy to an antibiotic. Clin Infect Dis 2002;35:26-31.)

The cross-reactivity of second- or third-generation cephalosporin (excluding cefamandole) with penicillins is probably not higher than that of any other class of antibiotic.[58,63] In a prospective study,[53] 128 patients with a history of allergic reactions to penicillin and positive skin test results were then skin tested with cephalothin, cefamandole, cefuroxime, ceftazidime, ceftriaxone, and cefotaxime. Of these, 10.9% had positive skin test results for cephalosporins (mostly the first-generation cephalothin and the second-generation cefamandole), and skin test results for the minor determinants were positive in 71.4% with cross-reactivity and 38.6% without cross-reactivity, leading the study authors to conclude that avoiding cephalosporins with a history of positive skin test results for penicillin is prudent.[53]

REFERENCES

1. Jain P, Parada JP, David A, et al: Overuse of the indwelling urinary catheter in hospitalized medical patients. Arch Intern Med. 1995;155:1425-1429. **III**

2. Hartstein AI, Garber SB, Ward TT, et al: Nosocomial urinary tract infection: A prospective evaluation of 108 catheterized patients. Infect Control 1981;2: 380-386. **III**

3. Warren JW: Catheter associated urinary tract infections. Infect Dis Clin North Am 1997;11:609-622. V

4. Kunin C: Nosocomial urinary tract infections and indwelling catheter: What is new and what is true? Chest 2001;120:10-12. V

5. Warren JW: Catheter-associated urinary tract infections. Int J Antimicrob Agent 2001;17:299-303. V

6. Wagenlehner FME, Naber KG: Hospital-acquired urinary tract infections. J Hosp Infect 2000;46:171-181. V

7. Platt R, Polk BF, Murdock B, Rosner B: Risk factors for nosocomial urinary tract infection. Am J Epidemiol 1986;124:977-985. III

8. Guidelines for preventing infections associated with the insertion and maintenance of short-term indwelling urethral catheters in acute care. J Hosp Infect 2001;47(Suppl):39-46. IV

9. Ouslander JG, Greengold B, Chen S: Complications of chronic indwelling urinary catheters among male nursing home patients: A prospective study. J Urol 1987; 138:1191-1195. III

10. Ouslander JG, Greengold B, Chen S. External Catheter use and urinary tract infections among incontinent male nursing home patients. J Am Geriatr Soc 1987; 35:1063-1070. III

11. King RB, Carlson CE, Mervine J, et al: Clean and sterile intermittent catheterization methods in hospitalized patients with spinal cord injury. Arch Phys Med Rehabil 1992;73:798-802. II

12. Shapiro J, Hoffman J, Jersky J: A comparison of suprapubic and transurethral drainage for postoperative urinary retention in general surgical patients. Acta Chir Scand 1982;148:323-327. III

13. Rupp ME, Fitzgerald T, Marion N, et al: Effect of silver-coated urinary catheters: Efficacy, cost-effectiveness, and antimicrobial resistance. Am J Infect Control 2004;32:445-450. III

14. Riley DK, Classen DC, Stevens LE, Burke JP: A large randomized clinical trial of a silver-impregnated urinary catheter: Lack of efficacy and staphylococcal superinfection. Am J Med 1995;98:349-356. II

15. Saint S, Elmore JG, Sullivan SD, et al: The efficacy of silver alloy-coated urinary catheters in preventing urinary tract infection: A meta-analysis. Am J Med 1998;105:234-236. I

16. Tambyah PA: Catheter-associated urinary tract infections: Diagnosis and prophylaxis. Int J Antimicrob Agent 2004;24S:S44-S48. V

17. Lai KK, Fontecchio SA: Use of silver-hydrogel catheters on the incidence of catheter-associated urinary tract infections in hospitalized patients. Am J Infect Control 2002;30:221-225. III

18. DiFilippo A, DeGaudio AR: Device-related infections in critically ill patients. Part II. Prevention of ventilator-associated pneumonia and urinary tract infections. J Chemother 2003;15:536-542. V

19. Saint S, Wiese J, Amory JK, et al: Are physicians aware which of their patients have an indwelling catheter? Am J Med 2000;160:678-682. III

20. Huang WC, Wann SR, Lin SL, et al: Catheter-associated urinary tract infections in intensive care units can be reduced by prompting physicians to remove unnecessary catheters. Infect Control Hosp Epidemiol 2004; 25:974-978. III

21. Wong ES, Hooton TM: Guidelines for prevention of catheter-associated urinary tract infections. Am J Infect Control 1983;11:28-36. IV

22. Garibaldi RA, Mooney BR, Epstein BJ, et al: An evaluation of daily bacteriologic monitoring to identify preventable episodes of catheter-associated urinary tract infection. Infect Control 1982;3:466-470. VI

23. Harding GKM, Nicolle LE, Ronald AR, et al: How long should catheter acquired urinary tract infection in women be treated. Ann Intern Med 1991;114: 713-719. II

24. Mangram AJ, Horan TC, Pearson ML, et al: Guideline for prevention of surgical site infection, 1999. Hospital Infection Control Practices Advisory Committee. Infect Control Hosp Epidemiol 1999;20:250-278. IV

25. Sessler DI, Akca O: Nonpharmacologic prevention of surgical wound infections. Clin Infect Dis 2002;35: 1397-1404. V

26. Kurz A, Sessler DI, Lenhardt RA: Perioperative normothermia to reduce the incidence of surgical-wound infection and shorten hospitalization. N Engl J Med 1996;334:1209-1215. II

27. Kotani N, Hashimoto H, Sessler DI, et al: Supplemental intraoperative oxygen augments antimicrobial and proinflammatory responses of alveolar macrophages. Anesthesiology 2000;93:15-25. III

28. Greif R, Akca O, Horn E-P, et al: Supplemental perioperative oxygen to reduce the incidence of surgical wound infection. N Engl J Med 2000;342:161-167. II

29. McCray E, Martone WJ, Wise RP, Culver DH: Risk factors for wound infections after genitourinary reconstructive surgery. Am J Epidemiol 1986;123:1026-1032. III

30. Seropian R, Reynolds BM: Wound infections after preoperative depilatory versus razor preparation. Am J Surg 1971;121:251-254. II

31. van den Berghe G, Wouters P, Wcekers F, et al: Intensive insulin therapy in the critically ill patients. N Engl J Med 2001;345:1359-1367. II

32. Furnary AP, Zerr K, Grunkemeier GL, Starr A: Continuous intravenous insulin infusion reduces the incidence of deep sternal wound infection in diabetic patients after cardiac surgical procedures [see discussion]. Ann Thorac Surg 1999;67:352-362. II

33. Bratzler D, Houck PM, for the Surgical Infection Prevention Guidelines Writers Workgroup: Antimicrobial prophylaxis for surgery: An advisory statement from the National Surgical Infection Prevention Project. Clin Infect Dis 2004;38:1706-1715. IV

34. Bratzler D, Houck PM, Richards C, et al: Use of antimicrobial prophylaxis for major surgery. Baseline results from the National Surgical Infection Prevention Project. Arch Surg 2005;140:174-182. III

35. American Society of Health-System Pharmacists: ASHP therapeutic guidelines on antimicrobial prophylaxis in surgery. Am J Health Syst Pharm 1999; 56:1839-1888. IV

36. Page CP, Bohnen JM, Fletcher JR, et al: Antimicrobial prophylaxis for surgical wounds: Guidelines for clinical care. Arch Surg 1993;128:79-88. IV

37. Perl TM, Cullen JJ, Wenzel RP, et al: Intranasal mupirocin to prevent postoperative *Staphylococcus aureus* infections. N Engl J Med 2002;346:1871-7187. II

38. Reagan DR, Doebbeling BN, Pfaller MA, et al: Elimination of coincident *Staphylococcus aureus* nasal and hand carriage with intranasal application of mupirocin calcium ointment. Ann Intern Med 1991;114:101-106. II

39. Doebbeling BN, Breneman DL, Neu HC, et al: Elimination of *Staphylococcus aureus* nasal carriage in health care workers: Analysis of six clinical trials with calcium mupirocin ointment. The Mupirocin

Collaborative Study Group. Clin Infect Dis 1993; 17:466-474. **II**

40. Kluytmans JA, Mouton JW, Van den Bergh MF, et al: Reduction of surgical site infections in cardiothoracic surgery by elimination of nasal carriage of *Staphylococcus aureus*. Infect Control Hosp Epidemiol 1996;17:780-785. **III**

41. Cimochowski GE, Harostock MD, Brown R, et al: Intranasal mupirocin reduces sternal wound infection after open heart surgery in diabetics and nondiabetics. Ann Thorac Surg 2001;71:1572-1579. **III**

42. Usry G, Johnson L, Weems J, Blackhurst D: Process improvement plan for the reduction of sternal surgical site infections among patients undergoing coronary artery bypass graft surgery. Am J Infect Control 2002;30: 434-436. **III**

43. Gernaat-van der Sluis AJ, Hoogenboom-Verdegaal AM, Edixhoven PJ, Spies-van Rooijen NH: Prophylactic mupirocin could reduce orthopedic wound infections: 1,044 patients treated with mupirocin compared with 1,260 historical controls. Acta Orthop Scand 1998;69:412-414. **III**

44. Suzuki Y, Kamigaki T, Fujino Y, et al: Randomized clinical trial of preoperative intranasal mupirocin to reduce surgical-site infection after digestive surgery. Br J Surg 2003;90:1072-1075. **II**

45. Yu VL, Goetz A, Wagener M, et al: *Staphylococcus aureus* nasal carriage and infection in patients on hemodialysis: efficacy of antibiotic prophylaxis. N Engl J Med 1986;315:91-96. **II**

46. Roberts GJ, Gardner P, Simmons NA: Optimum sampling time for detection of dental bacteraemia in children. Int J Cardiol 1992;35:311-315. **III**

47. van der Meer JTM, van Wijk W, Thompson J, et al: Efficacy of antibiotic prophylaxis for prevention of native-valve endocarditis. Lancet 1992;339:135-139. **III**

48. Dajani AS, Taubert KA, Wilson W, et al: Prevention of bacterial endocarditis. Recommendations by the American Heart Association. JAMA 1997;277:1794-1801. **IV**

49. Durack DT: Prevention of infective endocarditis. N Engl J Med 1995;332:38-44. **V**

50. Gadde J, Spence M, Wheeler B, Adkinson NF: Clinical experience with penicillin skin testing in a large inner-city STD clinic. JAMA 1993;270:2456-2463. **III**

51. Sogn DD, Evans R, Shepherd GM, et al: Results of the National Institute of Allergy and Infectious Diseases

Collaborative Clinical Trial to test the predictive value of skin testing with major and minor penicillin derivatives in hospitalized adults. Arch Intern Med 1992;152: 1025-1032. **III**

52. Salkind AR, Cuddy PG, Foxworth JW: The rational clinical examination. Is this patient allergic to penicillin? An evidence-based analysis of the likelihood of penicillin allergy. JAMA. 2001;285:2498-2505. **I**

53. Romano A, Gueant-Rodriguez R, Viola M, et al: Cross-reactivity and tolerability of cephalosporins in patients with immediate hypersensitivity to penicillins. Ann Intern Med 2004;141:16-22. **III**

54. Harris AD, Sauberman L, Kabbash L, et al: Penicillin skin testing: A way to optimize antibiotic utilization. Am J Med 1999;107:166-168. **III**

55. Puchner TC Jr, Zacharisen MC: A survey of antibiotic prescribing and knowledge of penicillin allergy. Ann Allergy Asthma Immunol 2002;88:1-3. **III**

56. Solensky R, Earl HS, Gruchalla RS: Clinical approach to penicillin-allergic patients: A survey. Ann Allergy Asthma Immunol 2000;84:329-333. **III**

57. Golembiewski JA: Allergic reactions to drugs: Implications for perioperative care. J Perianesth Nurs 2002;17:393-398. **V**

58. Robinson J, Hameed T, Carr S: Practical aspects of choosing an antibiotic for patients with a reported allergy to an antibiotic. Clin Infect Dis 2002;35:26-31. **V**

59. Weiss ME, Adkinson NF: Immediate hypersensitivity to penicillins and related antibiotics. Clin Allergy 1988;18:515-540. **III**

60. Adkinson NF Jr, Thompson WL, Maddrey WC, Lichtenstein LM: Routine use of penicillin skin testing on an inpatient service. N Engl J Med. 1971;285:22-24. **III**

61. Warrington RJ, Simons FER, Ho HW, et al: Diagnosis of penicillin allergy by skin testing: The Manitoba experience. CMAJ 1978;118:787-791. **III**

62. Anne S, Reisman RE: Risk of administering cephalosporin antibiotics to patients with histories of penicillin history. Ann Allergy Asthma Immunol 1995;74:167-170. **III**

63. Kelkar PS, Li JT: Cephalosporin allergy. N Engl J Med 2001;345:804-809. **I**

64. Dykewitz M. Adverse reactions to drugs. Clin Rev Allergy Immunol 2003;24:200-219. **V**

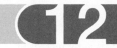

Psychiatric Issues in Medical Consultation

Melissa Reimel Cognetti, Colleen M. Crumlish, and Kendal Williams

1. What is the evidence for screening for and treating depression after myocardial infarction?

Search Date: April 2005

Search Strategy: *PubMed, clinical queries: systematic reviews: "depression AND myocardial infarction." Limited to English, 1990-2005; 46 citations retrieved. Separate search of "depression AND myocardial infarction OR postmyocardial infarction OR acute coronary syndrome OR post-MI AND mortality." Limited to humans, English language, 1990-2005; 465 citations retrieved. Separate search of "depression" and "myocardial infarction OR postmyocardial infarction OR acute coronary syndrome OR post-MI." Limited to human, English language, and randomized, controlled trials, 1990-2005; 179 citations retrieved. Titles and abstracts scanned, with relevant citations selected. Bibliographies of all relevant citations reviewed. Search of practice guidelines from the American College of Cardiology.*

Depression after acute myocardial infarction (MI) is common. Approximately one in six patients recovering from acute MI suffers from major depression, and at least twice as many experience depressive symptoms that do not fulfill criteria for major depression.[1] Several studies have shown that depression increases morbidity and mortality after acute MI.[2] Frasure-Smith and colleagues[3] found that patients with major depression during admission for acute MI have a threefold to fourfold increase in mortality within the first 6 months after MI compared with those who were not depressed. Patients with mild to moderate symptoms of depression based on the Beck

Depression Inventory also have a significantly increased mortality risk within the first 18 months after MI.[4] Although much of the literature in this area cites post-MI depression as an accepted independent predictor of increased mortality, a few studies failed to show a link between post-MI depression and cardiovascular outcomes.[5,6]

A meta-analysis performed by van Melle and coworkers[7] reviewed 22 prospective studies that addressed the association between depression after MI and cardiovascular prognosis. These studies described the post-MI follow-up (average, 13.7 months) of 6367 patients (16 cohorts). Post-MI depression was associated with a 2- to 2.5-fold increased risk of poor cardiovascular outcomes (OR for cardiac mortality = 2.59 [95% CI: 1.77 to 3.77]; OR for all-cause mortality = 2.38 [95% CI: 1.76 to 3.22]). The association was more pronounced in studies conducted before 1992 (OR = 3.22) than in later studies (OR = 2.01).[7]

In a systematic review, Sorensen and colleagues[8] called into question the validity of many of the studies linking post-MI depression with increased mortality. Thirty-one articles were reviewed and scored for quality, with only seven studies scoring above a predefined level of acceptable quality. The prevalence rates of depression ranged from 1.6% to 50%. A significant positive association was shown between depression and post-MI mortality in 15 studies, a nonsignificant association was seen in 14 studies, and association was not reported in 2 studies. The investigators concluded that many of the studies were not of acceptable quality, citing lack of sufficient power to show differences; use of nonvalidated instruments to assess depression, leading to wide variations in prevalence; and failure to provide sufficient details about the study populations.[8]

Aside from the possible role of depression increasing mortality risk after MI, it has been shown that depression is a predictor of poor quality of life in the first year after MI and that depressed patients are less likely to adhere to recommended lifestyle changes and medication regimens to reduce cardiac risk.[2,9] For these reasons, screening for depression in the post-MI setting is recommended. Ziegelstein[2] recommends screening for depression during hospitalization after MI as a way of predicting those at particular risk for nonadherence. In evaluating 153 post-MI patients older than 65 years, Romanelli and colleagues[10] found that older depressed patients are at greater risk for death, are prescribed fewer medications known to reduce cardiovascular risk, and have greater difficulty adhering to recommendations to reduce risk, concluding that more attention needs to be placed on identifying depression and making efforts to improve adherence in older adults. A study of 896 post-MI patients found that the level of depressive symptoms during admission is more closely linked to long-term survival than the level at 1 year, which also suggests that hospitalization is the best time to screen.[11] The absence of social support is also a risk factor for cardiac morbidity and mortality after MI, whereas high levels of social support seem to buffer the effect of depression on survival and predict improvement in depression during the first year after MI.[12] In their executive summary of the management of patients with ST segment elevation MI, the American College of Cardiology/American Heart Association (ACC/AHA) recommend that the psychosocial status of the patient be evaluated assessing for symptoms of depression, anxiety, sleep disorders, and low perceived level of social support. The guidelines recommend assessing post-MI patients for depression during hospitalization and during the first month after MI and performing yearly reassessments for depression in the first 5 years after MI as necessary.[13]

Although there seems to be a consensus regarding the importance of recognizing depression in the post-MI period, there is limited data regarding the optimal mode of treatment in terms of psychotherapy versus antidepressants, safety of antidepressants in post-MI patients, and whether treating depression decreases cardiac risk and improves survival.

The existing literature on depression pharmacotherapy for the post-MI patient is limited but suggests that selective serotonin reuptake inhibitors (SSRIs) are safer than tricyclic antidepressants (TCAs). TCAs should be avoided in patients with ischemic heart disease because of their tendency to increase heart rate, produce orthostatic hypotension, interfere with cardiac conduction, and increase susceptibility to ventricular arrhythmias.[1] In a study comparing the efficacy and safety of paroxetine with nortriptyline in 81 patients with ischemic heart disease and major depression, both medications improved symptoms of depression, but nortriptyline was associated with a significantly higher rate of serious adverse cardiac events.[14]

The Sertraline Antidepressant Heart Attack Randomized Trial (SADHART) was a randomized, controlled trial of 369 patients with depression after hospitalization for MI or unstable angina who were treated (initiated on average 34 days after MI) with sertraline (50 to 200 mg) or placebo for 24 weeks.[15] Sertraline was not superior to placebo with respect to measures of cardiovascular safety, including the primary outcome of left ventricular ejection fraction or secondary outcomes of heart rate, blood pressure, electrocardiographic parameters, Holter recordings for premature ventricular contractions, and heart rate variability. The incidence of cardiovascular events was less in the sertraline group, but it was not statistically significant, and this study was not sufficiently powered to assess risk reduction for cardiovascular mortality. Given that the course of post-MI depression often resembles that of an adjustment disorder with high rates of spontaneous recovery and placebo response, it was predetermined that sertraline efficacy would be assessed in a subset of patients with higher depression severity and history of prior depression. Sertraline was found to be superior to placebo in that subset of patients. Limitations of the SADHART study include failure to establish safety of SSRIs in the immediate post-MI period because treatment was initiated an average of 34 days after MI. Patients with significant medical comorbidities were excluded, leading to problems with generalizibility.[15] Another study with the same cohort found that sertraline therapy was associated with clinically meaningful improvement in multiple quality-of-life domains for patients with acute coronary syndrome and recurrent depression.[16]

There have been mixed results from studies evaluating the effect of psychosocial interventions on cardiovascular outcomes and mortality after MI. Two meta-analyses addressed this question and reported that psychosocial interventions after MI reduce all-cause mortality and cardiac morbidity.[17,18] However, a Cochrane systematic review analyzed 36 trials, many of which were of poor quality, and concluded that psychological interventions had no effect on total or cardiac mortality and produced small reductions in anxiety and depression.[19]

The Enhancing Recovery in Coronary Heart Disease Patients (ENRICHD) randomized trial is the latest and largest clinical trial that addresses whether mortality and recurrent infarction are reduced by treating depression and low perceived social support (LPSS) early (within 28 days) after MI.[20] A total of 2481 post-MI patients with depression (39%), LPSS (26%), or both (34%) were randomly assigned to usual care or cognitive-behavioral therapy (CBT) intervention for 6 months. SSRI medication (50 to 200 mg of sertraline) was added for those scoring higher than 24 on the Hamilton Rating Scale for Depression or having less than a 50% reduction in the Beck Depression Inventory score after 5 weeks of CBT. There was a statistically significant improvement in depression and perceived social support at 6 months, although the relative improvement compared with usual care was less than expected and diminished over time. At a median follow-up of 29 months, there was no significant difference in event-free survival between usual care (75.9%) and psychosocial intervention (75.8%). Potential confounding factors include spontaneous remission in the usual care group and a large percentage of patients in the usual care group being treated with pharmacotherapy for depression outside of the study, potentially masking the effect of CBT. In a post hoc analysis of this study, the risk of death or nonfatal MI was significantly lower in patients taking SSRIs (adjusted HR = 0.57; 95% CI: 0.38 to 0.85). The study authors conclude that this finding may result from chance or reflect a beneficial effect of pharmacotherapy on cardiac end points not mediated by change in depression. This effect is consistent with observational studies that have shown that SSRIs are associated with a reduced risk of MI, perhaps due to the inhibitory effects of SSRIs on platelets or combinations of other effects of SSRIs independent of treating depression.[21]

In summary, evidence exists to warrant screening for post-MI depression during hospitalization and follow-up. Sertraline is the only SSRI that has demonstrated safety in a randomized trial of post-MI patients. There is no evidence that antidepressant treatment improves cardiovascular mortality, and decisions therefore must be tailored to the individual patient. Additional randomized trials are needed to determine the optimal timing and duration of psychosocial interventions, evaluate the safety of antidepressants in post-MI patients, and determine the effects of antidepressants on cardiac end points. The ongoing study Myocardial Infarction and Depression-Intervention Trial (MIND-IT) is a randomized, placebo-controlled trial evaluating treatment of post-MI depression with mirtazapine and its effect on cardiac prognosis.[22]

2. What is the recommended medical evaluation for patients undergoing electroconvulsive therapy?

Search Date: April 2005

Search Strategy: PubMed, search of "electroconvulsive therapy OR ECT" and " medical evaluation OR medical consultation OR risk factors OR cardiovascular complications OR beta blockers OR pacemakers OR defibrillators." Limited to humans, English language, 1980-2005; 382 citations retrieved. Separate search strategy using PubMed: clinical queries: systematic reviews, search of "electroconvulsive therapy." Limited to human and English language; 98 citations retrieved. Titles and abstracts scanned, with relevant citations selected. Bibliographies of all relevant citations reviewed.

Electroconvulsive therapy (ECT) is a commonly performed procedure with established efficacy for psychiatric disorders, including major depression, mania, bipolar disorder, and psychotic disorders such as schizophrenia.[23] ECT is generally thought to be a low-risk procedure, with medical consultation primarily sought in cases that require clarification of medical status or management of known medical conditions. The mortality rate associated with ECT is 0.2 to 0.4 per 10,000 treatments, which is not higher than the mortality rate for general anesthesia.[24] The role of the medical consultant in ECT is to identify medical conditions that put the patient at increased risk, propose strategies for risk reduction, and manage complications during and after the procedure. Performing a preprocedural evaluation for ECT requires some knowledge of the physiologic responses that occur during the procedure.

The goal of ECT is to induce a 30- to 60-second tonic-clonic seizure. The procedure is performed under general anesthesia with the use of short-acting intravenous agents, most commonly methohexital or propofol. A neuromuscular agent is given before the procedure to prevent injury or fracture.[25] Delivery of the ECT stimulus is associated with an immediate increase in parasympathetic activity that may cause bradycardia and may rarely progress to asystole. An anticholinergic agent (i.e., atropine or glycopyrrolate) is given before the procedure to minimize this effect. The transient vagal discharge is followed by sympathetic stimulation that causes tachycardia and hypertension and results in an increase in myocardial oxygen demand equivalent to that of moderate exercise. These hemodynamic responses usually return to baseline within 3 to 20 minutes after the seizure.[26,27]

There are no absolute medical contraindications to ECT. The American Psychiatric Association (APA) states that the following conditions are associated with increased risk[23]:

- Unstable or severe cardiovascular conditions such as recent MI, unstable angina, poorly compensated congestive heart failure (CHF), and severe valvular disease
- Aneurysm or vascular malformation that may be susceptible to rupture with increased blood pressure
- Increased intracranial pressure, as may occur with some brain tumors or other space-occupying cerebral lesions
- Recent cerebral infarction
- Pulmonary conditions such as severe chronic obstructive pulmonary disease, asthma, or pneumonia
- Patient status rated as American Society of Anesthesiologists (ASA) level 4 or 5

The cornerstone of the pre-ECT evaluation is a careful medical history and examination focusing primarily on the cardiovascular, pulmonary, and neurologic systems in addition to inquiring about previous complications with anesthesia or ECT. There is minimal evidence available regarding the utility of laboratory testing before ECT. A study by Lafferty and colleagues[28] assessed the utility of electrocardiogram (ECG); serum levels of sodium, potassium, and creatinine; chest radiograph, hemoglobin concentration, and white blood cell count in the evaluation for ECT. These investigators concluded that measuring serum sodium and potassium levels and reviewing an ECG are useful screening tests because they detected correctable conditions that are relevant to the risk of the procedure and that would not be detected by history and physical examination. Hemoglobin and white blood cell count abnormalities did not predict ECT complications. The serum creatinine level and chest radiograph predicted a poor medical prognosis that appeared unrelated to administration of ECT and may only be useful in those older than 55 years.[28] The APA reports that no specific laboratory tests are routinely required in the pre-ECT evaluation, but they do state that it is common practice to perform a minimum battery of tests, including a complete blood cell count, serum potassium and sodium levels, and an ECG.[23] In general, the use of pre-ECT laboratory testing should be prompted by specific information obtained from the history and examination or from medical conditions or medications that increase the likelihood of an abnormality. For example, levels of serum electrolytes should be checked in patients on diuretics or with renal dysfunction.[23]

3. How does cardiovascular disease affect the medical evaluation before electroconvulsive therapy?
Cardiovascular complications represent the most common cause of ECT-related morbidity and mortality.[23] There are limited data that examine the cardiac complications from ECT in patients with established cardiovascular disease. One study of 40 patients found cardiac complications in 30%, but most were transient arrhythmias that have also been observed in patients without cardiovascular disease.[29] Zielinski and colleagues[30] performed a small, prospective study that also found an increased rate of cardiac complications among those with cardiac disease, particularly those with coronary artery

disease (CAD), but most of the complications were transitory and did not prevent the completion of the course of ECT. It is recommended that all patients with suspected CAD have a chest radiograph and ECG before ECT.[30] ECT is a low-risk procedure according to the AHA/ACC guidelines for noncardiac surgery. The guidelines state that extensive evaluation is unnecessary in most patients, except those with major clinical predictors of cardiovascular risk (i.e., unstable coronary syndromes, decompensated CHF, severe valvular disease, and significant arrhythmias).[25] More information on cardiovascular preoperative assessment can be found in Chapter 4.

4. Should prophylactic beta blockers be used during electroconvulsive therapy?

The use of prophylactic beta blockers for ECT is controversial. Data from the perioperative literature suggest that initiating beta-blocker therapy before surgery reduces cardiovascular risk and decreases overall mortality, but it is not clear whether these data can be extrapolated to ECT. No studies have documented that use of beta blockers before ECT reduces cardiac complications. Castelli and coworkers[31] compared esmolol and labetalol with placebo in patients at increased cardiac risk and found that beta blockers did reduce ECT-induced hemodynamic elevations, but no evidence was found with respect to reduction of cardiac complications. The APA reports that the decision to use beta blockers requires clinical judgment but makes no specific recommendation regarding their use. However, they do suggest that indiscriminant use of beta blockers should be avoided for the following reasons[23]:

1. Beta blockers may increase risk of asystole (less of a risk if atropine used).
2. Patients with baseline tachycardia and hypertension have the least dramatic increases after seizure induction and therefore preprocedural lowering may be unnecessary.
3. There is a theoretical risk that blunting the hemodynamic response may reduce the necessary cerebral

blood flow and oxygen supply and lead to short-ened seizure length and the potential for greater cognitive side effects.

Some investigators recommend use of short-acting prophylactic beta blockers in conjunction with atropine in patients with established CAD or multiple coronary risk factors.[26]

5. How should electroconvulsive therapy be managed in patients with specific medical conditions?

There is a general lack of prospective trials focused on the effectiveness, safety, and optimal management strategies for patients with significant medical illnesses who undergo ECT. Most reviews and guidelines regarding the medical evaluation before ECT are generated from case reports and case series.

CORONARY ARTERY DISEASE

For patients with CAD, the primary focus should be on optimal stabilization of cardiac status before treatment. Cardiac medications, including nitrates and beta blockers, should be continued in patients who are already taking them and should be given on the morning of ECT.[32] Diuretics should be held on the morning of ECT because of the risk of a full bladder and potential rupture. All lidocaine-type agents should be held because they can block seizure elicitation.[23,32] There are no clear guidelines on a safe interval to initiate ECT after MI, and the decision must take into account the severity of depression and cardiac stability of the patient.[32]

DYSRHYTHMIAS

Patients with asymptomatic, uncomplicated cardiac conduction delays, such as first-degree heart block or bundle branch block, can be safely treated with ECT.[32] Patients with atrial fibrillation should be adequately rate controlled before ECT, and because conversion to normal sinus occasionally occurs with ECT, pretreatment anticoagulation is optimal.[33] Malignant ventricular arrhythmias place patients at increased risk for hemodynamic instability and require consultation with cardiology for risk management.[32,34]

PACEMAKERS AND IMPLANTABLE DEFIBRILLATORS

ECT is thought to be safe in patients with cardiac pacemakers (PMs) and implantable cardiac defibrillators (ICDs) despite a paucity of evidence. Before 2004, there were only 11 case reports of patients with PMs or ICDs receiving ECT. Dolenc and colleagues[35] conducted a review of a significantly larger series of 26 patients with PMs and 3 with ICDs who received ECT and concluded that ECT could be safely used in these patients. Guidelines for monitoring patients with PMs and ICDs during ECT treatments suggest using multi-lead ECG monitoring and having equipment available in case central access or transvenous pacing is required. Skeletal muscle potentials that occur during ECT may trigger the activity of the PM or inhibit demand PMs. It is recommended that a magnet be available to place over the pulse generator to convert from demand to asynchronous mode if inhibition causes bradycardia or asystole.[25,35] PMs and ICDs should be interrogated to document programmed parameters before the first treatment and again after completion of the course of ECT. There is some controversy regarding the management of ICDs during ECT. The risk of deactivating an ICD during ECT is the occurrence of tachyarrhythmias that would not be treated. The risk of leaving an ICD in active mode is inappropriate firing, which can cause a ventricular arrhythmia that may not be detected due to simultaneous electromagnetic interference from the ECT. Pending further study, it is recommended that ICDs be temporarily deactivated before each ECT treatment and that careful cardiac monitoring take place during ECT with an external defibrillator available.[35]

HYPERTENSION

Optimal blood pressure control should be attained in hypertensive patients before ECT initiation. ECT causes transient increases in blood pressure in the peri-ictal period but does not result in sustained increases in blood pressure. Antihypertensive medications should be continued with the exception of diuretics, which should be held on the morning of ECT. If there are significant risks to elevations in blood pressure (e.g., vascular or cardiac aneurysms, severe left ventricular or valvular compromise), patients should be premedicated with short-acting agents most appropriate for the clinical situation.[32]

CONGESTIVE HEART FAILURE OR VALVULAR HEART DISEASE

Scant data exist regarding the specific risks of ECT in patients with CHF or valvular disease. ECT should be delayed in patients with decompensated heart failure or severe valvular disease. Patients with a history of CHF without a recent assessment of left ventricular function and those who have evidence of valve disease or heart failure on history and examination should undergo an echocardiogram before proceeding with ECT.[34] Cardiac status should be optimized with medications before ECT initiation. Laboratory testing for patients with CHF should include electrolytes. Large volumes of fluids should be avoided, and efforts to prevent hemodynamic stress should be attempted.[34]

ANTICOAGULATION

Patients who are on chronic anticoagulation for deep venous thrombosis, valvular heart disease, atrial fibrillation, or another strong indication should continue it during ECT.[23]

NEUROLOGIC DISEASE

Patients with elevated intracranial pressure (ICP) are at increased risk for neurologic deterioration with ECT. Small or chronic space-occupying lesions without evidence of increased ICP pose minimal risk, but in cases of a known intracranial tumor, consultation with a neurologist or neurosurgeon is indicated. Patients at risk for hemorrhagic cerebrovascular events should avoid hypertension through the use of periprocedural blood pressure agents. In contrast, care should be taken to avoid hypotension in those with ischemic cerebrovascular disease. Cognitive dysfunction during and immediately after ECT may be worse in patients with Parkinson's disease, dementia, multiple sclerosis, and brain trauma, but these diagnoses are not contraindications for ECT. Patients who have a history of neuroleptic malignant syndrome can undergo ECT.[23]

DIABETES

Patients with diabetes should hold oral hypoglycemic agents on the morning of ECT because patient usually do not eat before the procedure.[32] More information on insulin management in the fasting patient can be found in Chapter 10.

PULMONARY DISORDERS

The two most common pulmonary disorders among patients undergoing ECT are chronic obstructive pulmonary disease and asthma. There is little data about the efficacy and safety of ECT in these populations. The APA Committee on ECT recommends that these patients receive prescribed bronchodilators before ECT and that special attention be given to oxygenation. It is also recommended that theophylline be discontinued before ECT or, if medically necessary, that it be maintained at the lowest therapeutic level because of the risk of status epilepticus with ECT and theophylline. Patients who must continue theophylline should have a level obtained and any necessary dose adjustments made before ECT.[23,32]

6. **What are the screening recommendations and management strategies for hypothyroidism associated with lithium therapy?**

Search Date: April 2005

Search Strategy: *PubMed, search for "lithium" AND "thyroid OR hypothyroid." Limited to humans, English language, 1990-2005; 210 citations retrieved. Titles and abstracts scanned, with relevant citations selected. Bibliographies of all relevant citations reviewed. Search of practice guidelines from the American Association of Clinical Endocrinologists and the American Psychiatric Association.*

Lithium is known to increase the risk for thyroid dysfunction, most commonly causing goiter or hypothyroidism. In patients taking lithium, the prevalence of overt hypothyroidism ranges from 8% to 19%, compared with a prevalence of 0.5% to 1.8% in the general population. Subclinical hypothyroidism, which is defined as an elevated serum thyroid-stimulating hormone (TSH) level with normal serum level of free thyroxine (FT_4), has been reported in up to 23% of patients on lithium therapy, compared with rates of up to 10.4% in the general population.[36]

Lithium interferes with thyroid hormone synthesis and release through several mechanisms. When lithium therapy is initiated, there may be a compensatory rise in TSH during the first year of treatment that is usually transient.[36,37] Several prospective studies have revealed that many patients with one abnormal set of thyroid function test results after initiation of lithium therapy revert to a euthyroid state within the first 1 to 2 years of treatment.[37,38] However, the risk of progression of lithium-induced thyroid dysfunction may be increased in those with a history of prior thyroid dysfunction or a history of antithyroid antibodies indicative of autoimmune thyroiditis. Patients who are positive for antithyroid antibodies before lithium therapy have higher rates of lithium-associated thyroid dysfunction. It has also been suggested that lithium promotes development of autoimmune thyroiditis, but prospective studies have failed to show a greater incidence of thyroid antibody formation in those receiving lithium.[36] A study by Kupka and colleagues[39] found thyroid autoimmunity to be highly prevalent in those with bipolar disorder but unrelated to lithium treatment. They concluded that thyroid autoimmunity and lithium are independent but cumulative risk factors for hypothyroidism. In a retrospective study of 695 patients on lithium therapy for an average duration of 7 years, Johnston and Eagles[40] found that the primary risk factor for development of clinical hypothyroidism was female gender (14% of women versus 4.5% of men). Women were at highest risk during the first 2 years of treatment, and women between the ages of 40 and 59 years had the highest overall prevalence.

There is limited evidence regarding the optimal screening algorithm for hypothyroidism in those on lithium, and most recommendations are based on expert opinion and clinical guidelines. In their practice guideline for the treatment of patients with bipolar disorder, the APA recommends that patients undergo a thyroid function evaluation before initiating lithium therapy and that thyroid function be assessed once or twice during the first 6 months of therapy and every 6 months to 1 year thereafter unless indicated earlier due to clinical symptoms or signs.[41] Kleiner and colleagues[36] recommend that laboratory tests before initiation of lithium should include TSH, FT_4, antiperoxidase antibody, and antithyroglobulin antibody. They recommend the antibody tests as a means of identifying those at higher risk for lithium-induced subclinical hypothyroidism. The TSH assay should be repeated 3 months into therapy and then every 6 to 12 months.[36] If the TSH level is elevated at any point, a FT_4 level should be checked and the TSH test repeated. If the patient has overt hypothyroidism based on an elevated TSH and a subnormal FT_4 level, thyroxine therapy is indicated.[36] T_4 (levothyroxine) rather than T_3 (levotriiodothyronine) supplementation is recommended. Hypothyroidism is not a contraindication to continuing lithium therapy.[41]

If the patient has subclinical hypothyroidism based on an elevated TSH and a normal FT_4 level, the decision concerning whether to treat is more complicated. The scenario is similar to the decision analysis required for those with subclinical hypothyroidism who are not taking lithium.[42] If the TSH concentration is between 5 and 10 mU/L and the patient has no symptoms, thyroid replacement is not immediately necessary, and the TSH level should be rechecked in 1 to 2 months while monitoring for symptoms. If the TSH level is between 5 and 10 mU/L and the patient has symptoms that could be attributable to depressed thyroid function, thyroxine therapy should be initiated at a dose of 25 to 50 µg/day, increasing by 25 µg every 6 weeks until the serum TSH concentration is within normal range.[36] In bipolar patients exhibiting depressive symptoms associated with subclinical hypothyroidism, treatment with thyroxine should precede a trial of antidepressant medication, which may induce mania. Figure 12-1 provides a general approach to subclinical hypothyroidism.

For overt hypothyroidism (i.e., elevated TSH and subnormal FT_4 levels), thyroxine should be initiated regardless of whether a patient is symptomatic. The optimal dose of thyroxine is related to body weight and is 1.6 to 1.8 µg/kg/day in otherwise healthy adults. For older adults or those with mild hypothyroidism, dosing of 0.5 µg/kg/day is usually sufficient.[43] Because thyroxine can exacerbate myocardial ischemia through increased sympathetic tone, patients with ischemic heart disease

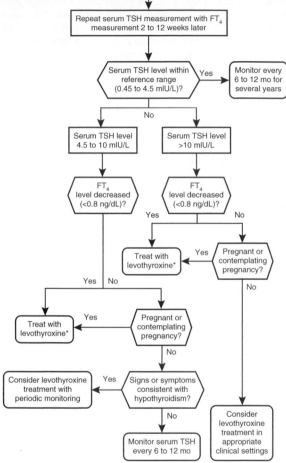

Figure 12-1. Suggested approach to the diagnosis and management of subclinical hypothyroidism. The normal range of free T_4 (FT_4) is 0.8 to 2.0 ng/dL (10 to 25 pmol/L); the normal range of thyroid-stimulating hormone (TSH) is 0.45 to 4.5 mIU/L. In rare instances *(asterisk)*, a slightly elevated serum TSH level represents hypothalamic-pituitary disease. In these situations, the FT_4 value is extremely low when the TSH level is only slightly elevated, in contrast to primary hypothyroidism, in which the TSH level

increases exponentially with small decreases in the serum FT_4 concentration. (Adapted from Col NF, Surks MI, Daniels GH: Subclinical thyroid disease: Clinical applications. JAMA 2004;291:239-243.)

should be started at lower doses (i.e., 25 µg/day with titration by 12.5 to 25 µg every 4 to 6 weeks, regardless of the degree of hypothyroidism).[43] After a maintenance dose is determined, TSH levels should be checked every 6 to 12 months or at any point if symptoms arise that suggest thyroid hormone excess or deficiency.[44]

7. How is delirium diagnosed?

Search Date: May 2005

Search Strategy: PubMed, clinical queries: systematic reviews: "delirium" or "acute confusional state." Limited to human and English language; 131 citations retrieved. Search of "delirium" OR "acute confusional state." Limited to randomized, controlled trial or meta-analysis, human and English language; 156 citations retrieved. Search of "delirium or acute confusional state" AND "pharmacotherapy." Limited to clinical trials, human and English language, 1990-2005; 85 citations retrieved. Titles and abstracts scanned with relevant citations selected. Bibliographies of all relevant citations reviewed. Search of practice guidelines from the American Psychiatric Association.

Delirium is a clinical diagnosis. The symptoms of delirium are wide ranging, but the essential features include disturbances of consciousness, attention, cognition, and perception. The disturbance develops over a short period and tends to fluctuate during the course of the day. The *Diagnostic and Statistical Manual of Mental Disorders*, fourth edition (DSM-IV) provides the following criteria for delirium[45]:

A. Disturbance of consciousness (i.e., reduced clarity of awareness of the environment) with reduced ability to focus, sustain, or shift attention

B. A change in cognition (e.g., memory deficit, disorientation, language disturbance) or the development of a perceptual disturbance (e.g., misinterpretations, illusions, hallucinations) that is not better accounted for by a preexisting, established, or evolving dementia

C. Disturbance developing over a short period (usually hours to days) and tending to fluctuate during the course of the day

D. Evidence from the history, physical examination, or laboratory tests that the disturbance is a direct physiologic consequence of a general medical condition, substance intoxication or withdrawal, use of a medication, toxin exposure, or a combination of these factors

Other commonly associated features of delirium include disturbances of sleep, psychomotor activity, and emotion. Subtypes of delirium based on psychomotor activity and arousal levels include the *hyperactive* (agitated, hyperalert) subtype, the *hypoactive* (lethargic, hypoalert) subtype, and *mixed* subtype.[45]

8. How common is delirium in hospitalized patients?
Delirium, or acute confusional state, is common, occurring in 10% to 60% of the older hospitalized population.[46] According to the APA practice guidelines on delirium, the prevalence of delirium in the hospitalized medically ill ranges from 10% to 40%.[45] In a meta-analysis of prospective studies of delirium, the prevalence of delirium superimposed on dementia ranged form 22% to 89%.[47] The authors observe that this wide variation likely reflects differences in measurement, inconsistent criteria for diagnosis, and various study populations. Up to 80% of patients with terminal illnesses, 25% of hospitalized cancer patients, 30% to 40% of hospitalized AIDS patients, and 50% of postoperative patients develop delirium.[45,48] Despite its prevalence, delirium often goes unrecognized. Nondetection rates of 33% to 66% have been reported.[49]

9. Is delirium associated with increased morbidity and mortality in hospitalized patients?

Existing evidence demonstrates that delirium is associated with increased morbidity and mortality in hospitalized patients. Medically ill patients, particularly the elderly, have a significantly increased risk of developing complications, such as falls, pneumonia, and pressure ulcers, resulting in longer hospital stays.[45,49] The development of delirium in non–intensive care unit (ICU) patients has an associated in-hospital mortality rate of 25% to 33%.[49] In a meta-analysis by Cole and associates[50], elderly patients with delirium had longer hospital stays, higher mortality rates at 1 month, and higher rates of institutional care at 1 and 6 months compared with unmatched control subjects. The study authors thought the results might have been confounded by the presence of concomitant dementia or severe physical illness.[50] In a multicenter, prospective, cohort study, Inouye and colleagues[51] concluded that delirium on admission is an independent prognostic determinant of hospital outcomes of institutionalization (adjusted OR = 3.0; 95% CI: 1.4 to 6.2) and functional decline (adjusted OR = 3.0; 95% CI: 1.6 to 5.8), even after controlling for age, gender, dementia, illness severity, and functional status. The associations between delirium and death alone and between delirium and length of stay were not statistically significant.[51]

Delirium has also been associated with increased mortality rates and length of hospitalization in ICU populations. In a prospective cohort study of 48 ICU patients that excluded patients with dementia, psychosis, mental retardation, or other neurologic diseases that could confound the diagnosis of delirium, 81% of patients developed delirium, and of these, 60% developed the complication while still in the ICU.[51] The duration of delirium was associated with length of stay in the ICU (r = .65; P = .0001) and in the hospital (r = .68; P < .0001) and the duration of benzodiazepine or narcotic use (r = .54; P = .0005).[51] Using multivariate analysis, delirium was the strongest predictor of length of hospital stay (P = .006), even after adjusting for confounders.[51] In a larger study of 275 ICU patients receiving mechanical ventilation, 19% had persistent coma and died in the hospital, and among the remaining patients, 82% developed delirium at some point during the ICU stay.[52] After adjusting for covariates (including age, severity of illness, comorbid conditions, coma, and use of sedatives or analgesic medications), delirium was independently associated with a higher 6-month mortality rate (adjusted HR = 3.2; 95% CI: 1.4 to 7.7) and longer hospital stay (adjusted HR = 2.0; 95% CI: 1.4 to 3.0).[52] In surgical populations, delirium is associated with a higher risk for postoperative complications, longer postoperative recuperation periods, longer hospital stays, and long-term disability.[45,46]

10. What are risk factors for developing delirium?

The cause of delirium is usually multifactorial and involves the interplay of predisposing and precipitating factors. Age, preexisting cognitive impairment, severe comorbidity, and exposure to medication are robust predictors of the risk of delirium.[49] Medications are implicated in 20% to 40% of cases; benzodiazepines, narcotics, and drugs with anticholinergic activity are common offenders.[49]

A systematic review by Elie and associates[53] analyzed 27 prospective studies—11 on medical patients, 9 on surgical patients, 2 on medical and surgical patients, and 5 on psychiatric patients—to identify risk factors associated with the development of delirium in hospitalized geriatric patients. In 1365 subjects with delirium, 61 different risk factors were examined; the five most common were dementia, medication, medical illness, age, and male gender.[53] The most strongly associated risk factors were dementia (OR = 5.2; 95% CI: 4.2 to 6.3), medical illness (OR = 3.8; 95% CI: 2.2 to 6.4), alcohol abuse (OR = 3.3; 95% CI: 1.9 to 5.5), and depression (OR = 1.9; 95% CI: 1.3 to 2.6).[53] Hearing impairment and visual impairment were moderate risk factors and produced combined odds ratios of 1.9 (95% CI: 1.4 to 2.6) and 1.7 (95% CI: 1.2 to 2.3), respectively.[53] Of 12 biochemical parameters studied, the blood urea nitrogen/creatinine ratio and sodium or potassium abnormalities were significant risk factors; the combined odds ratio for a sodium abnormality was 2.2 (95% CI: 1.3 to 4.0).[53] Although the combined odds ratio for medication use in delirium patients was 3.8, less than one half of the studies (6 of 13) found an association.[53] The investigators report overall study quality to be moderate in this systematic review, citing weaknesses in sample size necessary for significant association, blinding, statistical analysis, and control of confounding factors.

Inouye[46] demonstrated that the presence of more than one risk factor has a multiplicative rather than additive effect on delirium risk. A risk assessment model was developed based on prehospitalization risk factors (e.g., vision impairment, severe illness, cognitive impairment, blood urea nitrogen/creatinine ratio > 18) and precipitating stresses encountered during a hospital stay (e.g., use of physical restraints, malnutrition, > 3 medications added, use of bladder catheter, any iatrogenic event such as a hospital-acquired infection or fall).[46] According to this model, a patient with few predisposing factors at admission can develop delirium if subjected to severe stress during a hospital stay, whereas a patient with many risk factors is likely to become delirious even when subjected to mild stress during hospitalization.[46]

A prospective, randomized controlled trial comparing the effect epidural versus intravenous infusions of postoperative analgesia on the incidence of delirium after bilateral knee replacement surgery in elderly nondemented patients found age, male gender, and preoperative alcohol use to be predictors of delirium. There was no difference in the incidence of delirium when both forms of postoperative analgesia were compared.[54]

11. Can delirium be prevented?

Preliminary evidence indicates that risk factor modification and interventions that reduce sensory deficits, immobility, sleep disturbance, dehydration, and cognitive impairment can reduce the number of episodes of delirium and their duration.[49]

In a randomized, controlled trial, Mercantonio and coworkers[55] investigated whether a proactive geriatrics consultation on admission and subsequent daily visits making targeted recommendations based on a structured protocol could prevent delirium in a group of 126 patients 65 years or older admitted emergently for surgical repair of a hip fracture. The geriatrics consultation included recommendations regarding adequate oxygen delivery;

fluid-electrolyte balance; treatment of severe pain; elimination of unnecessary medications; regulation of bowel or bladder function; adequate nutritional intake; early mobilization and rehabilitation, prevention, early detection, and treatment of major postoperative complications; appropriate environmental stimuli; and treatment of agitated delirium. Delirium was diagnosed using the Confusion Assessment Method (CAM) algorithm, a reliable, sensitive (94% to 100%), specific (90% to 95%), and validated means for identifying delirium. Delirium occurred in 32% of intervention patients, compared with 50% of control patients, representing a relative risk of 0.64 (95% CI: 0.37 to 0.98) for the intervention group.[55] There was a greater reduction in cases of severe delirium (RR = 0.4; 95% CI: 0.18 to 0.89).[55] At baseline, prefracture dementia and activities of daily living (ADL) impairment were higher in the usual-care group compared with the intervention group (51% versus 37% and 31% versus 19%, respectively). Adjusting for this imbalance did not diminish the effect size of the intervention (OR for prevention of delirium = 0.6), but this was no longer statistically significant (95% CI: 0.3 to 1.3).[55] Length of stay or discharge disposition did not significantly differ between intervention and usual-care groups, and in a subgroup analysis, the intervention showed little or no benefit in patients with prefracture dementia or ADL impairment.[55]

In a nonrandomized, controlled trial of 852 general medical inpatients 70 years or older, Inouye and colleagues[56] tested the effectiveness of a multicomponent strategy, the Elder Life Program, for the prevention of delirium. This program consists of standardized protocols for the management of six risk factors for delirium: cognitive impairment, sleep deprivation, immobility, visual impairment, hearing impairment, and dehydration.[56] Many patients with dementia were included in the study. The incidence of delirium was 9.9% of the intervention group, compared with 15% of the usual-care group (matched OR = 0.60; 95% CI: 0.39 to 0.92).[56] The total number of days with delirium and the total number of episodes were significantly lower in the intervention group; however, the severity and recurrence rates were not significantly different.[56] In a subgroup analyses, the risk factor intervention significantly reduced the incidence of delirium in the group at intermediate risk for delirium at baseline (OR = 0.52; 95% CI: 0.0.29 to 0.92) but not in the high risk group (OR = 0.73; 95% CI: 0.38 to 1.38).[56]

12. How is delirium best managed in hospitalized patients?

The appropriate management of delirium involves identifying and treating underlying causes, providing supportive care, and relieving current symptoms.[45] An initial clinical assessment, review of medications, and appropriate laboratory and radiologic studies are needed. The APA guidelines identify hypoglycemia, hypoxia or anoxia, hyperthermia, hypertension, thiamine deficiency, withdrawal states, and anticholinergic-induced or other substance-induced delirium as readily identifiable and treatable disorders.[45]

Based on current clinical guidelines and expert opinion, initial investigation should include a complete blood count, blood chemistries (electrolytes, blood urea nitrogen, creatinine, liver injury tests), urinalysis, electrocardiogram, and chest radiography.[45] Additional testing should be directed by the history and physical exam. Neuroimaging should be reserved for patients with new focal neurologic signs or head trauma and can be considered when the history or neurologic examination cannot be completed.

NONPHARMACOLOGIC MANAGEMENT

There is some empirical evidence that environmental and cognitive-emotional interventions can reduce the severity of delirium and improve outcomes. Environmental interventions include providing an optimal level of environmental stimulation, reducing sensory impairments (e.g., restoring a patient's glasses or hearing aid), making environments more familiar, and providing environmental cues that facilitate orientation (e.g., clock, calendar).[45,49]

Cognitive-emotional measures include providing patients with reorientation, reassurance, and information concerning delirium that may reduce fear or demoralization. There have been no large clinical trials examining the efficacy of such measures.[45]

Cole and colleagues[58] randomized 227 general medical patients with prevalent or incident delirium based on the CAM model to usual care or evaluation by a geriatric specialist consultant with daily follow-up by an intervention nurse addressing the patient's environment, orientation, familiarity, communication, and activities. The primary outcome measure was time to improvement in the MMSE score. The Cox proportional hazards ratio for a shorter time to improvement with the intervention versus usual care was 1.1 (95% CI: 0.74 to 1.63) after adjustment for age, gender, and marital status.[58] There were no significant differences within 8 weeks after enrollment between the groups in time to and rate of improvement of the Delirium Index (measuring the severity of the delirium), length of hospital stay, rate of discharge to the community, or survival.[58] The study authors concluded that this intervention to detect and manage delirium was not more beneficial than usual care for older patients admitted to medical services.[58]

PHARMACOLOGIC MANAGEMENT

Pharmacologic therapy should be reserved for agitated patients whose symptoms threaten their own safety or the safety of others and/or interfere with medical treatment plans. Antipsychotic medications are the agents of choice in the pharmacologic treatment of delirium, but this is an off-label indication. Evidence for their efficacy in improving symptoms has come from numerous case reports, uncontrolled trials, and clinical experience.[45] Haloperidol is most frequently used because it has been the most studied, has few anticholinergic side effects, has few active metabolites, and has a low likelihood of causing sedation and hypotension.[45] It may be administered orally, intramuscularly, or intravenously. There have been few studies to determine the optimal doses of antipsychotic medications in the treatment of delirium. Based on doses used in several studies, the APA guidelines suggest dosing haloperidol at 1 to 2 mg every 2 to 4 hours, as needed (0.25 to 0.50 mg every 4 hours as needed for elderly patients), with titration to higher doses based upon peak effect for patients who continue to be agitated.[45] The peak effect of oral haloperidol is 4 to 6 hours; the peak effect of IM/IV haloperidol is 20 to 40 minutes.[45] Patients receiving antipsychotic medications for delirium should have their ECGs monitored for QT prolongation. Haloperidol should be avoided in patients with Parkinson's disease or Lewy body dementia.

Breitbart and coworkers[59] randomized 30 delirious AIDS patients to treatment with haloperidol, chlorpromazine, or lorazepam. Outcome measures were delirium severity and side effects. Treatment with haloperidol or chlorpromazine resulted in significant improvements in delirium with a very low prevalence of extrapyramidal side effects.[59] No improvement in delirium symptoms was found in the lorazepam group, and all patients developed treatment-limiting adverse effects (e.g., sedation, increased confusion, ataxia, disinhibition).[59] Benzodiazepine treatment is generally reserved for delirium caused by withdrawal of alcohol or sedative-hypnotics.[45]

There has been interest in the treatment of delirium with atypical neuroleptics because of their more favorable side-effect profile, including less sedation and fewer extrapyramidal side effects. Several small, open-label trials have supported the safety and efficacy of low-dose risperidone in the treatment of delirium in medically hospitalized patients.[60-62] In a small, double-blind study of 28 Korean patients, Han and colleagues[63] compared the clinical efficacy of risperidone with haloperidol for the treatment of delirium and found no significant differences in efficacy or response rates between the two agents. Several small, open-label trials have also supported the safety and efficacy of olanzapine and quetiapine in the treatment of delirium.[63a,b,c] Skrobik and coworkers[64] randomized 73 predominantly surgical ICU patients with delirium to receive olanzapine or haloperidol. Both medications were effective in reducing delirium and benzodiazepine use, but the haloperidol group developed more adverse effects (6 versus 0 patients) due to extrapyramidal side effects.[64]

In a prospective study by Gagnon and associates,[65] 14 patients with advanced cancer and hypoactive delirium that could not be explained by an underlying cause (i.e., metabolic or drug-induced) were treated with methylphenidate, and changes in their cognitive function were measured using the MMSE.[65] All patients showed improvement in their cognitive function; the median pretreatment MMSE score was 21 (mean ± SD = 20.9 ± 4.9), which improved to a median of 27 (mean ± SD = 24.9 ± 4.7) after the first dose ($P < .001$).[65]

PHYSICAL RESTRAINTS

Restraints can increase agitation and injury and should be considered only when other means of control are not effective or appropriate.[23] Whenever possible, nonrestraint measures, such as bedside companions or medications, should be used to prevent the delirious patient or others from harm.

13. How is opioid withdrawal best managed in the inpatient setting?

Search Date: May, 2005

Search Strategy: PubMed, search of "opioid withdrawal OR opioid detoxification," limited to meta-analysis, human, and English language; 14 citations retrieved. Search of "opioid withdrawal OR opioid detoxification" and "treatment," limited to randomized, controlled trial, adults 19+ years, human, English language; 201 citations retrieved. Search of "acute opioid withdrawal OR acute opioid detoxification," limited to clinical trial, human, English language; 66 citations retrieved. Titles and abstracts scanned with relevant citations selected. Bibliographies of all relevant citations reviewed. Search of Cochrane Collaboration "opioid withdrawal"; 5 citations retrieved.

The symptoms of opiate withdrawal include pupillary dilatation, lacrimation, rhinorrhea, piloerection, yawning, sneezing, anorexia, nausea, vomiting, and diarrhea.[66] Time to onset of peak withdrawal symptoms and duration after abrupt discontinuation depend on the half-life of the drug involved. For heroin, symptoms peak within 36 to 72 hours and last for 7 to 10 days, compared with methadone, for which symptoms peak at 72 to 96 hours but last for 14 days or longer.[66]

Hospitalization of opioid-dependent individuals for acute and chronic illness often interrupts their substance use and can result in withdrawal. Although usually not life threatening, treatment of opioid withdrawal is justified to ameliorate symptoms, avoid confounding medical assessment, and increase compliance with inpatient medical care.[67] Managed withdrawal (i.e., detoxification) is an essential step before longer-term drug-free treatment. Evidence exists for the efficacy of temporary substitution with a long-acting opioid (i.e., methadone or buprenorphine) and a_2-adrenergic agonists (i.e., clonidine and lofexidine) in the treatment of opioid withdrawal. Antagonist-induced (i.e., naloxone or naltrexone) withdrawal with symptom management using adjuvant medications is another approach to detoxification. Evidence is limited in general by small studies and heterogeneous comparisons and outcomes. Most inpatient studies are investigated in special detoxification facilities in otherwise medically stable patients.

In the *Cochrane Database of Systematic Reviews*, Amato and colleagues[68] reviewed 20 studies comparing methadone with adrenergic agonists, different modalities of methadone detoxification, methadone with other opioid agonists, one study of methadone compared with chlordiazepoxide, and one study of methadone compared with placebo. The conclusion was that the existing data were not comparable given the variability in study duration, design, and treatment objectives. The studies included in this review confirm that slow tapering with temporary substitution of long-acting opioids, accompanied by medical supervision and ancillary medications, can reduce withdrawal severity.[68] Regardless of which medication was selected for heroin detoxification, most patients in these studies relapsed.[68]

Few studies have evaluated pharmacologic treatments of opioid withdrawal in patients hospitalized for an acute illness. In a study by Welsh and coworkers,[69] 30 heroin-dependent patients hospitalized for medical reasons were given intravenous buprenorphine for the management of opioid withdrawal. Patients received 0.3 to 0.9 mg every 6 to 12 hours, based on severity of withdrawal symptoms and pain. No respiratory depression was observed, and no patients reported feeling a "high" or "rush." The investigators suggest that intravenous buprenorphine appears to be a safe and effective means to manage opioid withdrawal in medically ill, hospitalized, opioid-dependent patients.[69]

A study by Umbricht and associates[67] evaluated the impact of opioid detoxification medications (i.e., clonidine, methadone, and buprenorphine) on the signs and symptoms of withdrawal and pain severity in heroin-dependent patients with human immunodeficiency virus (HIV) who were hospitalized for medical reasons. Fifty-five patients were randomized to receive a 3-day taper with intramuscular buprenorphine (0.6 mg every 4 hours on day 1, 0.6 mg every 6 hours on day 2, and 0.6 mg every 8 hours on day 3), oral clonidine (loading dose of 0.2 mg, followed by 0.1 mg every 4 hours on day 1, 0.1 mg every 6 hours on day 2, and 0.1 mg every 8 hours on day 3), or oral methadone (30 mg on day 1, 20 mg on day 2, and 10 mg on day 3), followed by a clonidine transdermal patch on the fourth day. Observer- and subject-rated opiate withdrawal scores decreased significantly after the first dose of medication and overall during treatment. Among all subjects, self-reported and observer-reported pain decreased after treatment. Although the sample size was small, there were no significant differences in pain decline and other measures of withdrawal for the three treatment groups.[67]

14. What is the evidence for using buprenorphine in the treatment of opiate withdrawal?

Buprenorphine, as a partial mu opioid receptor agonist with kappa opioid receptor antagonist action, has the ability to reduce opiate craving and alleviate withdrawal, but it also has the potential to precipitate withdrawal symptoms in patients with physiologic dependence on opioids.[70] Due to high receptor affinity but low intrinsic activity, buprenorphine can antagonize the action of morphine and other high-efficacy mu agonists. It has a *ceiling effect*; after a certain point, increases in dose produce no increase in euphoric effects.[71] No serious side effects such as severe respiratory depression or sedation occur at high doses. Buprenorphine has a long duration of action due to its long plasma half-life and its slow dissociation from the receptor.[71]

Several studies have compared buprenorphine with clonidine for heroin detoxification and consistently demonstrated buprenorphine's superiority in treating withdrawal symptoms.[70] This was supported in a Cochrane systematic review of 13 studies (10 randomized, controlled trials), which showed less severe withdrawal, fewer adverse effects, and more likely completion of withdrawal (RR = 1.35; 95% CI: 1.13 to 1.62) in groups treated with buprenorphine than in groups treated with clonidine.[72] In the same systematic review, when buprenorphine was compared with methadone, peak severity of symptoms and completion of withdrawal were similar, but withdrawal symptoms resolved more quickly with buprenorphine.[72]

The optimal dosing regimen and duration of detoxification with buprenorphine remains unknown. Uncontrolled studies have examined a wide range of doses from 0.6 to 6 mg per day.[70] A small, randomized, double-blind study by Oreskovich and colleagues[70] compared two 5-day buprenorphine sublingual tablet dosing strategies (high dose: 8-8-8-4-2 mg/day, low dose: 2-4-8-4-2 mg/day) with high-dose oral clonidine (0.2-0.3-0.3-0.2-0.1 mg/day given four times daily). Severity of opioid withdrawal was assessed using three withdrawal symptom assessment instruments: the Clinical Opiate Withdrawal Scale (COWS), the Adjective Rating Scale for Withdrawal (ARSW), and the Visual Analogue Craving Scale (VAS).[70] The study found that by three separate measures (i.e., time to suppression of withdrawal, COWS, and VAS), higher-dose buprenorphine was superior to clonidine, whereas lower-dose buprenorphine was superior to clonidine in time to suppression of withdrawal and in the change in severity of withdrawal as measured by the COWS.[70] The study was not able to detect a difference between higher-dose compared with lower-dose buprenorphine. Postural hypotension was identified in all groups, and a substantial proportion of active and placebo clonidine doses had to be withheld because of low diastolic pressures.[70]

In an investigation of shortening the duration of opioid detoxification for cost-effectiveness, Assadi and colleagues[71] randomized 40 treatment-seeking opioid dependents to receive high-dose (12 mg in eight divided doses) intramuscular buprenorphine in 24 hours or conventional doses (starting at 3 mg/day) of intramuscular buprenorphine tapered over 5 days. There were no significant differences between the two groups in treatment retention or rate of successful detoxification (90%), the primary outcomes of interest.[71] There were also no significant differences in craving scores or severity of subject-rated opioid withdrawal using the Subjective Opiate Withdrawal Scale (SOWS).[71]

15. What is the evidence for using α_2-agonists in the treatment of opiate withdrawal?

The efficacy of clonidine, an α_2-adrenergic agonist, in the treatment of opioid withdrawal was demonstrated by Gold and coworkers[73] in 1978, when a single oral dose arrested the acute withdrawal discomfort experienced by 11 methadone-dependent patients after abrupt discontinuation of methadone. A meta-analysis of 22 studies (18 randomized, controlled trials) assessed the effectiveness of α_2-adrenergic agonists (e.g., clonidine, lofexidine [available in the UK], guanfacine) to manage opioid withdrawal in terms of withdrawal signs and symptoms, completion of withdrawal, and adverse effects.[74] When comparing α_2-adrenergic agonists with methadone, there were insufficient data for statistical analysis, but withdrawal intensity appeared similar over a period of about 10 days, whereas signs and symptoms of withdrawal occurred and resolved earlier in treatment with α_2-agonists.[74] Participants stayed in treatment longer with methadone. Clonidine is associated with more adverse effects (e.g., hypotension, dizziness, dry mouth, lack of energy) than methadone. Lofexidine was similar to clonidine in its effects on opiate withdrawal, but it did not reduce blood pressure to the same extent as clonidine.[74]

Lofexidine and clonidine were compared directly in a double-blind, randomized trial involving 28 opiate-dependent inpatients who had been stabilized on methadone.[75] There was no significant difference in withdrawal symptoms between treatment groups over 18 days, but lofexidine resulted in significantly less hypotension and less sedation.[75]

In a randomized, double-blind study, lofexidine was found to be clinically equivalent to methadone in the inpatient treatment of opioid withdrawal.[76] Self-rated withdrawal symptoms were more severe in the lofexidine-treated group during the early phase of abstinence, but thereafter, both groups showed similar progression of symptom decline.[76] In another study, 74 opioid-dependent male inmates in Britain were randomized to receive lofexidine or a methadone protocol (30 mg divided twice daily on day 1, followed by 25 mg on days 2 and 3, 20 mg on days 4 and 5, and tapered to zero by day 10).[77] The primary outcome was withdrawal symptom severity measured using the Withdrawal Problems Scale (WPS) and the SOWS, two self-rating scales that have been shown to be reliable measures of the opiate withdrawal syndrome.[77] There were no significant differences in withdrawal scores between the two groups at the beginning of the trial (i.e., the maximum withdrawal scores) and the two groups showed similar trends of a small progressive decrease in withdrawal scores during the 10 days of the trial.[77] The findings support prior evidence that lofexidine has comparable efficacy to methadone in ameliorating the effects of the opioid withdrawal syndrome.

16. What is the evidence for using opioid antagonists in the treatment of opiate withdrawal?

Rapid and ultra-rapid detoxifications consist of the administration of opioid antagonists such as naloxone and naltrexone to precipitate opioid withdrawal.[71] In rapid opioid detoxification, clonidine is prescribed simultaneously to inhibit autonomic hyperactivity associated with the withdrawal. Ultra-rapid opioid detoxification involves the administration of opioid antagonists under heavy sedation or general anesthesia.[66,71] In a Cochrane review of 10 studies (5 randomized, 5 nonrandomized trials) to assess the effectiveness of opioid antagonists in the treatment of opiate withdrawal, antagonist-induced withdrawal was associated with similar or less overall withdrawal severity compared with withdrawal with an α_2-adrenergic agonist.[78] Peak severity is likely to be higher and require the use of additional adjunct medications (e.g., antiemetics, benzodiazepines, nonsteroidal anti-inflammatory drugs).[78] The studies varied significantly enough in treatment protocols to preclude a description of the most effective approach.

Studies of ultra-rapid detoxification are limited by small numbers of patients, variable protocols, different patient characteristics, and limited follow-up. Withdrawal symptoms persisting for a week or longer, risks of sedation and anesthesia, and costs are noteworthy concerns.[66] The authors of a Cochrane review conclude that more research is needed before any conclusions can be drawn regarding the use of ultra-rapid detoxification with opioid antagonists for opiate withdrawal.[78]

17. Are there nonpharmacologic treatments for opiate withdrawal?

Acupuncture is one nonpharmacologic adjuvant therapy for opioid detoxification. In a study of 40 adult males undergoing rapid opiate detoxification with naloxone, acupuncture reduced the severity of withdrawal symptoms.[79] Psychosocial treatments should also be considered in conjunction with pharmacologic treatment for opioid detoxification. In a systematic review of randomized, controlled trials, the benefits of psychosocial interventions in addition to detoxification treatment are supported.[80]

18. How is the alcohol withdrawal syndrome defined?

Search Date: February 2005

Search Strategy: PubMed, 1990 to 2005, search of "alcohol withdrawal." Limited to randomized, controlled trial or meta-analysis or practice guideline. Limited to human and English language; 237 citations retrieved. Titles and abstracts scanned with relevant citations selected. Bibliographies of all relevant citations reviewed. Search of practice guidelines from the American Society of Addiction Medicine.

The alcohol withdrawal syndrome can range from minor symptoms to a severe, even fatal condition. Diagnostic criteria for alcohol withdrawal include two or more of the following signs or symptoms developing within several hours to a few days after the cessation or reduction in alcohol use that has been heavy and prolonged that are not due to another mental or medical condition: insomnia, tremulousness, anxiety, nausea or vomiting, diaphoresis or tachycardia, psychomotor agitation, grand mal seizures, and transient visual, tactile, or auditory hallucinations.[81] Alcohol withdrawal delirium or delirium tremens, is the most serious and potentially lethal alcohol withdrawal complication. Current diagnostic criteria for delirium tremens include disturbance of consciousness, change in cognition (e.g., memory deficit, disorientation, or language disturbance) or perceptual disturbance developing in a short period, and the emergence of symptoms during or shortly after withdrawal from heavy alcohol intake.[81] The classic clinical presentation of delirium tremens also includes hyperpyrexia, tachycardia, hypertension, and diaphoresis. Delirium typically does not develop until 2 to 3 days after cessation of drinking and usually lasts 48 to 72 hours, but cases of longer duration have been reported.[81]

19. What is the treatment for alcohol withdrawal?

BENZODIAZEPINES

The evidence for benzodiazepines in the treatment of alcohol withdrawal is well established. A meta-analysis of 11 trials comparing benzodiazepines with placebo or with an active control drug showed that there was more often a clinically significant reduction of symptoms within 2 days with benzodiazepines than with placebo (OR = 3.28; 95% CI: 1.30 to 8.28).[82] Nine of the trials compared benzodiazepines with other drugs (i.e., bromocriptine, carbamazepine, chlorpromazine, clonidine, doxepin, ethanol, hydroxyzine, paraldehyde, propranolol, and thiamine). The heterogeneity of measured efficacy outcomes in these trials precluded the combination of data, but there was no evidence of overall superiority of any agent over benzodiazepines in these small trials.[82] In addition to reducing the signs and symptoms of withdrawal, a meta-analysis of six prospective, placebo-controlled trials demonstrates a significant reduction of seizures (risk reduction of 7.7 seizures per 100 patients treated; 95% CI: −12.0 to −3.5; $P = .003$) and delirium (risk reduction of 4.9 cases of delirium per 100 patients treated; 95% CI: −9.0 to −0.7; $P = .04$).[83] A major limitation to the established evidence is that most studies investigating treatment of alcohol withdrawal have been conducted in inpatient alcohol detoxification units, where the participants are typically younger men with few or no comorbidities.

BARBITURATES

Barbiturates (e.g., phenobarbital) are used to reduce the signs and symptoms of alcohol withdrawal, but there is insufficient evidence to draw conclusions about their use in preventing seizures and delirium.[83] Barbiturates have a risk of respiratory depression in higher doses or when combined with alcohol and therefore have a lower safety profile compared with benzodiazepines.

TREATMENT OF ALCOHOL WITHDRAWAL DELIRIUM

In the treatment of alcohol withdrawal delirium, sedative-hypnotic agents are recommended to control agitation because they have been shown to reduce the duration of symptoms and mortality compared with neuroleptic agents in controlled trials (relative risk of mortality with neuroleptics in two trials = 6.6; 95% CI: 1.2 to 34.7).[81] The effectiveness of different sedative-hypnotic agents (i.e., diazepam, chlordiazepoxide, pentobarbital, paraldehyde, and barbital) in reducing mortality was evaluated in five controlled trials, but given the small number of deaths, no statistically significant differences were detected.[81] Benzodiazepines are most commonly used because of their favorable therapeutic to toxic effect index.

OTHER DRUGS

β-Adrenergic antagonists, carbamazepine, and centrally acting α-adrenergic agonists, such as clonidine, can ameliorate the symptoms of withdrawal, but insufficient evidence exists to support their use, therefore, they should be reserved as adjuvant therapy.[82,83] Neuroleptic agents, including phenothiazines and the butyrophenone haloperidol, demonstrate some effectiveness in reducing signs and symptoms of withdrawal, but they are less effective than benzodiazepines in preventing delirium and seizures (phenothiazines actually lower the seizure threshold).[83] They are associated with higher mortality, longer duration of delirium, and more complications in the treatment of delirium tremens.[81] Small case series describing oral or intravenous ethyl alcohol to alleviate withdrawal symptoms have been published but do not use objective or quantitative assessment of withdrawal severity, and no controlled trials exist evaluating its safety or relative efficacy compared with placebo or benzodiazepines.[83]

Magnesium levels are frequently low during alcohol withdrawal. A double-blind, placebo-controlled, randomized trial studying intramuscular administration of magnesium as a supplement to benzodiazepines showed no significant difference in severity of withdrawal symptoms or in the incidence of seizures or delirium.[83]

Patients with alcohol dependence are frequently thiamine deficient. In one large trial, thiamine did not reduce delirium or seizures.[83] Despite the weak evidence for its replacement, the administration of thiamine (given before the administration of intravenous fluids containing glucose) is recommended given its low cost, lack of side effects, and the risk of precipitating Wernicke's encephalopathy without its replacement.

20. Which benzodiazepine should be used in the treatment of alcohol withdrawal?

All benzodiazepines appear similarly efficacious in reducing the signs and symptoms of alcohol withdrawal.[82,83] Studies that compared benzodiazepines directly (i.e., chlordiazepoxide versus clobazam, diazepam versus lorazepam, and alprazolam versus chlordiazepoxide) do not show significant differences in efficacy.[82,84] A summary of prospective, controlled trials demonstrates that longer-acting agents may be more effective in preventing seizures, but this trend is not statistically significant (risk reduction of 6.7 cases of seizures/100 seizures; 95% CI: −13.0 to −0.0; $P = .07$).[83] The agent of choice can be guided by the following considerations[81,83]:

1. Long-acting agents may be more effective in preventing withdrawal seizures.
2. Long-acting agents can contribute to a smoother withdrawal with fewer rebound symptoms.

3. Short-acting agents may have a lower risk when there is concern about prolonged sedation, such as in the elderly and those with liver disease.

4. Lorazepam and oxazepam undergo less hepatic metabolism.

5. Agents with a rapid onset of action (e.g., diazepam) control agitation more quickly.

6. Cost varies considerably for the different agents.

21. What is the evidence for symptom-triggered versus a fixed-schedule of benzodiazepine administration?

Different dosing schedules of benzodiazepines have been compared for efficacy: fixed-schedule, symptom-triggered, and front-loaded therapy. Fixed-schedule dosing is defined as a fixed amount of medication given at specified intervals for several days in tapering doses, even if symptoms are absent. In this dosing schedule, additional medication can be given if withdrawal symptoms develop. In symptom-triggered dosing, patients are monitored, and medication is administered only when withdrawal symptoms cross a threshold of severity. Front-loaded therapy involves administering high doses of a long-acting benzodiazepine, after which the elimination of the drug proceeds slowly enough to avoid the recurrence of withdrawal.

The Clinical Institute Withdrawal Assessment–Alcohol, revised (CIWA-Ar) is a reliable, reproducible, and validated measure of the current severity of alcohol withdrawal (Table 12-1). The composite score, ranging from 0 to 67, is the sum of the scores of 10 individual assessment items: nausea and vomiting, sweats, anxiety, agitation, tremor, headache, auditory, visual, and tactile disturbances, and disorientation.[85] High scores predict the development of seizures and delirium.[83]

Two prospective, randomized, controlled trials have demonstrated the symptom-triggered approach to be as effective as fixed-dose therapy and that symptom-triggered therapy results in the administration of significantly less medication and a significantly shorter duration of treatment.[85,86] One of these studies randomized

Table 12-1. Ten-Item Clinical Institute Withdrawal Assessment
Scale for Alcohol

Nausea and Vomiting (Questioning and Observation)

0	No nausea and vomiting
1	Mild nausea with no vomiting
2	
3	Intermittent nausea with dry heaves
4	
5	
6	
7	Constant nausea, frequent dry heaves/vomiting

Tremor (Observation)

0	No tremor
1	Not visible, but can be felt at fingertips
2	
3	
4	Moderate when patient's arms extended
5	
6	
7	Severe, even with arms not extended

Paroxysmal Sweats (Observation)

0	No sweat visible
1	Barely perceptible sweating, palms moist
2	
3	
4	Beads of sweat obvious on forehead
5	
6	
7	Drenching sweats

Anxiety (Questioning And Observation)

0	No anxiety, at ease
1	Mildly anxious
2	
3	
4	Moderately anxious, guarded
5	
6	
7	Acute panic attack state

Continued

Table 12-1. Ten-Item Clinical Institute Withdrawal Assessment Scale for Alcohol—cont'd

Agitation (Observation)

0	Normal activity
1	Somewhat more than normal activity
2	
3	
4	Moderately fidgety and restless
5	
6	
7	Pacing or thrashing

Headache (Questioning)

0	Not present
1	Very mild
2	Mild
3	Moderate
4	Moderately severe
5	Severe
6	Very severe
7	Extremely severe

Tactile Disturbances (Questioning and Observation)

0	None
1	Very mild itching or paresthesias
2	Mild itching or paresthesias
3	Moderate itching or paresthesias
4	Moderately severe hallucinations
5	Severe hallucinations
6	Extremely severe hallucinations
7	Continuous hallucinations

Auditory Disturbances (Questioning and Observation)

0	Not present
1	Very mild harshness or ability to frighten
2	Mild harshness or ability to frighten
3	Moderate harshness or ability to frighten
4	Moderately severe hallucinations
5	Severe hallucinations
6	Extremely severe hallucinations
7	Continuous hallucinations

Table 12-1. Ten-Item Clinical Institute Withdrawal Assessment Scale for Alcohol—cont'd	
Visual Disturbances (Questioning and Observation)	
0	Not present
1	Very mild photosensitivity
2	Mild photosensitivity
3	Moderate photosensitivity
4	Moderately severe hallucinations
5	Severe hallucinations
6	Extremely severe hallucinations
7	Continuous hallucinations
Orientation/Sensorium (Questioning)	
0	Oriented and can do serial additions
1	Cannot do serial additions or uncertain about date
2	Disoriented for date by no more than 2 days
3	Disoriented for date by more than 2 days
4	Disoriented for place and/or person
Total Score	
Total score is a simple sum of each item score. The maximum score is 67.	
Adapted from Sullivan JT, Syora K, Schneiderman J, et al: Assessment of alcohol withdrawal: The Revised Clinical Institute Withdrawal Assessment for Alcohol scale (CIWA-Ar). Br J Addict 1989;84:1357.	

101 patients admitted to an inpatient detoxification unit in a Veterans Affairs medical center to standard fixed-schedule therapy of chlordiazepoxide (50 mg every 6 hours for four doses, followed by 25 mg every 6 hours for eight doses) or to symptom-triggered therapy (25 to 100 mg of chlordiazepoxide hourly when the CIWA-Ar score was 8 or higher). The median duration of treatment in the symptom-triggered group was 9 hours, compared with 68 hours in the fixed-schedule group ($P < .001$), and the former group received a median amount of 100 mg of chlordiazepoxide compared with 425 mg in the latter group ($P < .001$).[85] There were no significant differences in the severity of withdrawal during treatment or in the incidence of seizures or delirium tremens.[85] Important exclusion criteria included concurrent acute

or psychiatric illness requiring acute care hospitalization and a history of seizures of any cause.

Another controlled, double-blind trial randomly assigned 117 patients entering an alcohol treatment program to receive oxazepam on a fixed schedule every 6 hours (with additional medication as needed) or on a symptom-triggered protocol.[86] There were no significant differences in the incidence of seizures or DTs or in the severity of withdrawal symptoms between the two treatment groups. The mean oxazepam dose administered in the symptom-triggered group was 37.5 mg, compared with 231.4 mg in the fixed-schedule group ($P < .001$); 61% of patients in the former group did not require any oxazepam.[86] The mean duration of treatment was 20.0 hours in the symptom-triggered group and 62.7 hours in the fixed-schedule group ($P < .001$).[86] Exclusion criteria included a major cognitive, psychiatric, or medical comorbidity.

Although alcohol withdrawal severity and the amount of medication needed to control symptoms can vary greatly, the symptom-triggered approach has been validated only in alcohol detoxification units with frequent assessment by nursing staff trained in using the CIWA-Ar. In a retrospective analysis, the efficacy of a symptom-triggered approach for alcohol withdrawal in medical inpatients was supported, but it did not result in less medication or shorter duration of treatment.[87]

Ideally, treatment should be individualized to reduce administration of unnecessary medication. Symptom-triggered therapy using structured assessment scales such as the CIWA-Ar allows for objective titration of doses to individual need, but it requires frequent monitoring by trained personnel. This approach is best suited for substance abuse treatment programs. Realistically, the fixed-schedule approach may be the safer alternative on psychiatric and general medical and surgical wards in higher-risk patients (i.e., history of seizures, DTs, or prolonged, heavy alcohol consumption). The scales need to be used with caution for patients with concomitant medical or psychiatric illness because they rate signs and symptoms that may be caused by conditions other than alcohol withdrawal.[83]

22. In patients taking atypical antipsychotic agents, what is the risk for the development of the metabolic syndrome?

Search Date: November 30, 2005

Search Strategy: PubMed, 1996-2005, search for "antipsychotic agents AND obesity, hyperlipidemia, hypertension"; 701 documents retrieved. Limited to human and English language, resulting in 580 documents. Titles scanned. Further limited to systematic reviews.

In February of 2004, a Consensus Development Conference on Antipsychotic Drugs published a statement warning physicians of the increased risk of diabetes and obesity in patients taking atypical antipsychotic medications.[88] This followed a decision in September 2003 by the U.S. Food and Drug Administration (FDA) that all atypical antipsychotic labels contain the recommendation that regular glucose testing be undertaken in all individuals at risk for diabetes.[89] The term *metabolic syndrome*, which consists of abdominal obesity, low levels of high-density lipoprotein cholesterol, hypertriglyceridemia, hypertension, and hyperglycemia, has been used to characterize the adverse effects of atypical antipsychotics.

DIABETES AND SCHIZOPHRENIA

The relationship between diabetes and schizophrenia has a long history, and a substantial amount of literature has suggested that the two have a biologic relationship regardless of treatment. However, this putative relationship is potentially confounded by lifestyle factors. Schizophrenic patients are more likely to exercise less, follow poor diets, and lead a sedentary lifestyle, and teasing out the true contribution of lifestyle versus inherent predisposition has been difficult. The absence of firm conclusions regarding these fundamental issues has made the added question of whether the therapy for schizophrenia itself induces diabetes particularly challenging.

Case Reports

Early evidence suggesting a relationship between atypical antipsychotics and diabetes came from case reports. These have been summarized in a series of articles by Koller and colleagues[90-92] based on their experience with the FDA's MedWatch program. For clozapine and olanzapine, 78% of new cases of diabetes mellitus (384 and 289, respectively) were reversible on discontinuation of the drug. Fewer cases were reported for risperidone (132), and there was less evidence of reversibility.

Epidemiological Studies

More evidence for a relationship can be found in the more than 20 analyses of various health care databases that have been published.[93],[94] These epidemiologic studies provide the backbone for the recommendation of the Consensus Development Conference and the FDA statements mentioned previously. All of these studies used ICD-9 codes or prescription listings as surrogates of disease status. They are potentially confounded by lack of patient specific data on baseline risk factors and duration of antipsychotic use. They also did not evaluate the newer atypical medications, ziprasidone and aripiprazole. Nevertheless, a consistent increased risk of diabetes mellitus is seen with olanzapine in particular, but also with clozapine and, in some cases, with typical antipsychotics. Risperidone was found to have no increased risk of diabetes mellitus in some studies, and in all studies, it had less of an increased risk of diabetes compared with olanzapine.[95]

Prospective Controlled Studies

Prospective data in the form of randomized, controlled trials supporting an association between diabetes and atypical antipsychotics are scarce, although a number of studies are ongoing.[96] An often cited randomized, controlled trial of 157 schizophrenic patients taking clozapine, haloperidol, olanzapine, or risperidone for an initial 8-week fixed-dose period, followed by a 6-week variable-dose period, found that patients taking clozapine and haloperidol had significant increases in mean blood glucose levels at 8 weeks and that olanzapine patients had an increase at 14 weeks. Patients taking risperidone did not have a significant increase at any time in the study.[97] The increased concern about diabetes mellitus with antipsychotics has led to increased attention to this element in the RCTs of the newer atypical antipsychotic agents. However, the clinical trials of ziprasidone and aripiprazole have not revealed any statistically significant increase in diabetes compared with placebo.[98]

In summary, there is a much evidence to suggest that atypical antipsychotics—particularly clozapine and olanzapine—cause diabetes, but there is little evidence to clearly prove it. The risk appears to be less with risperidone and has been found no evidence of increased risk with ziprasidone and aripiprazole.

ANTIPSYCHOTICS AND OBESITY

As opposed to atypical antipsychotics and diabetes risk, for which the evidence is primarily in the form of case reports and large epidemiologic database studies, the association between atypical agents and obesity is clearer and based on randomized, controlled trial data. Allison and colleagues[99] summarized the bulk of data in their 1999 systematic review, from which Figure 12-2 is derived. After a 10-week period, patients taking most atypical agents experienced a statistically significant weight gain. Olanzapine and clozapine caused the most weight gain (approximately 5 kg). Ziprasidone had no associated weight gain, a finding that also has been confirmed in later trials.[100] Aripiprazole was not available at the time of Allison's 1999 review, but clinical trials with this agent suggest that weight gain is minimal if present.[100]

This has led to an ordering of weight gain risk as follows: olanzapine > quetiapine > risperidone > ziprasidone > aripripazole.[100] This ordering mirrors the risk of diabetes from the observational data mentioned previously.

ANTIPSYCHOTICS AND DYSLIPIDEMIA

The other component of the metabolic syndrome that has received significant attention is the risk of dyslipidemia associated with the atypical antipsychotics. Meyer and Koro[102] published a comprehensive review of the evidence in 2004. Case reports and retrospective studies of clozapine suggest that it causes an increase in triglyceride levels more than cholesterol, with some concerning reports of severe triglyceride elevations in individual patients. Case reports, retrospective studies, and small, prospective studies suggest a similar pattern of lipid elevation with olanzapine. Risperidone, ziprasidone, and aripiprazole have very little effect on serum lipids based on a similar evidence base.

In summary, schizophrenic patients eligible for antipsychotic therapy should be regarded as a high-risk group for

95% confidence interval for weight change (kg)

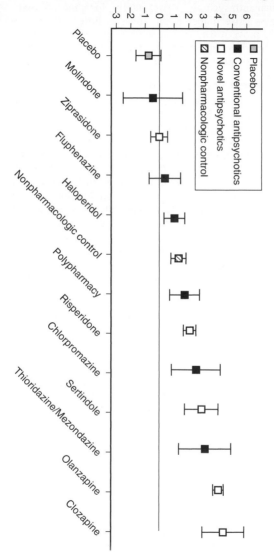

Figure 12-2. Weight change associated with antipsychotic drugs. (Adapted from Allison DB, Mentore JL. Heo M, et al: Antipsychotic induced weight gain: A comprehensive research synthesis. Am J Psychiatry 1999;156: 1686-1696.)

the development of the metabolic syndrome. Based on the accumulated evidence, it is very likely that atypical antipsychotics contribute to this risk. The evidence base implicating olanzapine and clozapine is substantial, but there is less evidence against risperidone and very little for aripiprazole and ziprasidone. The Consensus Development Conference on antipsychotics recommends baseline measurement of weight, waist circumference, blood pressure, fasting plasma glucose levels, and a fasting lipid profile in all patients started on antipsychotics. Weight should be monitored at 4-week intervals and thereafter, with repeat tests of lipids, fasting glucose levels, and blood pressure at 12 weeks and then annual measurements of waist circumference, blood pressure, and fasting glucose.[103]

23. What is the significance of QT interval prolongation in the use of antipsychotic drugs?

Search Date: September 2005

Search Strategy: PubMed, 1966 to 2005, search "QT interval" or "torsades de pointes" and "antipsychotic agents." Limited to human and English language; 154 citations retrieved. Titles and abstracts scanned, with relevant citations selected. Bibliographies of all relevant citations reviewed.

The QT interval is measured on an ECG from the beginning of the QRS complex to the end of the T wave. The interval depends on heart rate, and various corrections for heart rate have been developed. The most common correction used in clinical practice and the one used in the automated reading of most ECG machines is the Bazett formula, in which the corrected QT interval (QTc) = QT/vRR interval.

There is a recognized association between the length of the corrected QT interval and the development of the malignant polymorphic ventricular arrhythmia torsades de pointes. Torsades can lead to sudden cardiac death. It has not been determined the exact threshold above which the risk of torsades increases, but a QT interval longer than 450 msec in men and longer than 460 msec in women is considered prolonged. Intervals longer than 500 msec generally warrant the discontinuation of any drug known to prolong the QT interval.[103]

The significance of QT interval prolongation lies in its association with torsades de pointes and sudden cardiac death, but it should only be regarded as a marker of such risk. Not all drugs that prolong the QT interval have been associated with ventricular arrhythmia; amiodarone is the most prominent example. The significance of the QT interval prolongation can be determined only by considering other associated risk factors for malignant arrhythmia (Table 12-2).[104] Basic and clinical research studies suggest

Table 12-2. **Risk Factors for Ventricular Arrhythmia**
Congenital QT syndrome
Individual predisposition (not otherwise defined)
Ventricular hypertrophy
Congestive heart failure
Bradycardia
Hypokalemia or hypomagnesemia
Hypocalcemia
Female sex
Physical restraint or agitation
Substance abuse
Renal and hepatic impairment
Pharmacokinetic factors that lead to higher drug concentration (co-prescribed drugs)
Pharmacodynamic factors (co-prescription with other QT prolonging medication)
From Haddad P, Anderson IM: Antipsychotic-related QTc prolongation, torsades de pointes, and sudden death. Drugs 2002;62:1649-1671.

that the genesis of malignant arrhythmias in the setting of QT interval prolongation is multifactorial, with environmental factors serving to induce arrhythmias in susceptible patients under certain conditions.[88] Minimization of the risk of sudden death in the clinical setting involves identifying patients with an increased risk for arrhythmia, considering alternative therapies, and eliminating modifiable risk factors in susceptible patients when possible. No formal guidelines exist for the management of antipsychotic-induced QT prolongation in the clinical setting, but individual experts advise weighing the risk and benefits on an individual basis.[88,105]

ANTIPSYCHOTICS AND MALIGNANT VENTRICULAR ARRHYTHMIAS

The association between drug-induced prolongation of the QT interval and torsades de pointes has been most clearly described for the class IA (i.e., quinidine, disopyramide, and procainamide) and class III antiarrhythmic agents. Data from randomized, controlled trials support a dose-related increased incidence of torsades with the class III agents sotalol, dofetilide, ibutilide, and azimilide, but not with amiodarone.[106] Antipsychotic drugs have been proved to prolong the QT interval to various degrees. Table 12-3 illustrates the best data available on the extent of prolongation for antipsychotic agents.[107] Empirical support for an association between antipsychotic

Table 12-3. **Antipsychotics and Mean Changes in the QTc Interval**

Antipsychotic Drug	QTc Interval	
	Baseline Mean	Mean Change
Thioridazine (Mellaril)	395.9	35.6
Ziprasidone (Geodon)	402.1	20.3
Quetiapine (Seroquel)	398.0	14.5
Risperidone (Risperdal)	396.3	11.6
Olanzapine (Zyprexa)	397.9	6.8
Haloperidol (Haldol)	394.7	4.7

Adapted from Koller EA, Doraiswamy PM: Olanzapine-associated diabetes mellitus. Pharmacotherapy 2002;22:841-852.

use and sudden cardiac death, however, is uncompelling. Mehtonen and colleagues[108] published an observational study of autopsy-negative sudden deaths in Finland and found an increased odds of phenothiazine use compared with the general population. A case-control study by Reilly and coworkers[109] of psychiatric inpatients dying suddenly found an increased odds ratio for current thioridazine use. A retrospective cohort study of Medicaid enrollees from 1988 to 1993 looked at 1487 confirmed sudden deaths and found the risk was 2.39 times higher for patients on a moderate dose of antipsychotic medication.[110]

All of these studies predate the widespread use of atypical antipsychotic agents and mostly implicate the now less used thioridazine. They also largely lack appropriate control for confounding and can only be regarded as suggestive. A later retrospective, cohort study of U.S. Medicaid programs that controlled for many potential confounders found increased relative risks for cardiac arrest and ventricular arrhythmia for Haldol (RR = 2.4; range, 1.5 to 3.9), thioridazine (RR = 2.4; range, 1.4 to 3.9), and risperidone (RR = 3.2; range, 1.9 to 5.4) compared with a control population. The study authors thought that the higher risk found with risperidone may have been confounded by the fact that patients with more or more severe overall risk factors may have been preferentially given this drug.[111] A case-control study from the Netherlands, whose investigators had broader access to patient-specific data, found an increased risk of sudden death with antipsychotics that was threefold that of controls.[112] This collection of studies, in addition to multiple case reports and case series of various agents, raises concern that the QT interval prolongation associated with certain antipsychotic medications may precipitate sudden cardiac death in susceptible patients.

HALDOL AND ATYPICAL ANTIPSYCHOTICS

Over the past 10 years, atypical antipsychotics have gradually superseded many of the older antipsychotics for the treatment of schizophrenia and their various off-label uses. Haldol continues to have a niche in the ICU and hospitalized patients as a drug used to reduce aggression and agitation. As shown in Table 12-4, although atypical antipsychotics can slightly prolong the QT to various degrees, there have been no reports of torsades de

Table 12-4. Summary of the Evidence—Antipsychotics and the Risk of Malignant Arrhythmia

Antipsychotic Drug	Evidence for Torsades de Pointes or Sudden Death
Thioridazine	Case reports, cross-sectional study, case-control, cohort
Haldol	Case reports, case series, case-control, retrospective cohort
Pimozide	Case reports
Chlorpromazine	Case reports
Sulpiride	Case report
Clozapine	One case report
Risperidone	One case report, potentially confounded association in cohort study
Olanzapine	No case reports
Ziprasidone	No case reports
Quetiapine	No case reports

Data from Haddad PM, Anderson IM: Antipsychotic-related QTc prolongation, torsades de pointes and sudden death. Drugs 2002;62:1649-1671; Titier K, Girodet PO, Verdoux H, et al: Atypical antipsychotics: From potassium channels to torsades de pointes and sudden death. Drug Saf 2005;28:35-51; Straus SM, Bleumink GS, Dieleman JP, et al: Antipsychotics and the risk of sudden cardiac death. Arch Intern Med 2004;164:1293-1297.

pointes or sudden cardiac death, or both, with the exception of a single report on the use of risperidone.[113] Haldol, because it has historically been used in ECG-monitored settings, has an extensive history of case reports and case series alleging it as the cause of ventricular arrhythmia. The risk of torsades with Haldol appears considerably less than with thioridazine. The studies cited earlier suggest that despite a lesser degree of QT prolongation, the risk of torsades may be greater with Haldol than the atypical antipsychotics.

In summary, antipsychotic medications clearly cause prolongation of the QT interval to some degree, with the older typical agent thioridazine causing the most prolongation and the atypical agents causing the least. Modest epidemiologic evidence supports the proposition that this

QT interval prolongation can result in sudden cardiac death in susceptible patients, particularly with the older agent thioridazine and, to a lesser degree, with Haldol. There is little empirical evidence that the risk is increased with atypical antipsychotics. Prudence requires that we seriously consider the risk of QT prolongation and sudden death in otherwise susceptible patients, proactively reduce all associated risk factors, and use the lowest dose of antipsychotic necessary to achieve the therapeutic goal.

24. In agitated patients with dementia, what is the evidence for the effectiveness of antipsychotic agents in improving behavior?

Search Date: September 2005

Search Strategy: PubMed, 1996 to 2005, search "antipsychotic agents AND dementia." Limited to human and English language; 528 citations retrieved. Titles and abstracts scanned, with relevant citations selected. Bibliographies of all relevant citations reviewed.

In hospital and nursing home settings, physicians frequently encounter demented patients who manifest behavioral and psychological symptoms of dementia (BPSD), including agitation, aggressiveness, wandering, and delusions. Historically, the typical antipsychotic haloperidol has been used in the management of these patients, but antidepressants, mood stabilizers, and cholinesterase inhibitors are also prescribed, despite little evidence for their effectiveness.[114] The effectiveness of haloperidol for agitation in dementia was the subject of a Cochrane systematic review.[115] Five randomized, controlled trials were reviewed. The studies collectively included outpatients and institutionalized patients, ranged from 3 to 16 weeks, and used haloperidol doses from 0.5 to 6 mg daily. No study clearly demonstrated that haloperidol was effective in the overall management of the agitated patient, as measured by well-validated scales of behavioral assessment. The three studies that assessed *aggression* as a subtype of agitation did find haloperidol to be significantly better than placebo. Patients treated with haloperidol also experienced increasing somnolence, extrapyramidal symptoms, and fatigue compared with controls. Haloperidol therefore appears to have a role in the management of aggressive behavior in demented patients, but there is no evidence for its use in patients with dementia and agitation, when agitation is defined broadly.

The atypical antipsychotics—clozapine, aripiprazole, olanzapine, quetiapine, risperidone, and ziprasidone—have emerged as first-line agents in the treatment of psychotic disorders because of a favorable side-effect profile, particularly a decreased incidence of extra-pyramidal side effects compared with the older, typical antipsychotic agents. The first atypical antipsychotic clozapine represented a significant advance in psychopharmacology, but the risk of agranulocytosis limited its off-label use. Two newer atypical antipsychotics, risperidone (Risperdal) and Olanzapine (Zyprexa), are frequently used off label for a variety of indications,[116] including controlling the behavioral and psychological symptoms of dementia. Antipsychotics, most commonly atypical agents, have become the most costly drugs for the Medicaid program. An observational study showed that approximately 20% of nursing home patients receive them, frequently for off-label indications such as the management of agitated, demented patients.[117]

The effectiveness of the atypical antipsychotics for BPSD has been reviewed in two systematic reviews.[118,119] Both reviews cite three drug company–sponsored trials that compared risperidone with placebo, with the behavioral outcome measured by well-validated scoring systems. However, the trials did not use the same measurement scale and could not be formally combined. Katz and colleagues[120] randomized patients to three different doses of risperidone and attempted to demonstrate a more than 50% reduction in the BEHAVE-AD total score; 45% of patients in the 1-mg risperidone group achieved it, and only 33% of subjects in the placebo arm did. The 2-mg dose was equally effective as the 1-mg dose, but it resulted in increased extrapyramidal side effects. Brodaty and coworkers[121] demonstrated a significant reduction in CMAI aggression scores with risperidone compared with placebo. However, this trial also raised serious concerns about stroke risk by finding an almost doubling of the risk of serious adverse events with risperidone, including six cerebrovascular events (discussed later). DeDeyn and associates[122] failed to show the 1-mg dose of risperidone was superior to placebo in reducing the BEHAVE-AD score by 30%—the study's predetermined definition of clinical improvement. However, risperidone did reduce the overall BEHAVE-AD score by more than placebo and demonstrated a significant impact on aggression. Based on initial trials, it appears that risperidone may be effective in reducing the behavioral and psychological symptoms of dementia.

Olanzapine has also been studied in drug company–sponsored trials. Street and colleagues[123] found that 5- and 10-mg doses of oral olanzapine were effective in reducing agitation, aggression, hallucinations, and delusions, as measured by a Neuropsychiatric Inventory (NPI), but they were clearly associated with increases in somnolence and gait disturbance. A second larger and longer trial[124] failed to demonstrate a difference between oral olanzapine and placebo in NPI score, but there was also no significant increase in adverse events. It is unclear whether oral olanzapine is effective for BPSD.

Only one small study has been performed with the intention of comparing haloperidol with an atypical antipsychotic, risperidone. Chan and colleagues[125] reported after a 12-week trial that both haloperidol and risperidone significantly reduced BPSD as measured by well-validated scales, although there was no statistically significant difference between them.

POTENTIAL RISKS OF ANTIPSYCHOTICS

The clinical decision to use haloperidol or an atypical antipsychotic for the treatment of BPSD must also involve weighing the risk of such therapy. Serious concerns have been raised by the unexpected finding in multiple trials involving atypical antipsychotic use in the elderly that patients are at increased risk for cerebrovascular events and death. In May 2005, the FDA reported its analyses of 17 placebo-controlled trials (published and unpublished) of atypical antipsychotics used in elderly patients, including risperidone, olanzapine, aripiprazole, and quetiapine, which demonstrated a 4.5% mortality rate compared with a rate of 2.6% for placebo.[125] Deaths were caused by cardiovascular disease or infection. Much of the reported data came from unpublished studies performed under the auspices of the drug manufacturer.

The 11 studies that specifically compared risperidone with placebo in elderly patients found a combined stoke risk of 3.3% compared with a 1.1% risk for placebo.[126] The five studies that compared olanzapine with placebo in elderly patients found a stroke risk of 1.3% compared with a risk of 0.4% for placebo.[127] The potential causative mechanism of this finding has not been identified, but the FDA subsequently required that a black box warning be placed on all antipsychotic agents regarding the potential for increased mortality when used in elderly patients.

In conclusion, the evidence supports a small potential benefit for the use of risperidone and olanzapine in moderating the behavioral and psychological symptoms of dementia, but this benefit may come at an increased risk for serious side effects, including stroke, infection, and even death. Haloperidol continues to have a role in managing aggressive behavior associated with dementia, but this is counterbalanced by its less favorable side-effect profile, specifically increased somnolence and the occurrence of extrapyramidal symptoms.

REFERENCES

1. Ziegelstein RC: Depression in patients recovering from a myocardial infarction. JAMA 2001;286:1621-1627. **V**

2. Ziegelstein RC: Depression after myocardial infarction. Cardiol Rev 2001;9:45-51. **V**

3. Frasure-Smith N, Lesperance F, Talajic M: Depression following myocardial infarction. Impact of 6-month survival. JAMA 1993;270:1819-1825. **III**

4. Frasure-Smith N, Lesperance F, Talajic M: Depression and 18-month prognosis after myocardial infarction. Circulation 1995;91:999-1005. **III**

5. Lane D, Carroll D, Ring C, et al: Mortality and quality of life 12 months after myocardial infarction: Effects of depression and anxiety. Psychosom Med 2001; 63:221-230. **III**

6. Mayou RA, Gill D, Thompson DR, et al: Depression and anxiety as predictors of outcome after myocardial infarction. Psychosom Med 2000;62:212-219. **III**

7. van Melle JP, de Jonge P, Spijkerman TA, et al: Prognostic association of depression following myocardial infarction with mortality and cardiovascular events: A meta-analysis. Psychosom Med 2004;66:814-822. **I**

8. Sorensen C, Friis-Hasche E, Haghfelt T, Bech P: Postmyocardial infarction mortality in relation to depression: A systematic critical review. Psychother Psychosom 2005;74:69-80. **I**

9. Beck CA, Joseph L, Belisle P, Pilote L, for the QOLAMI Investigators: Predictors of quality of life 6 months and 1 year after acute myocardial infarction. Am Heart J 2001;142:271-279. **III**

10. Romanelli J, Fauerbach JA, Bush DE, Ziegelstein RC: The significance of depression in older patients after myocardial infarction. J Am Geriatr Soc 2002;50:817-822. **III**

11. Lesperance F, Frasure-Smith N, Talajic M, Bourassa MG: Five-year risk of cardiac mortality in relation to initial severity and one-year changes in depression symptoms after myocardial infarction. Circulation 2002;105: 1049-1053. **III**

12. Frasure-Smith N, Lesperance F, Gravel G, et al: Social support, depression, and mortality during the first year after myocardial infarction. Circulation 2000;101; 1919-1924. **III**

13. American College of Cardiology/American Heart Association (ACC/AHA): Guidelines for the management of patients with ST-elevation myocardial infarction— Executive summary. J Am Coll Cardiol 2004;44: 671-719. **IV**

14. Roose SP, Laghrissi-Thode F, Kennedy JS, et al: Comparison of paroxetine and nortriptyline in depressed patients with ischemic heart disease. JAMA 1998;279:287-291. **II**

15. Glassman AH, O'Connor CM, Califf RM, et al, for the Sertraline Antidepressant Heart Attack Randomized Trial (SADHART) Group: Sertraline treatment of major depression in patients with acute MI or unstable angina. JAMA 2002;288:701-709. **II**

16. Swenson JR, O'Connor CM, Barton D, et al, for the Sertraline Antidepressant Heart Attack Randomized Trial (SADHART) Group: Influence of depression and effect of treatment with Sertraline on quality of life after hospitalization for acute coronary syndrome. Am J Cardiol 2003;92:1271-1276. **II**

17. Linden W, Stossel C, Maurice J: Psychosocial interventions for patients with coronary artery disease:a meta-analysis. Arch Intern Med 1996;156:745-752. **I**

18. Dusseldorp E, van Elderen T, Maes S, et al: A meta-analysis of psychoeducational programs for coronary heart disease patients. Health Psychol 1999;18:506-519. **I**

19. Rees K, Bennett P, West R, et al: Psychological interventions for coronary heart disease. The Cochrane Database Syst Rev 2004;(2):CD002902. **I**

20. Berkman LF, Blumenthal J, Burg M, et al: Effects of treating depression and low perceived social support on clinical events after myocardial infarction: The Enhancing Recovery in Coronary Heart Disease Patients (ENRICHD) Randomized Trial. JAMA 2003;289: 3106-3116. **II**

21. Sauer WH, Berlin JA, Kimmel SE. Selective serotonin reuptake inhibitors and myocardial infarction. Circulation 2001;104:1894-1898. **III**

22. van den Brink RHS, van Melle JP, Honig A, et al, for the MIND-IT investigators: Treatment of depression after myocardial infarction and the effects on cardiac prognosis and quality of life: Rationale and outline of the Myocardial Infarction and Depression-Intervention Trial (MIND-IT). Am Heart J 2002;144: 219-225. **II**

23. American Psychiatric Association, Committee on Electroconvulsive Therapy: The Practice of Electroconvulsive Therapy: Recommendations for Treatment, Training, Privileging, 2nd ed. Washington, DC, APA Press, 2001. **IV**

24. Abrams R: The mortality rate with ECT. Convuls Ther 1997;13:125-127. **V**

25. Dolinski SY, Zvara DA: Anesthetic considerations of cardiovascular risk during electroconvulsive therapy. Convuls Ther 1997;13:157-164. **V**

26. Applegate RJ: Diagnosis and management of ischemic heart disease in the patient scheduled to undergo electroconvulsive therapy. Convuls Ther 1997;13: 128-144. **V**

27. Abrams R: Electroconvulsive Therapy, 2nd ed. New York, Oxford University Press, 1992. **V**

28. Lafferty JE, North CS, Spitznagel E, Isenberg K: Laboratory screening prior to ECT. J ECT 2001;17: 158-165. **III**

29. Gerring JP, Shields HM: The identification and management of patients with a high risk for cardiac arrhythmias during modified ECT. J Clin Psychiatry 1982;43: 140-143. **III**

30. Zielinski RJ, Roose SP, Devanand DP, et al: Cardiovascular complications of ECT in depressed patients with cardiac disease. Am J Psychiatry 1993;150:904-909. III

31. Castelli I, Steiner LA, Kaufman MA, et al: Comparative effects of esmolol and labetalol to attenuate hyperdynamic states after electroconvulsive therapy. Anesth Analg 1995;80:557-561. III

32. Rasmussen KG, Rummans TA, Richardson JW: Electroconvulsive therapy in the medically ill. Psychiatr Clin North Am 2002;25:177-193. V

33. Petrides G, Fink M: Atrial fibrillation, anticoagulation, and electroconvulsive therapy. Convuls Ther 1996;12:91-98. V

34. Rayburn BK: Electroconvulsive therapy in patients with heart failure or valvular heart disease. Convuls Ther 1997;13:145-156. V

35. Dolenc TJ, Barnes RD, Hayes DL, Rasmussen KG: Electroconvulsive therapy in patients with cardiac pacemakers and implantable cardioverter defibrillators. PACE 2004;27:1257-1263. VI

36. Kleiner J, Altshuler L, Hendrick V, Hershman JM: Lithium-induced subclinical hypothyroidism: Review of the literature and guidelines for treatment. J Clin Psychiatry 1999;60:249-255. V

37. Bocchetta A, Bernardi F, Burrai C, et al: The course of thyroid abnormalities during lithium treatment: A two-year follow-up study. Acta Psychiatr Scand 1992; 86:38-41. III

38. Smigan L, Wahlin A, Jocobsson L, et al: Lithium therapy and thyroid function test: A prospective study. Neuropsychobiology 1984;11:39-43. III

39. Kupka RW, Nolen WA, Post RM, et al: High rate of autoimmune thyroiditis in bipolar disorder: Lack of association with lithium exposure. Biol Psychiatry 2002;51:305-311. III

40. Johnston AM, Eagles JM: Lithium-associated clinical hypothyroidism. Prevalence and risk factors. Br J Psychiatry 1999;175:336-339. III

41. American Psychiatric Association (APA): Practice guideline for the treatment of patients with bipolar disorder (revised). Am J Psychiatry 2002;159(Suppl): 1-50. IV

42. Surks MI, Ortiz E, Daniels GH, et al: Subclinical thyroid disease. Scientific review and guidelines for diagnosis and management. JAMA 2004;291:228-238. V

43. Roberts CG, Ladenson PW: Hypothyroidism. Lancet 2004;363:793-803. Ⓥ

44. American Association of Clinical Endocrinologists (AACE) Thyroid Task Force: AACE medical guidelines for the clinical practice for the evaluation and treatment of hyperthyroidism and hypothyroidism. Endocr Pract 2002;8:457-469. Ⓘⱽ

45. American Psychiatric Association (APA): Practice guidelines for the treatment of patients with delirium. Am J Psychiatry 1999;156:1-20. Ⓘⱽ

46. Inouye SK: Delirium in hospitalized older patients: Recognition and risk factors. J Geriatr Psychiatry Neurol 1998;11:118-125. Ⓘ

47. Fick DM, Agostini JV, Inouye SK: Delirium superimposed on dementia: A systematic review. J Am Geriatr Soc 2002;50:1723-1732. Ⓘ

48. Weber JB, Coverdale JH, Kunik ME: Delirium. Current trends in prevention and treatment. Intern Med J 2004;34:115-121. Ⓥ

49. Meagher DJ. Delirium: Optimizing management. BMJ 2001;322:144-149. Ⓥ

50. Cole MG, Primeau FJ: Prognosis of delirium in elderly hospital patients. CMAJ 1993;149:41-46. Ⓘ

51. Inouye SK, Rushing JT, Foreman MD, et al: Does delirium contribute to poor hospital outcomes? A three-site epidemiologic study. J Gen Intern Med 1998;13:234-242. Ⓘⱽ

52. Ely EW, Shintani A, Truman B, et al: Delirium as a predictor of mortality in mechanically ventilated patients in the intensive care unit. JAMA 2004;291: 1753-1762. Ⓘⱽ

53. Elie M, Cole MG, Primeau FJ, Bellavance F: Delirium risk factors in elderly hospitalized patients. J Gen Intern Med 1998;13:204-212. Ⓘ

54. Williams-Russo P, Urquhart BL, Sharrock NE, Charlson ME: Post-operative delirium: Predictors and prognosis in elderly orthopedic patients. J Am Geriatr Soc 1992;40:759-767. Ⓘ

55. Marcantonio ER, Flacker JM, Wright RJ, Resnick NM: Reducing delirium after hip fracture: A randomized trial. J Am Geriatr Soc 2001;49:516-522. Ⓘ

56. Inouye SK, Bogardus ST, Charpentier PA, et al: A multicomponent intervention to prevent delirium in hospitalized older patients. N Engl J Med 1999;340: 669-676. Ⓘⱽ

57. Naughton BJ, Saltzman S, Ramadan F, et al: A multifactorial intervention to reduce prevalence of delirium and shorten hospital length of stay. J Am Geriatr Soc 2005;53:118-123. III

58. Cole MG, McCusker J, Bellavance F, et al: Systematic detection and multidisciplinary care of delirium in older medical inpatients: A randomized trial. CMAJ 2002;167:753-759. II

59. Breitbart W, Marotta R, Platt MM, et al: A double-blind trial of haloperidol, chlorpromazine, and lorazepam in the treatment of delirium in hospitalized AIDS patients. Am J Psychiatry 1996;153:231-237. II

60. Horikawa N, Yamazaki T, Miyamoto K, et al: Treatment for delirium with risperidone: Results of a prospective open trial with 10 patients. Gen Hosp Psychiatry 2003;25:289-292. III

61. Parellada E, Baeza I, de Pablo J, Martinez G: Risperidone in the treatment of patients with delirium. J Clin Psychiatry 2004;65:348-353. III

62. Mittal D, Jimerson NA, Neely EP, et al: Risperidone in the treatment of delirium: Results from a prospective open-label trial. J Clin Psychiatry 2004;65:662-667. III

63. Han C, Kim Y: A double-blind trial of Risperidone and Haloperidol for the treatment of delirium. Psychosomatics 2004;45:297-301. II

63a. Breitbart W, Tremblay A, Gibson C: An open trial of Olanzapine for the treatment of delirium in hospitalized cancer patients. Psychosomatics 2002;43:175-182. III

63b. Kim KY, Bader GM, Kotlyar V, Gropper D: Treatment of delirium in older adults with quetiapine. J Geri Psych Neurol 2003;16:29-31. III

63c. Sasaki Y, Matsuyama T, Inoue S, et al: A prospective open-label, flexible-dose study of quetiapine in the treatment of delirium. J Clin Psychiatry 2003;64:1316-1321. III

64. Skrobik YK, Bergeron N, Dumont M, Gottfried SB: Olanzapine vs haloperidol: Treating delirium in a critical care setting. Intensive Care Med 2004;30:444-449. II

65. Gagnon B, Low G, Schreier G: Methlyphenidate hydrochloride improves cognitive function in patients with advanced cancer and hypoactive delirium: A prospective clinical study. J Psychiatry Neurosci 2005;30:100-107. III

66. Kosten TR, O'Connor PG: Management of drug and alcohol withdrawal. N Engl J Med 2003;348:1786-1795. V

67. Umbricht A, Hoover DR, Tucker MJ, et al: Opioid detoxification with buprenorphine, clonidine, or methadone in hospitalized heroin-dependent patients with HIV infection. Drug Alcohol Depend 2003; 69:262-272. **II**

68. Amato L, Davoli M, Ferri M, Ali R: Methadone at tapered doses for the management of opioid withdrawal. Cochrane Database Syst Rev 2004;(4):CD003409. **II**

69. Welsh CJ, Suman M, Cohen A, et al: The use of intravenous buprenorphine for the treatment of opioid withdrawal in medically ill hospitalized patients. Am J Addictions 2002;11:135-140. **III**

70. Oreskovich MR, Saxon AJ, Ellis MK, et al: A double-blind, double-dummy, randomized, prospective pilot study of the partial mu opiate agonist, buprenorphine, for acute detoxification from heroin. Drug Alcohol Depend 2005;77:71-79. **II**

71. Assadi SM, Hafezi M, Mokri A, et al: Opioid detoxification using high doses of buprenorphine in 24 hours: A randomized, double blind, controlled clinical trial. J Subst Abuse Treat 2004;27:75-82. **II**

72. Gowing L, Ali R, White J: Buprenorphine for the management of opioid withdrawal. Cochrane Database Syst Rev 2004;(4):CD002025. **I**

73. Gold MS, Redmond DE Jr, Kleber HD: Clonidine blocks acute opiate-withdrawal symptoms. Lancet 1978; 2:599-602. **II**

74. Gowing L, Farrell M, Ali R, White J: Alpha 2 adrenergic agonists for the management of opioid withdrawal. Cochrane Database Syst Rev 2004;(4):CD002024. **I**

75. Kahn A, Mumford JP, Rogers GA, Beckford H: Double-blind study of lofexidine and clonidine in the detoxification of opiate addicts in hospital. Drug Alcohol Depend 1997;44:57-61. **II**

76. Bearn J, Gossop M, Strang J: Randomised double-blind comparison of lofexidine and methadone in the in-patient treatment of opiate withdrawal. Drug Alcohol Depend 1996;43:87-91. **II**

77. Howells C, Allen S, Gupta J, et al: Prison based detoxi-cation for opioid dependence: A randomized double blind controlled trial of lofexidine and methadone. Drug Alcohol Depend 2002;67:169-176. **II**

78. Gowing L, Ali R, White J: Opioid antagonists under heavy sedation or anaesthesia for opioid withdrawal. Cochrane Database Syst Rev 2005;2:CD00202. **I**

79. Montazeri K, Farahnakian M, Saghaei M: The effect of acupuncture on the acute withdrawal symptoms from rapid opiate detoxification. Acta Anaesthesiol Sin 2002;40:173-177. III

80. Amato L, Minozzi S, Davoli M, et al: Psychosocial and pharmacological treatments for opioid detoxification. Cochrane Database Syst Rev 2004;4: CD005031. I

81. Mayo-Smith MF, Beecher LH, Fischer TL, et al: Management of alcohol withdrawal delirium: An evidence-based practice guideline. American Society of Addiction Medicine Working Group on the Management of Alcohol Withdrawal Delirium. Arch Intern Med 2004;164:1405-1412. IV

82. Holbrook AM, Crowther R, Lotter A, et al: Meta-analysis of benzodiazepine use in the treatment of acute alcohol withdrawal. CMAJ 1999;160:649-655. I

83. Mayo-Smith MF: Pharmacologic management of alcohol withdrawal: A meta-analysis and evidence-based practice guideline. American Society of Addiction Medicine Working Group on Pharmacologic Management of Alcohol Withdrawal. JAMA 1997;278:144-151. I

84. Wilson A, Vulcano BA: Double-blind trial of alprazolam and chlordiazepoxide in the management of the acute ethanol withdrawal syndrome. Alcohol Clin Exp Res 1985;9:23-27. II

85. Saitz R, Mayo-Smith MF, Roberts MS, et al: Individualized treatment for alcohol withdrawal: A randomized double-blind controlled trial. JAMA 1994;272:519-523. II

86. Daeppen JB, Gache P, Landry U, et al: Symptom-triggered vs fixed-schedule doses of benzodiazepine for alcohol withdrawal: A randomized treatment trial. Arch Intern Med 2002;162:1117-1121. II

87. Jaeger TM, Lohr RH, Pankratz VS: Symptom-triggered therapy for alcohol withdrawal syndrome in medical inpatients. Mayo Clin Proc 2001;76:695-701. III

88. American Diabetes Association, American Psychiatric Association, American Association of Clinical Endocrinologists, North American Association for the Study of Obesity: Consensus development conference on antipsychotic drugs and obesity and diabetes. Diabetes Care 2004;27:596-601. IV

89. Rosack J: FDA to require diabetes warning on antipsychotics. Psychiatr News 2003;38:1. VI

90. Koller EA, Doraiswamy PM: Olanzapine-associated diabetes mellitus. Pharmacotherapy 2002;22: 841-852. **VI**

91. Koller E, Schneider B, Bennett K, Dubitsky G: Clozapine-associated diabetes. Am J Med 2001;111: 716-723.

92. Koller E, Cross JT, Doraiswamy PM, Schneider BS: Risperidone associated diabetes mellitus: A pharmacovigilance study. Pharmacotherapy 2003;23: 735-744. **VI**

93. Bellantuono C, Tentoni L, Donda P: Antipsychotic drugs and risk of type 2 diabetes: An evidence-based approach. Hum Psychopharmacol Clin Exp 2004; 19:549-558. **III**

94. Haddad PM: Antipsychotics and diabetes: Review of non-prospective data. Br J Psychiatry 2004;184 (Suppl 47):S80-S84. **III**

95. Jin H, Meyer JM, Jeste DV: Atypical antipsychotics and glucose dysregulation: A systematic review. Schizophr Res 2004;71:95-212. **I**

96. Bushe C, Leonard B: Association between atypical antipsychotic agents and type 2 diabetes: Review of prospective clinical data. Br J Psychiatry 2004;184 (Suppl 47):S87-S93. **I**

97. Lindenmayer JP, Czobor P, Volavka J, et al: Changes in glucose and cholesterol levels in patients with schizophrenia treated with typical or atypical antipsychotics. Am J Psychiatry 2003;160:290-296. **III**

98. Newcomer JW: Abnormalities of glucose metabolism associated with atypical antipsychotic drugs. J Clin Psychiatry 2004;65(Suppl 18):36-46. **II**

99. Allison DB, Mentore J, Heo M, et al: Antipsychotic induced weight gain: A comprehensive research synthesis. Am J Psychiatry 1999;156:1686-1696. **I**

100. Wirshing DA: Schizophrenia and obesity: Impact of antipsychotic medications. J Clin Psychiatry 2004;65(Suppl 18):13-26. **V**

101. Allison DB, Casey DE: Anti-psychotic induced weight gain: A review of the literature. J Clin Psychiatry 2001;62(Suppl 7):22-31. **V**

102. Meyer JM, Koro CE: The effects of antipsychotic therapy on serum lipids: A comprehensive review. Schizophr Res 2004;70:1-17. **I**

103. Al-Khatib S, Lapointe NM, Kramer JM, Califf RM: What clinicians should know about the QT interval. JAMA 2003;289:2120-2127. **V**

104. Zareba W, Lin D: Antipsychotic drugs and QT interval prolongation. Psychiatr Q 2003;74:291-306. Ⓥ

105. Center for Education and Research on Therapeutics: Available at www.torsades.org Ⓥ

106. Yap YG, Camm AJ: Drug induced QT prolongation and torsades de pointes. Heart 2003;89:1363-1372. Ⓥ

107. U.S. Food and Drug Administration (FDA): Psychopharmacological drugs advisory committee. Zeldox, Pfizer, 2000. Available at www.fda.gov/ohrms/dockets/ac/00/backrgrd/3619b1.htm

108. Mehtonen OP, Aranko K, Malkonen L, Vapaatalo H: A survey of sudden death associated with the use of antipsychotic or antidepressant drugs: 49 cases in Finland. Acta Psychiatr Scand 1991;84:58-64. ⒾⒾ

109. Reilly JG, Ayis SA, Ferrier IN, et al: Thioridazine and sudden unexplained death in psychiatric inpatients. Br J Psychiatry 2002;180:515-522. Ⓘ

110. Ray WA, Meredith S, Thapa PB, et al: Antipsychotics and the risk of sudden cardiac death. Arch Gen Psychiatry 2001;58:1161-1167. Ⓘ

111. Hennessy S, Bilker W, Knauss JS, et al: Cardiac arrest and ventricular arrhythmia in patients taking antipsychotic drugs: Cohort using administrative data. BMJ 2002;325:1070. Ⓘ

112. Straus S, Bleumink G: Antipsychotics and the risk of sudden cardiac death. Arch Intern Med. 2004;164:1293-1297. Ⓘ

113. Ravin DS, Levenson JW: Fatal cardiac event following initiation of risperidone therapy. Ann Pharmacother 1997;31:867-870. Ⓥ

114. Haddad P, Anderson IM: Antipsychotic-related QTc prolongation, torsades de pointes, and sudden death. Drugs 2002:62:1649-1671. Ⓥ

115. Sink KM, Holden KF, Yaffe K: Pharmacological treatment of neuropsychiatric symptoms of dementia: A review of the evidence. JAMA 2005;293:596-608. Ⓘ

116. Lonergan E, Luxenberg J, Colford J: Haloperidol for agitation in dementia. Cochrane Database Syst Rev 2002;(2):CD002852. Ⓘ

117. Glick ID, Murray SR, Vasudevan P, et al: Treatment with atypical antipsychotics: New indications and new populations. J Psychiatr Res 2001;35:187-191. Ⓘ

118. Briesacher BA, Limcangco MR, Simoni-Wastila L, et al: The quality of antipsychotic drug prescribing in nursing homes. Arch Intern Med 2005;165:1280-1285. III

119. Lee P, Gill SS, Freedman M, et al: Atypical antipsychotic drugs in the treatment of behavioral and psychological symptoms of dementia: Systematic review. BMJ 2004;329:75. I

120. Katz I, Jeste DV, Mintzer JE, et al: Comparison of risperidone and placebo for psychosis and behavioural disturbances associated with dementia: A randomized double blind trial. J Clin Psychiatry 1999;60: 107-115. II

121. Brodaty H, Ames D, Snowdon J, et al: A randomized placebo controlled trial of risperidone for the treatment of aggression, agitation, and psychosis in dementia. J Clin Psychiatry 2003;64:134-143. II

122. De Deyn PP, Rabheru K, Rasmussen A, et al: A randomized trial of risperidone, placebo, and haloperidol for behavioural symptoms of dementia. Neurology 1999:53:946-955. II

123. Street JS, Clark WS, Gannon KS, et al: Olanzapine treatment of psychotic and behavioral symptoms in patients with Alzheimer disease in nursing care facilities: A double-blind, randomized, placebo-controlled trial. The HGEU study group. Arch Gen Psychiatry 2000;57:968-976. II

124. DeDeyn PP, Carrasco MM, Deberdt W, et al: Olanzapine versus placebo in the treatment of psychosis with or without associated behavioral disturbance in patients with Alzheimer's disease. Int J Geriatr Psychiatry 2004;19:115-126. II

125. Chan W, Lam LC, Choy CN, et al: A double-blind randomized comparison of risperidone and haloperidol in the treatment of behavioral and psychological symptoms in Chinese dementia patients. Int J Geriatric Psychiatry 2001;16:1156-1162. II

126. Kuehn BM: FDA warns antipsychotic drugs may be risky for elderly. JAMA 2005;293:2462. I

127. Herrmann N, Lanctot KL: Do atypical antipsychotics cause stroke? CNS Drugs 2005;19:91-103. I

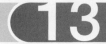

Selected Medical Problems Encountered During Pregnancy

Aba Barden-Maja, C. Jessica Dine,
Laura M. Kosseim, Jodi Savitz, and
Daniel I. Steinberg

1. Which routine immunizations are safe to administer during pregnancy?

Search Date: June 2005

Search Strategy: *PubMed, 1988 to 2005, search of "pregnancy AND immunization OR vaccine." Limited to human studies and English language; 782 citations retrieved. Titles and abstracts scanned, with relevant citations selected. Bibliographies of all relevant citations reviewed. Search of practice guidelines from the American College of Obstetricians and Gynecologists and the Centers for Disease Control and Prevention.*

Vaccinations in pregnant women should be considered on the basis of risks versus benefits. The Centers for Disease Control and Prevention (CDC) guidelines state that live-virus vaccines are generally contraindicated for pregnant women because of the theoretical risk of transmission of the vaccine virus to the fetus.[1] However, they also declare that if a live-virus vaccine is inadvertently given to a pregnant woman or if a woman becomes pregnant within 4 weeks of vaccination it is not an indication to terminate the pregnancy. The woman should instead be counseled about the potential effects on the fetus. The guidelines also report that there are no known risks to a fetus from immune globulin preparations administered to the mother.[2] Table 13-1 is adapted from the 2005 CDC guidelines.[1]

Table 13-1. Vaccine Safety During Pregnancy

Vaccine	Type	Vaccinate during Pregnancy if Indicated?	Notes, Recommendations, or Considerations
Hepatitis A	Inactivated	See notes in next column	Safety has not been determined in pregnancy, but an inactivated virus is theoretically low risk. Vaccine risk should be weighed against exposure risk.[3]
Hepatitis B	Recombinant	Yes	
Human Papillomavirus (HPV)	Recombinant	Not recommended	Data are limited, though so far the vaccine has not been associated with poor pregnancy outcomes. Vaccination should be delayed until after pregnancy.[1]
Influenza	Inactivated	Yes	Given an increased risk for influenza-related complications, this vaccine is recommended to all women who will be pregnant during flu season, and it can be safely administered during any trimester.[4]
Influenza	Live	Contraindicated	Live attenuated influenza vaccine (LAIV)
Measles	Live	Contraindicated	Women should avoid becoming pregnant for 28 days after vaccination.[2]
Mumps	Live	Contraindicated	Women should avoid becoming pregnant for 28 days after vaccination.[5]
Pneumococcal	Inactivated, PPV23	See notes in next column	Safety has not been evaluated in the first trimester of pregnancy, but no adverse outcomes have been reported in mothers inadvertently vaccinated during pregnancy.[6] Two randomized, controlled trials involving women in their third trimester have revealed no serious adverse reactions in the pregnant women or the fetuses or infants of the women who received PPV23.[7,8]

Continued

Table 13-1. Vaccine Safety During Pregnancy—cont'd

Vaccine	Type	Vaccinate during Pregnancy if Indicated	Notes, Recommendations, or Considerations
Polio	Inactivated, IVP	See notes in next column	Although it has not been documented to cause adverse effects in pregnant women or their fetuses, the CDC recommends avoidance of vaccination in pregnant women on theoretical grounds. However, if a pregnant woman is at increased risk for infection and requires immediate protection against polio, IPV can be administered in accordance with recommended schedules for adults.[9]
Rubella	Live	Contraindicated	Women should avoid becoming pregnant for 28 days after vaccination.[5,10] Infants born to 226 pregnant women who received the RA27/3 (the only rubella vaccine used in the United States) between 3 months before and 3 months after conception had no evidence of congenital rubella infection in a CDC registry.[11] ACOG guidelines state that rubella vaccination that occurs during pregnancy is not an indication to terminate the pregnancy.[12]
Tetanus/diphtheria	Inactivated	Yes	There is no evidence that tetanus and diphtheria toxoids are teratogenic, but waiting until the second trimester to give this vaccination is recommended to minimize theoretical risk.[13]
Varicella	Live	Contraindicated	Women should avoid becoming pregnant for 1 month after vaccination.[14]

ACOG, American College of Obstetricians and Gynecologists; CDC, Centers for Disease Control and Prevention; IPV, inactivated polio vaccine; LAIV, live attenuated influenza vaccine.
*Adapted from Centers for Disease Control and Prevention: Guidelines for vaccinating pregnant women: Recommendations of the Advisory Committee on Immunization Practices (ACIP). Available at http://www.cdc.gov/nip/publications/preg_guide.htm/ Accessed July 2005.

2. What are the risk factors and screening recommendations for toxoplasmosis in pregnancy?

Search Date: June 2005

Search Strategy: *PubMed, 1988 to 2005, search of "pregnancy AND toxoplasmosis." Limited to human studies and English language; 147 citations retrieved. Titles and abstracts scanned, with relevant citations selected. Bibliographies of all relevant citations reviewed. Search of practice guidelines from the American College of Obstetricians and Gynecologists and the Centers for Disease Control and Prevention.*

RISK FACTORS FOR TOXOPLASMA INFECTION

Toxoplasma gondii infection acquired during pregnancy can be transmitted transplacentally, causing congenital toxoplasmosis. Infections are less likely to be transmitted to the fetus if they occur earlier in the pregnancy, but earlier fetal infections are more likely to be severe than later ones.[15] Congenital toxoplasmosis can lead to complications such as miscarriage, mental retardation, and seizures. An estimated 400 to 4000 cases of congenital toxoplasmosis occur in the United States each year.[16] Pregnant women and their physicians need to be informed about risk factors for toxoplasmosis to help lower the risk of congenital infections.

A large, multicenter, European, case-control study revealed several independent risk factors for *Toxoplasma* seroconversion during pregnancy: contact with raw or undercooked beef (OR = 1.73; 95% CI: 1.1 to 7.2; *P* = .01), lamb (OR = 3.13; 95% CI: 1.4 to 7.2; *P* = .007), or other meat (OR = 4.12; 95% CI: 1.6 to 10.9; *P* = .004); contact with soil (OR = 1.81; 95% CI: 1.2 to 2.7; *P* = .005); and travel outside Europe, the United States, or Canada (OR = 2.33; 95% CI: 1.3 to 4.1; *P* = .003).[17] Contact with cats was not a risk factor in this study. A smaller study of 63 women in Norway revealed that cleaning the cat litter box was a risk factor for seroconversion during pregnancy in addition to other predictors, such as eating raw or undercooked mutton, washing kitchen knives infrequently after preparing raw meat before handling another food item, eating raw or undercooked minced meat products, eating raw or undercooked pork, and eating unwashed raw vegetables or fruits.[18] In a small case-control study in France, having a pet cat was also a risk factor for *Toxoplasma* seroconversion during pregnancy (adjusted OR = 4.5; 95% CI: 1.0 to 19.9).[19] Other risk factors in this study included consuming undercooked beef and raw vegetables eaten outside the home. There have been no studies in the United States assessing risk factors for *Toxoplasma* seroconversion during pregnancy.

SCREENING FOR TOXOPLASMA INFECTION DURING PREGNANCY

Whether pregnant women should be screened for primary *Toxoplasma* infection is controversial.[20] One reason for this is the estimated 1.3% false-positive rate of IgM detection during pregnancy.[21] Experts have expressed valid concerns about the effects of these false-positive test results on a woman's decision regarding pregnancy termination.[22] The incidence of maternal primary *Toxoplasma* infection is very low. Rates of maternal seroconversion vary from 0.15% in Norway to 0.5% in Hungary.[23] One study screening 5288 susceptible pregnant women from a large urban area in Italy did find a higher seroconversion rate of 3.5%.[24]

TOXOPLASMOSIS TREATMENT DURING PREGNANCY

The benefits of toxoplasmosis treatment during pregnancy are not clear. A systematic review of the evidence for efficacy in the treatment of congenital toxoplasmosis found conflicting results.[25] Four of the nine nonrandomized studies included in the review found no reduction of fetal infection in the patients treated for toxoplasmosis, whereas five of the studies reported significantly lower transmission rates in children born to treated mothers ($P < .01$). Another cohort study found that treatment for congenital toxoplasmosis had no impact on the maternal-fetal transmission rate but did significantly reduce the sequelae among the infected infants (OR = 0.30; 95% CI: 0.10 to 0.86; $P = .026$).[26] A later cohort study showed an increased risk of congenital toxoplasmosis if untreated: 21% of untreated (95% CI: 6 to 45.6) versus 5.6% of treated (95% CI: 2.4 to 10.6), with an odds ratio of 4.5 ($P = .04$).[24] But when these effects of therapy were adjusted for month of infection, the odds ratio from lack of therapy was not associated with sequelae

(OR = 0.4; P = .5). The investigators concluded that the timing of fetal infection is a much stronger predictor of fetal outcomes than the use of antibiotic treatment for congenital toxoplasmosis. Another study in Europe failed to find any difference in the risk of congenital infection with treatment compared with no treatment.[27]

GUIDELINES FOR TOXOPLASMOSIS DURING PREGNANCY

The 2000 ACOG practice guidelines do not recommend routine serologic screening of pregnant women for toxoplasmosis, but they point out that this is based primarily on consensus and expert opinion.[28] The guidelines do recommend treating women who acquire toxoplasmosis during pregnancy with spiramycin. If fetal toxoplasmosis is then diagnosed, treatment with pyrimethamine, sulfadiazine, and leucovorin (i.e., folinic acid) is recommended. Treatment options include 3-week courses of pyrimethamine, sulfadiazine, and leucovorin alternating with 3-week courses of spiramycin or alternatively treatment with only pyrimethamine, sulfadiazine, and leucovorin until delivery.

3. What are risk factors and screening recommendations for rubella in pregnancy?

Search Date: June 2005

Search Strategy: PubMed, 1988 to 2005, search of "pregnancy AND rubella." Limited to human studies and English language; 121 citations retrieved. Titles and abstracts scanned, with relevant citations selected. Bibliographies of all relevant citations reviewed. Search of practice guidelines from the American College of Obstetricians and Gynecologists and the Centers for Disease Control and Prevention.

Rubella is usually a mild illness, but it can cause serious complications when contracted by a pregnant woman, especially in the first trimester. The complications can include miscarriage, abortion, stillbirth, and congenital rubella syndrome, which can manifest as hearing loss and developmental delay in addition to cardiovascular and central nervous system defects.[29,30] Risk factors for rubella include settings where large numbers of young adults are gathered, such as military bases and colleges.[31]

The CDC recommends routinely screening all pregnant women with rubella IgG serology at their earliest prenatal visit.[32] The recommendations stress the importance of identifying susceptible women so they can be monitored for infection during the pregnancy and then vaccinated after delivery.

4. What are the recommended screening procedures and treatment options for urinary tract infections during pregnancy?

Search Date: June 2005

Search Strategy: PubMed, 1988 to 2005, search of "pregnancy AND urinary AND screen OR treat." Limited to human studies and English language; 558 citations retrieved. Titles and abstracts scanned, with relevant citations selected. Bibliographies of all relevant citations reviewed. Search of practice guidelines from the American College of Obstetricians and Gynecologists.

The most common bacterial infections during pregnancy are urinary tract infections (UTIs).[33] Any UTI in a pregnant woman is considered to be complicated and requires treatment.[34] Pregnancy-associated UTIs have been associated with an increased risk for pyelonephritis (and its complications) and may be associated with an increased risk for preterm delivery. The predisposition of pregnant women for UTIs and pyelonephritis is thought to be the result of the ureteral dilation and slowed urinary tract peristalsis that occurs during pregnancy as a result of increased progesterone and estrogen levels. These hormones also cause decreased bladder tone, resulting in increased urinary stasis and ureterovesical reflux. The ureters and bladder are affected by the mechanical compression of the growing uterus, and this may result in urinary stasis.[34,35] Unlike in the nonpregnant patient, bacteriuria (i.e., presence of bacteria in the urinary tract without significant evidence of infection as measured by urinary leukocytes) in the pregnant patient should always be treated.

TREATMENT OF BACTERURIA DURING PREGNANCY

The Cochrane Collaboration conducted a meta-analysis of 14 randomized, controlled trials comparing antibiotic treatment with placebo in pregnant women with asymptomatic bacteriuria.[36] The incidence of pyelonephritis was reduced (OR = 0.24; 95% CI: 0.19 to 0.32) in the treatment groups, and antibiotic treatment was effective in clearing asymptomatic bacteriuria (OR = 0.07; 95% CI: 0.05 to 0.10). Antibiotics also reduced the incidence of preterm delivery and low birth weight (OR = 0.60; 95% CI: 0.45 to 0.80). However, given the limitations related to individual study quality in this meta-analysis, the investigators concluded that the association between untreated urinary tract infections, bacteriuria, and preterm birth should be interpreted with caution.

The American College of Obstetricians and Gynecologists (ACOG) recommends routine screening for bacteriuria with a urine culture at all first prenatal visits and during the third trimester.[37] The U.S. Preventive Services Task Force recommends screening pregnant women with a urine culture at 12 to 16 weeks' gestation but states that the optimal frequency of subsequent urine testing during pregnancy is uncertain.[38,39]

ANTIBIOTIC MANAGEMENT OF BACTERURIA DURING PREGNANCY

To clarify treatment options, the Cochrane Collaboration conducted a meta-analysis of different durations of antibiotic treatment for asymptomatic bacteriuria in pregnancy.[40] Ten studies that compared single- dose treatment with 4- to 7-day treatments were evaluated. The analysis showed a trend toward improved effectiveness in the longer treatment duration group, but it was not statistically significant (RR = 1.25; 95% CI: 0.93 to 1.67). The World Health Organization is conducting a large trial to further investigate the optimal duration of treatment for pregnancy-associated UTIs.

The ACOG guidelines for the treatment of asymptomatic bacteriuria or symptomatic cystitis recommend an initial 3-day course of antibiotics.[37] The guidelines stress that it is not the duration of therapy that is most important, but the documentation of successful treatment by demonstrating the clearance of bacteriuria after therapy is completed.[37,41] Choice of antibiotic should be based on sensitivity test results while avoiding agents that are contraindicated during pregnancy, such as tetracycline and quinolones.[37]

To determine which antibiotics are most effective in successfully eradicating UTIs, a Cochrane review evaluated different antibiotic options for symptomatic urinary tract infections (including pyelonephritis) in pregnant women.[42] Many different antibiotic regimens were compared, including oral nitrofurantoin, oral ampicillin, oral cefuroxime, intramuscular cefazolin or ceftriaxone, intravenous cefazolin or cefuroxime, and intravenous ampicillin plus gentamicin. All eight trials included had small sample sizes, but there were no significant differences in cure rates, recurrent infections, incidence of preterm delivery, incidence of prolonged fever, admission to the neonatal intensive care unit, or in the need to change the antibiotic. The study authors concluded that no single antibiotic was superior to any other and that all were effective and had high cure rates.

PYELONEPHRITIS DURING PREGNANCY

Pyelonephritis during pregnancy is traditionally treated with hospitalization and intravenous antibiotics. The ACOG recommends inpatient intravenous therapy until the patient is afebrile and symptomatically improved, followed by outpatient oral antibiotics to complete 10 days of therapy.[37] Several studies have been done to explore the safety of outpatient pyelonephritis treatment in pregnant women. In one study, 120 women with a gestational age less than 24 weeks were randomized to receive intramuscular ceftriaxone as outpatients or intravenous cefazolin as inpatients.[43] Those to be treated as outpatients were observed for up to 24 hours or until clinically stable and were seen by home health nurses between 18 and 36 hours after discharge for a second intramuscular dose of antibiotics, followed by a course of oral cephalexin. Ten percent of the outpatients were hospitalized because of sepsis, recurrent pyelonephritis, or abnormal laboratory test results. Eleven outpatients (18%) and 12 inpatients (20%) had positive urine cultures at follow-up (RR = 0.9; 95% CI: 0.4 to 1.9; P = .82). No significant differences between the groups were found in rates of recurrent pyelonephritis, abortion, or preterm delivery. There were no serious complications or pregnancy losses from either treatment regimen.[35,42]

Another trial randomized women with pyelonephritis at a gestational age greater than 24 weeks to receive two doses of intramuscular ceftriaxone, followed by oral cephalexin in an inpatient or outpatient setting.[44] Those randomized to outpatient care were arranged to be discharged after 24 hours of observation if clinically stable, although almost 30% of those women remained as inpatients due to sepsis, preterm labor, or other medical complications. No significant differences were seen between the inpatient and outpatient groups in the numbers of repeat positive urine culture after treatment ($P = .44$), recurrent pyelonephritis ($P = .35$), or preterm delivery ($P = .75$). More than 60% (154 of 246) of the women initially eligible for the study were eliminated due to preterm labor, obvious sepsis, recurrent pyelonephritis, or other preexisting medical conditions. The evidence suggests that although it may be effective to treat some patients at a gestational age greater than 24 weeks as outpatients, only very select groups may be safely treated in this manner.[35,44] ACOG comments on the limited evidence in this area and emphasizes that if these patients are to be treated as outpatients, home health care should be provided.[37]

The ACOG states that all women treated for urinary tract infections should be rescreened periodically for infection with urine dipstick tests or cultures. If the infection recurs, the patient should be retreated, and chronic suppression should be considered.[37]

5. What is the incidence of developing hypertension during pregnancy?

Search Date: May 2005

Search Strategy: PubMed, 1988 to 2005, search of "incidence OR prevalence AND pregnancy AND hypertension." Limited to human studies and English language; 464 citations retrieved. Titles and abstracts scanned, with relevant citations selected. Bibliographies of all relevant citations reviewed.

The hypertensive disorders of pregnancy encompass several conditions, including pregnancy-induced hypertension, otherwise known as gestational hypertension; preeclampsia and eclampsia; chronic hypertension; and preeclampsia superimposed on chronic hypertension.[45] *Pregnancy-induced hypertension* is defined as a blood pressure elevation (systolic BP > 140 or diastolic BP > 90) that is first detected after mid-pregnancy and returns to normal 12 weeks postpartum. *Chronic hypertension* includes blood pressure elevations that occur before the 20th week of gestation. *Preeclampsia* is gestational blood pressure elevations after the 20th week of gestation in the presence of proteinuria. Other symptoms may be present in preeclampsia and can point to the diagnosis even if proteinuria is absent. *Eclampsia* is defined by the presence of seizures that cannot otherwise be explained in a woman with preeclampsia.

The hypertensive disorders often overlap, and their epidemiologic patterns are difficult to separate. Together, these disorders occur in 6% to 8% of pregnancies.[45] Because of the increasing prevalence and recognition of hypertension in adults, it is estimated that 5% of pregnant women will have chronic hypertension complicating their pregnancies in the future.[46]

6. What are the proposed causes of pregnancy-associated hypertension?

Search Date: May 2005

Search Strategy: *PubMed, 1988 to 2005, search of "risk factors AND pregnancy AND hypertension." Limited to human studies and English language; 322 citations retrieved. Titles and abstracts scanned, with relevant citations selected. Bibliographies of all relevant citations reviewed. Search of practice guidelines from the American College of Obstetricians and Gynecologists.*

The cause of pregnancy-induced hypertension remains unknown and is likely multifactorial. Calcium deficiency, insulin resistance, and imbalances of prostacyclins have been postulated to play a role in its development. A clinical trial of 4500 nulliparous women studied calcium supplementation to assess its effects on the development of hypertensive disorders of pregnancy. The trial showed no significant reduction in these disorders.[47] It has been suggested that pregnancy-associated insulin resistance may play a role in the pathogenesis of the hypertensive disorders of pregnancy. Although no cause-and-effect relationship has been established, women with hypertension during pregnancy have been found to have greater levels of insulin resistance.[48] Given the cyclooxygenase inhibitory properties of aspirin, it was postulated that aspirin could reverse the vasodilatory and vasoconstrictive effects of prostacyclins in pregnancy. A multicenter clinical trial of low-dose aspirin in nulliparous women showed a decreased incidence of preeclampsia in women who had a pregnancy-induced elevation in blood pressure but no decrease in perinatal morbidity or placental abruption.[49]

7. What are the risk factors for the hypertensive disorders of pregnancy?

Search Date: May 2005

Search Strategy: PubMed, 1988 to 2005, search of "risk factors AND pregnancy AND hypertension." Limited to human studies and English language; 322 citations retrieved. Titles and abstracts scanned, with relevant citations selected. Bibliographies of all relevant citations reviewed. Search of practice guidelines from the American College of Obstetricians and Gynecologists.

Risk factors for hypertensive disorders of pregnancy include maternal age (OR = 3.5 for women 26 to 30 years old [95% CI: 1.6 to 7.1] and 4.2 for women older than 30 years [95% CI: 1.9 to 8.8] compared with 20- to 25-year-old women) and nonpregnant body mass index (BMI). A BMI of 25 to 30 increased the risk of pregnancy-induced hypertension with an odds ratio of 1.7 (95% CI: 1.1 to 2.7), whereas a BMI of greater than 30 resulted in an odds ratio of 2.1 (95% CI: 1.3 to 3.6) compared with women with a BMI of less than 25. Women with prior births have a slightly increased risk for pregnancy-induced hypertension, with odds ratios of 0.7 for one prior birth (95% CI: 0.4 to 1.0) and 0.5 for two prior births (95% CI: 0.3 to 0.9) compared with nulliparous women.[50] Twin gestations have a relative risk of 1.2 to 2.7 of pregnancy-induced hypertension compared with singleton pregnancies.[51]

Smoking during pregnancy seems to mildly reduce the risk for developing pregnancy-induced hypertension. A multicenter cohort study followed 4589 nulliparous women for 3 years and found a reduced risk of pregnancy-induced hypertension in women who smoked at the time of enrollment compared with nonsmokers (RR = 0.8; 95% CI: 0.6 to 0.9), even after adjusting for maternal age, race, BMI, type of health insurance, and clinical center. Quitting before or during pregnancy negated this decreased relative risk.[52] Given the multitude of other possible adverse effects of smoking to both mother and fetus, smoking during pregnancy is not recommended.

Later studies have looked at the genetics of pregnancy-induced hypertension. Results of these studies suggest that molecular variants of angiotensinogen,[53] polymorphisms of reductase genes, and factor V Leiden mutations[54] may contribute to the development of pregnancy-induced hypertension.

8. What are the risks of adverse clinical outcomes to the mother and fetus in the pregnant hypertensive patient?

Search Date: May 2005

Search Strategy: PubMed, 1988 to 2005, search of "adverse effects OR adverse outcomes AND pregnancy AND hypertension." Limited to human studies and English language; 422 citations retrieved. Titles and abstracts scanned, with relevant citations selected. Bibliographies of all relevant citations reviewed. Search of practice guidelines from the American College of Obstetricians and Gynecologists.

As a group, the hypertensive disorders during pregnancy account for almost 15% of maternal deaths, making it the second leading cause of maternal morbidity in the United States.[45] Most of these complications can be attributed to preeclampsia or eclampsia, although the other hypertensive disorders do carry some risk for the mother and fetus.

Pregnancy-induced hypertension carries a good prognosis for the outcome of the pregnancy. The primary risk to the mother is its tendency to recur in subsequent pregnancies and its association with the development of chronic hypertension later in life.[55]

Chronic hypertension during pregnancy, however, carries a more substantial risk to the mother and fetus. First, it increases the risk of superimposed preeclampsia. In a multicenter, randomized trial, 763 women with chronic hypertension were randomly assigned to aspirin or placebo. There were no difference in outcomes between the aspirin-treated and placebo group, but the study was able to comment on risk factors for preeclampsia. The overall rate of superimposed preeclampsia was 25%, but it was even higher in women who had hypertension for at least 4 years (31% versus 22%), women with preeclampsia in a previous pregnancy (32% versus 23%), and women with diastolic blood pressures (DBPs) of 100 to 110 mm Hg compared with women with DBPs of less than 100 mm Hg (42% versus 24%). Women with chronic hypertension also have an increased risk of placental abruption (1.5%). This risk of abruption increased significantly to 3% ($P = .04$) in women with chronic hypertension and superimposed preeclampsia.

Chronic hypertension with and without superimposed preeclampsia affects neonatal outcomes. Preeclampsia alone has significant adverse neonatal risks, such as increased rates of preterm labor, neonatal intraventricular hemorrhage, small for gestational age (SGA) births, and overall higher rates of perinatal death.[56] However, even mild chronic hypertension (< 160/110 mm Hg), when superimposed on preeclampsia, triples the risk for perinatal mortality, as demonstrated in a systematic review[57] (OR = 3.4; 95% CI: 3.0 to 3.7). Chronic hypertension without superimposed preeclampsia increased the rate of SGA babies (10.9%) compared with the general population (4.1%) (OR = 2.9; 95% CI: 1.6 to 5.0). Severe hypertension, defined as a DBP of equal to or greater than 110, at less than 20 weeks was associated with a significant risk to the fetus. The risk of SGA babies (OR = 3.8; 95% CI: 1.0 to 13.7) and of delivery at less than 32 weeks (OR = 7.4; 95% CI: 1.9 to 29.5) were both increased in the pregnant patient with chronic hypertension.[58]

9. How is hypertension safely treated during pregnancy?

Search Date: May 2005

Search Strategy: PubMed, 1988 to 2005, search of "treatment AND pregnancy AND hypertension." Limited to human studies and English language; 1229 citations retrieved. Titles and abstracts scanned, with relevant citations selected. Bibliographies of all relevant citations reviewed. Search of practice guidelines from the American College of Obstetricians and Gynecologists.

The 2001 *ACOG Practice Bulletin* does not recommend treating uncomplicated mild chronic hypertension (i.e., SBP in the range of 140 to 179 mm Hg and a DBP in the range of 90 to 109 mm Hg) during pregnancy because it has no known beneficial effects on perinatal outcome.[59] Conversely, the National High Blood Pressure Education Program Working Group on High Blood Pressure in Pregnancy recommends starting or reinstituting antihypertensive therapy if the SBP exceeds 150 to 160 mm Hg, the DBP exceeds 100 to 110 mm Hg, or there are signs of end-organ damage, such as renal insufficiency or left ventricular hypertrophy.[45] A randomized, controlled trial of 263 women with hypertension during their 6th to 13th week of pregnancy found no difference in the rates of superimposed preeclampsia (15.6% with no treatment, 18.4% with methyldopa, and 16.3% with labetalol), placental abruption (2.2% without treatment, 1.1% with methyldopa, and 2.3% with labetalol), preterm delivery (10% without treatment, 12.5% with methyldopa, and 11.6% with labetalol), or perinatal mortality with methyldopa, labetalol, or no antihypertensive treatment.[60]

The *ACOG Practice Bulletin* recommendations for women with chronic treated or untreated hypertension are not as clear. ACOG recommends withholding the initiation of new antihypertensives in the absence of complications and to consider discontinuation or dose reduction of previously prescribed antihypertensives.[59] This is based on two meta-analyses. In the first meta-analysis, treatment of 623 women with mild chronic hypertension was found to decrease the incidence of severe hypertension in the mother but not affect perinatal outcomes.[61] In a follow-up meta-analysis that included the seven trials from the previous meta-analysis and 38 trials of women with late-onset (> 20 weeks) hypertension, an adverse effect on fetal growth in the antihypertensive treatment group was seen (i.e., 10-mm Hg fall in mean arterial pressure was associated with a 145-g decrease in birth weight).[62]

METHYLDOPA

The *ACOG Practice Bulletin* and the National High Blood Pressure Education Program Working Group on High Blood Pressure in Pregnancy recommend methyldopa as the first-line antihypertensive to use for chronic hypertension during pregnancy based on the reports that it does not alter uteroplacental blood flow or fetal hemodynamics.[59,63]

LABETOL AND OTHER BETA BLOCKERS

Labetalol can be used as a safe alternative to methyldopa. One randomized, controlled trial reported no differences in perinatal outcomes for labetalol, methyldopa, or no antihypertensive treatment in women with chronic hypertension.[60] A meta-analysis of beta blockers for hypertension in pregnancy showed an increase in SGA infants (OR = 2.46 [95% CI: 1.02 to 5.92] for women with mild hypertension; OR = 1.47 [95% CI: 0.96 to 2.2] for women with mild to moderate hypertension) in women receiving beta blockers during pregnancy.[64] Given these data, beta blockers are avoided during pregnancy if possible.

DIURETICS

The only meta-analysis looking at the safety of diuretics in treating hypertension during pregnancy is from 1985. This meta-analysis examined nine randomized, controlled trials that included almost 7000 patients. No negative effects of diuretics on perinatal mortality were found, but women treated with diuretics did have lower blood pressures compared with controls. A lower incidence of eclampsia was observed in the women treated with diuretics, perhaps because of the reduced blood pressure trend.[65] A later randomized study looked at the use of diuretics in pregnant women on diuretic therapy for chronic hypertension during the first trimester. Patients were randomized to continue or discontinue diuretic therapy. The study concluded that diuretics prevent normal plasma volume expansion (mean increase of 18% with diuretics versus 52% without diuretics) but do not affect perinatal outcomes.[66] The study is limited by its small sample size ($N = 20$). The National High Blood Pressure Education Program Working Group on High Blood Pressure in Pregnancy states that diuretics are contraindicated in settings in which uteroplacental perfusion is already reduced, such as in preeclampsia or intrauterine growth restriction. In the absence of these conditions, diuretics are considered safe to use during pregnancy.[45]

CALCIUM CHANNEL BLOCKERS

Calcium channel blockers have been studied in one randomized, controlled trial. There was no significant difference in preterm deliveries between women taking nifedipine compared with those receiving no antihypertensive treatment. The difference between cesarean sections and the percentage of babies weighing less than the 10th percentile in the two treatment groups was also not significant.[67] This is the only study to examine the effects and safety of calcium channel blockers in the treatment of hypertension during pregnancy.

ANGIOTENSIN-CONVERTING ENZYME INHIBITORS

Angiotensin-converting enzyme inhibitors are contraindicated in the second and third trimesters of pregnancy because of their teratogenic risk.[68] There is little data on using angiotensin receptor blockers during the first trimester, but they are not recommended in the second and third trimester based on theoretic risks.[69]

10. How many patients diagnosed with hypertension during pregnancy remain hypertensive after the pregnancy?

Search Date: May 2005

Search Strategy: PubMed, 1988 to 2005, search of "persistent hypertension OR postpartum hypertension AND pregnancy AND hypertension." Limited to human studies and English language; 172 citations retrieved. Titles and abstracts scanned, with relevant citations selected. Bibliographies of all relevant citations reviewed.

Women who are diagnosed with hypertension during pregnancy are at higher risk for developing hypertension and preeclampsia in their subsequent pregnancies and at higher risk for developing chronic hypertension. Some studies suggest that these women should also be considered to be at higher risk for developing coronary artery disease.

One case-control study described 406 women that had severe preeclampsia or eclampsia and assessed their risk for subsequent complications related to hypertension. The women in the preeclampsia-eclampsia group had an increased risk for developing preeclampsia in their second (46.8% versus 7.6%, $P < .0001$) and subsequent pregnancies (20.7% versus 7.7%, $P < .001$) and for developing chronic hypertension (14.8% versus 5.6%, $P < .001$) compared with controls.[70]

A prospective cohort study found that compared with women without a history of hypertension during pregnancy, women with a history of hypertension during pregnancy had an increased risk for chronic hypertension (RR = 2.35), acute myocardial infarction (RR = 2.24), chronic ischemic heart disease (RR = 1.74), angina (RR = 1.53), all ischemic heart disease (RR = 1.65), and venous thromboembolism (VTE) (RR = 1.62). The rates for cerebrovascular disease and peripheral vascular disease were not significantly increased.[71]

11. How common are pulmonary embolism and deep vein thrombosis in pregnancy, and what are the risk factors for venous thromboembolism in the pregnant patient?

Search Date: May 2005

Search Strategy: PubMed, 1988 to 2005, search of "pregnancy AND incidence OR prevalence OR risk factors AND deep vein thrombosis OR pulmonary embolism OR venous thromboembolism." Limited to human studies and English language; 244 citations retrieved. Titles and abstracts scanned, with relevant citations selected. Bibliographies of all relevant citations reviewed.

Pulmonary embolism (PE) is uncommon in pregnancy. Retrospective studies examining a total of more than 300,000 deliveries report only 65 cases of objectively diagnosed PE.[72,73] Large, retrospective studies also show that deep vein thrombosis (DVT) is rare in pregnancy, with only 162 cases reported in more than 300,000 births.[73,74]

Risk factors for venous thrombosis in pregnancy include maternal age older than 35 years, operative vaginal delivery, cesarean section, current multiple pregnancy, blood type A, delivery at gestational age less than 36 weeks, BMI greater than 25, previous VTE, thrombophilia, and family history suggestive of thrombophilia.[75,76] Multivariate analysis has shown that although thrombophilias such as factor V Leiden (heterozygous), prothrombin mutation (heterozygous), antithrombin deficiency, and protein C and protein S deficiency are associated with an increased risk for VTE, the absolute increase in risk is low when these disorders occur in isolation. For example, for prothrombin mutation, which incurs the highest risk (RR of VTE = 12.4; 95% CI: 7.1 to 22), the probability of VTE in pregnancy is estimated to be only 0.32%. However, in patients with both factor V Leiden and the prothrombin mutation, the risk is significantly greater (RR of VTE = 84; 95% CI: 19 to 369).[77]

12. What is the approach to diagnosis of pulmonary embolism in the pregnant patient?

Search Date: May 2005

Search Strategy: *PubMed, 1988 to 2005, search of "pregnancy AND venous thromboembolism OR deep vein thrombosis OR pulmonary embolism AND sensitivity AND specificity OR sensitivity OR diagnosis OR diagnostic use OR specificity." Limited to human studies and English language; 234 citations retrieved. Titles and abstracts scanned, with relevant citations selected.*

Bibliographies of all citations reviewed. Search of practice guidelines from the American College of Obstetricians and Gynecologists and the American College of Chest Physicians.

Diagnosis begins with an estimation of the pretest probability of disease. The clinical prediction rules used for diagnosing PE in the nonpregnant population are not applicable to pregnant patients. The prevalence of PE in pregnant patients presenting with suspected PE (i.e., the patient group encountered in practice) is not well defined, because pregnant patients have been excluded from most prospective trials of DVT or PE. One retrospective study of 120 consecutive pregnant patients with suspected PE reported a prevalence range of 3.3% to 8.0%.[78,79] Retrospective data indicate that common presenting symptoms of VTE during pregnancy include dyspnea (63%), pleuritic chest pain (55.3%), and cough (23.7%).[74] The presence of risk factors for VTE, as outlined in Question 11, should also be considered when estimating pretest probability. The low reported prevalence of PE must be weighed against the fact that symptoms are notoriously unreliable in the diagnosis of PE and that the consequences of a missed diagnosis can be grave. Objective testing is indicated for all patients with suspected PE.

Diagnostic testing for PE in the pregnant patient relies on expert opinion and extrapolation from studies of nonpregnant patients. No diagnostic algorithms or individual tests have been studied prospectively in pregnant patients. The need for accurate diagnosis outweighs concern about the effects of radiation exposure of the fetus and radiation exposure from standard tests used to evaluate PE, such as ventilation-perfusion $\dot{V}/\dot{Q}$ scans, is minimal.[79,80]

Because the D-dimer level can be elevated during pregnancy for various reasons, a positive test result is nonspecific. A negative test result would seem to argue against VTE, although none of the D-dimer assays has been evaluated in pregnant patients.

Computed tomography (CT) should be avoided if possible because of the relatively large amount of radiation involved and lack of safety data.[81] Although no studies of contrast CT have included pregnant patients, one meta-analysis found that single-slice spiral CT ($-LR =$ 0.08; 95% CI: 0.05 to 0.13) and multidetector-row CT ($-LR = 0.15$; 95% CI: 0.05 to 0.43) were helpful in excluding clinically relevant VTE at the 3-month follow-up.[82] Although test results must always be interpreted in combination with the pretest probability of disease, it is reassuring that VTE event rates after a negative contrast CT result appear similar to those after a normal conventional angiogram. If necessary, CT scans should be done with abdominal screening.

$\dot{V}/\dot{Q}$ scans have been examined retrospectively in pregnant patients suspected of PE. Withholding anticoagulation in patients with nondiagnostic or normal $\dot{V}/\dot{Q}$ scan results correlated with no reported episodes of VTE during 20-month follow-up.[83] This is consistent with data from nonpregnant patients indicating that a normal $\dot{V}/\dot{Q}$ scan result excludes PE. In the absence of prospective diagnostic trials, an algorithm based on expert opinion presents a reasonable approach (Fig. 13-1).

13. How is deep vein thrombosis diagnosed in the pregnant patient?

Search Date: May 2005

Search Strategy: *PubMed, 1988 to 2005, search of "pregnancy AND venous thromboembolism OR deep vein thrombosis OR pulmonary embolism AND diagnosis." Limited to human studies and English language; 226 citations retrieved. Titles and abstracts scanned, with relevant citations selected. Bibliographies of all citations reviewed. Search of practice guidelines from the American College of Obstetricians and Gynecologists and the American College of Chest Physicians.*

The pretest probability of DVT in a particular patient can be estimated by combining data on prevalence with clinical judgment, findings from the history and physical examination, and determination of risk factors (see Question 11). Clinical prediction rules developed for nonpregnant patients cannot be applied to pregnant patients. In one prospective study of 152 patients with suspected DVT who were referred to a thrombosis specialty center,

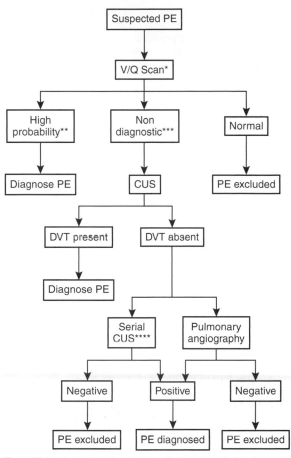

Figure 13-1. Approach to the diagnosis of pulmonary embolism in pregnancy. CUS, compression ultrasonography; DVT, deep venous thrombosis; PE, pulmonary embolism. (From Bates SM, Ginsberg JS: How we manage venous thromboembolism during pregnancy. Blood 2002;100:3470-3478.)

* Can substitute CUS and, if abnormal, diagnose PE; if normal further testing is required.

** At least one segmental perfusion mismatch.

*** Neither normal nor high probability.

**** Can substitute sensitive D-dimer test and, if negative, exclude PE.

DVT was objectively diagnosed in 8.5%.[84] The applicability of these data to patients in other settings is unclear, but the low reported prevalence is consistent with other data and may serve as a rough initial estimate of pretest probability. These data support the theory that because symptoms of leg swelling and pain are very common in pregnancy, most patients with these symptoms will not have DVT. However, a meta-analysis found that the incidence of DVT was highest in the third trimester, when benign leg swelling and pain are most frequent.[85]

Meta-analysis shows that in pregnant patients, DVT is more common in the left leg,[85] and symptoms in this leg therefore should raise the pretest probability. Retrospective data show that common signs and symptoms include pain (91%), tenderness on palpation (70%), and an "enlarged leg" on physical examination (75%).[86] Because the diagnostic power of the history and physical examination alone is likely to be low and the need for diagnostic certainty is high, further objective testing is indicated for all patients.

The only diagnostic modality that has been rigorously evaluated in pregnant patients with suspected DVT is impedance plethysmography. A prospective study showed that withholding anticoagulation in patients with negative IPG is safe, with no reported DVT on follow-up to 3 months postpartum.[84] However, IPG is not widely used anymore.

Compression ultrasonography (CUS) is the initial test of choice, and withholding anticoagulation in nonpregnant patients with low to intermediate pretest probability of DVT has been shown to be safe. Because the prevalence of DVT in symptomatic patients is likely to be low or intermediate (see Question 14) and because there are no other available data, a reasonable approach is to employ serial CUS if the initial ultrasound result is negative and to use venography for equivocal cases (Fig. 13-2).

14. How is the pregnant patient with venous thromboembolism treated?

Search Date: May 2005

Search Strategy: PubMed, 1988 to 2003, search of "pregnancy AND venous thromboembolism OR deep

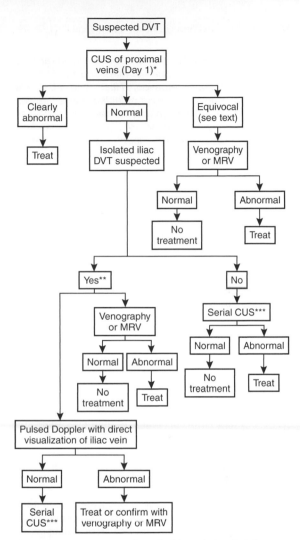

Figure 13-2. Approach to the diagnosis of deep vein thrombosis in pregnancy. CUS, compression ultrasonography; DVT, deep venous thrombosis; MRV, magnetic resonance venogram. (From Bates SM, Ginsberg JS: How we manage venous thromboembolism during pregnancy. Blood 2002;100:3470-3478.)

* IPG is a substitute for CUS.

** D-dimer testing can be performed and, if needed, further testing witheld; if abnormal, investigate further.

*** Repeat days 2 and 3 and 6 to 8; if highly suspicious, MRV or venography.

vein thrombosis OR pulmonary embolism AND treatment OR therapy." Limited to human studies and English language; 335 citations retrieved. Titles and abstracts scanned, with relevant citations selected. Bibliographies of all citations reviewed. Search of practice guidelines from the American College of Obstetricians and Gynecologists and the American College of Chest Physicians.

There is a paucity of data on the use of medications during pregnancy. Guidelines are primarily based on consensus opinion and extrapolation of data from the nonpregnant patient. There is debate regarding the use of unfractionated heparin (UFH) versus low-molecular-weight heparin (LMWH) during pregnancy.[80] There is more clinical experience using UFH. A retrospective cohort study of 100 pregnancies concluded that maternal heparin therapy is safe for the fetus and is associated with an acceptable bleeding rate in the mother.[87] A systematic review of 486 patients treated with LMWH concluded that the risk of using LMWH was comparable to that in a normal population.[88] There are no randomized, controlled trials comparing UFH versus LMWH in the pregnant patient.

The acute management of venous thromboembolic disease in the pregnant patient is similar to that for the nonpregnant patient. Initial anticoagulation is done with UFH or LMWH. Anticoagulation is then continued for 3 months with adjusted-dose UFH or once- or twice-daily injections of UFH. UFH and LMWH do not cross the placenta. Coumadin can cross the placenta and is a known teratogen. It should therefore be avoided in the pregnant patient.[89]

Risks of UFH include increased bone loss in the mother and the risk of heparin-induced thrombocytopenia (HIT). Use of LMWH has a lower incidence of osteoporosis and HIT.[90,91]

The partial thrombin time (PTT) is followed in the patient using UFH. The PTT is not altered with LMWH, but some experts recommend following factor Xa levels during pregnancy. After the initial 3 months of anticoagulation, some experts continue the anticoagulation through the end of pregnancy, and others advise a lower dose of heparin for the remainder of the pregnancy.[92-94]

15.   In the pregnant patient with a first deep venous thrombosis or pulmonary embolism, what workup should be done for thrombophilia?

Search Date: May 2005

Search Strategy: *Pub Med, 1988 to 2005, search of "pregnancy AND venous thromboembolism OR deep vein thrombosis OR pulmonary embolism AND thrombophilia." Limited to human studies and English language; 72 citations retrieved. Titles and abstracts scanned, with relevant citations selected. Bibliographies of all citations reviewed. Search of practice guidelines from the American College of Obstetricians and Gynecologists and the American College of Chest Physicians.*

Although there are multiple predisposing factors related to pregnancy that increase a woman's risk for developing VTE (see Question 11), there are convincing data that more than 50% of women who develop pregnancy-related VTE or have a personal or family history of VTE have a genetic predisposition.[95]

Gerhardt and colleagues[96] reviewed coagulation defects in a case-control study of 119 women with a history of VTE in pregnancy and 233 age-matched controls. The prevalences of factor V Leiden mutation, prothrombin G20210A, MTHFR 677TT, antithrombin III deficiency, protein C deficiency, protein S deficiency, and antiphospholipid Ab were analyzed. The factor V Leiden mutation was the most common, affecting more than 40% of the VTE group and only 7.7% of the control group.[96]

A reasonable approach to screening pregnant patients with a first DVT or PE should include evaluation for protein C deficiency, protein S deficiency, antithrombin III deficiency, factor V Leiden, prothrombin G20210A, anticardiolipin antibodies, and the lupus anticoagulant.[97] The clinician should be aware that testing for several of these disorders is not possible during active anticoagulant treatment. The thrombophilia tests that are not affected by antithrombotic drugs are anticardiolipin antibodies and the polymerase chain reaction (PCR) assays for factor V Leiden and the prothrombin G20210A mutation. All of the other tests mentioned must be postponed until after antithrombotic therapy has been discontinued.

16. What are the treatment recommendations for a pregnant patient with a history of thromboembolic disease?

Search Date: May 2005

Search Strategy: Pub Med, 1988 to 2003, search of "pregnancy and venous thromboembolism OR deep vein thrombosis OR pulmonary embolism AND thromboprophylaxis OR prevention OR prophylaxis." Limited to human studies and English language; 177 citations retrieved. Titles and abstracts scanned, with relevant citations selected. Bibliographies of all citations reviewed. Search of practice guidelines from the American College of Obstetricians and Gynecologists and the American College of Chest Physicians.

Women with prior VTE are believed to be at higher risk for VTE in a subsequent pregnancy, although that risk depends on whether the patient has a thrombophilia or the prior VTE was associated with a transient risk factor.

A prospective cohort study of women with a single prior episode of VTE was designed to calculate the risk of recurrent VTE during pregnancy while withholding heparin. Patients with a known thrombophilia or DVT within the past 3 months were excluded. For patients whose prior VTE was associated with a transient risk factor (e.g., oral contraceptive pill use, surgery, pregnancy, trauma, immobility, chemotherapy) and who had a negative evaluation for thrombophilia, the rate of recurrent VTE was 0 (95% CI: 0 to 8.0). The group with the highest rate of recurrence was the subgroup of patients with an idiopathic condition and abnormal blood work for thrombophilia (20% recurrence rate [95% CI: 2.5 to 55.6]).[98] Table 13-2 provides suggested approaches to prophylaxis in pregnant women with a history of VTE.[94]

17. What is the incidence of the HELLP syndrome, and what are the risk factors for developing it?

Search Date: May 2005

Search Strategy: PubMed, 1988 to 2005, search of "pregnancy AND hellp AND prevalence OR incidence

Table 13-2. **Suggested Management Strategies for Venous Thromboembolism Prophylaxis in Pregnancy in Various Clinical Situations**

Clinical Situation	Suggested Management*
Single previous VTE associated with a temporary risk factor that is no longer present and no additional current risk factors such as obesity	Antenatal: Surveillance or prophylactic doses of LMWH are indicated (e.g., 40 mg of enoxaparin or 5000 IU of dalteparin daily) ± graduated elastic compression stockings. Discuss decision regarding antenatal LMWH with the woman. Postpartum: Anticoagulant therapy is indicated for at least 6 weeks (e.g., 40 mg of enoxaparin or 5000 IU of dalteparin daily or coumarin [target INR, 2 to 3] with LMWH overlap until the INR is ≥ 2.0.) ± graduated elastic compression stockings.
Single previous idiopathic VTE or single previous VTE with underlying thrombophilia and not on long-term anticoagulant therapy or a single previous VTE and additional current risk factors (e.g., obesity, nephrotic syndrome)	Antenatal: Prophylactic doses of LMWH are indicated (e.g., 40 mg of enoxaparin or 5000 IU of dalteparin daily) ± graduated elastic compression stockings. There is strong support for more intense LMWH therapy in antithrombin deficiency (e.g., 0.5 to 1 mg/kg 12 hourly of enoxaparin or 50 to 100 IU/kg 12 hourly of dalteparin). Postpartum: Anticoagulant therapy is indicated for at least 6 weeks (e.g., 40 mg of enoxaparin or 5000 IU of dalteparin daily or coumarin [target INR, 2 to 3] with LMWH overlap until the INR is ≥ 2.0.) ± graduated elastic compression stockings.
More than one previous episode of VTE, with no thrombophilia and not on long-term anticoagulant therapy	Antenatal: Prophylactic doses of LMWH are indicated (e.g., 40 mg of enoxaparin or 5000 IU of dalteparin daily) + graduated elastic compression stockings.

Continued

Table 13-2. Suggested Management Strategies for Venous Thromboembolism Prophylaxis in Pregnancy in Various Clinical Situations—cont'd

Clinical Situation	Suggested Management*
	Postpartum: Anticoagulant therapy is indicated for at least 6 weeks (e.g., 40 mg of enoxaparin or 5000 IU of dalteparin daily or coumarin [target INR, 2 to 3] with LMWH overlap until the INR is ≥ 2.0.) + graduated elastic compression stockings.
Previous VTE in women receiving long-term anticoagulants (e.g., with underlying thrombophilia)	Antenatal: A switch should be made from oral anticoagulants to LMWH therapy (e.g., 0.5 to 1 mg/kg 12 hourly of enoxaparin or 50 to 100 IU/kg 12 hourly of dalteparin) by 6 weeks' gestation + graduated elastic compression stockings. Postpartum: Long-term oral anticoagulants should be resumed with LMWH overlap until the INR is in the pre-pregnancy therapeutic range + graduated elastic compression stockings.
Thrombophilia (confirmed abnormality) but no prior VTE	Antenatal: Surveillance or prophylactic LMWH is indicated ± graduated elastic compression stockings. The indication for pharmacologic prophylaxis in the antenatal period is stronger in AT-deficient women than in the other thrombophilias, in symptomatic kindred when compared with asymptomatic kindred, and when additional risk factors are present. Postpartum: Anticoagulant therapy is indicated for at least 6 weeks (e.g., 40 mg of enoxaparin or 5000 IU of dalteparin daily or coumarin [target INR, 2 to 3] with LMWH overlap until the INR is ≥ 2.0.) ± graduated elastic compression stockings.

Table 13-2. Suggested Management Strategies for Venous Thromboembolism Prophylaxis in Pregnancy in Various Clinical Situations—cont'd

Clinical Situation	Suggested Management*
After cesarean section or vaginal delivery	Carry out risk assessment for VTE. If additional risk factors such as emergency section in labor, age older than 35 years, or a high BMI, consider LMWH thromboprophylaxis (e.g., 40 mg of enoxaparin or 5000 IU of dalteparin) ± graduated elastic compression stockings.

*Specialist advice for individualized management of patients is advisable in many of these situations.

AT, antithrombin; BMI, body mass index; INR, international normalized ratio; LMWH, low-molecular-weight heparin; VTE, venous thromboembolism.

Adapted from Greer IA: Prevention and management of venous thromboembolism in pregnancy. Clin Chest Med 2003;24:123-137.

OR risk factor." Limited to human studies and English language; 109 citations retrieved. Titles and abstracts scanned, with relevant citations selected. Bibliographies of all citations reviewed. Search of practice guidelines from the American Gastroenterology Association.

HELLP syndrome (*h*emolysis, *e*levated *l*iver enzymes, and *l*ow *p*latelet count) is thought to be part of the spectrum of disease that includes hypertension of pregnancy, preeclampsia, and eclampsia. HELLP syndrome has been thought of as a rare complication of pregnancy. Preeclampsia affects 3% to 10% of pregnancies, and HELLP syndrome affects 4% to 12% of women with severe preeclampsia. These figures are based on a retrospective analysis of 442 patients at a single tertiary care center.[99] However a prospective study of 4,77 patients in Wales reported that the incidence of HELLP was 22%.[100] The diagnostic criteria for HELLP used in both studies were an aspartate aminotransferase (AST) level higher than 70, platelet count less than 100, and lactate dehydrogenase (LDH) level higher than 600.

Sibai and colleagues[99] found that 70% of HELLP cases in their tertiary care center in Memphis, Tennessee, occurred between 27 and 36 weeks' gestation. In this study, mean maternal age was 24.4 5 years, and white women were more likely to develop HELLP than black women.[99] Little is known about the risk factors that predispose a woman to HELLP.

18. How is HELLP diagnosed and treated?

Search Date: May 2005

Search Strategy: PubMed, 1988 to 2005, search of "pregnancy and hellp AND diagnostic OR treatment." Limited to human studies and English language; 155 citations retrieved. Titles and abstracts scanned, with relevant citations selected. Bibliographies of all citations reviewed. Search of practice guidelines from the American Gastroenterology Association.

HELLP syndrome is suspected when a woman in her second or third trimester has abnormal liver function test results. Abdominal pain is the most common symptom, affecting 60% of patients diagnosed, and 85% of patients may have hypertension or proteinuria, or both.[101] Up to 30% of patients with HELLP are diagnosed after delivery.

There are no consensus guidelines from ACOG on laboratory values for diagnosing HELLP. Practice guidelines from the American Gastroenterology Association also do not identify specific values for laboratory results but rather describe a constellation of laboratory test results, including an elevated AST level, thrombocytopenia, and a peripheral smear with schistocytes. Hepatic function remains intact, and the prothrombin time should be normal. Liver biopsy shows findings typical of preeclampsia with periportal hemorrhage and fibrin deposition.[102]

Treatment for HELLP is delivery. Expert recommendations for the management of HELLP include the following.[101]

1. Intravenous magnesium sulfate to prevent seizures
2. Medications to lower blood pressure if indicated
3. Delivery if gestational age is 34 weeks or more
4. Delivery if evidence of fetal distress
5. Delivery if evidence of severe maternal disease (i.e., eclampsia, disseminated intravascular coagulation,

liver infarction, renal failure, respiratory distress, or abruptio placenta)

There is debate about the benefits of corticosteroids in the treatment of HELLP. There is some evidence that steroids may help temporarily improve platelet counts and hypertension.[103] Because steroids can help enhance fetal lung maturity, it is reasonable to give steroids in a pregnancy of less than 34 weeks' gestation but within the limits of viability.[101]

19. What are the risks of adverse clinical outcomes to the mother and fetus in the pregnant patient with HELLP?

Search Date: May 2005

Search Strategy: PubMed, 1988 to 2005, search of "pregnancy AND hellp AND outcome." Limited to human studies and English language; 216 citations retrieved. Titles and abstracts scanned, with relevant citations selected. Bibliographies of all citations reviewed.

Determining the risk of adverse outcomes from HELLP is difficult because of issues related to study design. Many studies of HELLP are retrospective, have inadequate sample sizes, or describe HELLP outcomes from single, tertiary care institutions, thereby limiting the generalizability of the findings. Patients are often referred to tertiary care centers because of the complexity of the HELLP syndrome. Mortality and morbidity rates from these centers may not reflect accurate risks of adverse clinical outcomes. Sibai and coworkers[104] performed a prospective cohort study on 442 pregnancies with HELLP syndrome managed at a large tertiary care hospital in the United States from 1977 through 1992. Eighty percent of the cases developed at term. The maternal mortality rate was 1.1%. Serious maternal morbidity included disseminated intravascular coagulation (21%), abruptio placentae (16%), acute renal failure (7.7%), pulmonary edema (6%), subcapsular liver hematoma (0.9%), and retinal detachment (0.9%). Fifty-five percent of patients required blood product transfusions, and 2% required laparotomies for major abdominal bleeding.[104]

Gul and associates[105] performed a prospective analysis of 106 patients with HELLP syndrome detected in 2786 admissions to a hospital in Istanbul. Overall, there were 17 deaths (16.8% mortality rate). Seventy-five percent of the deaths were among women who presented at less than 32 weeks. There was a 6% overall neonatal mortality rate.[105] The study authors attribute their high mortality rates to the lack of prenatal care in their study population.

For the woman with a history of HELLP, there are two studies that look at outcomes in subsequent pregnancies. The risk of preeclampsia in a subsequent pregnancy is 19% to 22%, and the risk of recurrent HELLP syndrome is 3% to 19%.[106,107]

One study retrospectively reviewed outcomes for subsequent pregnancies of women who had HELLP diagnosed before 28 weeks' gestation. For this select group of 48 women with subsequent pregnancies, their risk of preeclampsia was 55%, and risk of recurrent HELLP was 6%.[108] HELLP syndrome is associated with significant risk of morbidity and mortality for the mother and significant morbidity for the fetus, especially in situations of poor prenatal care. Women with a history of HELLP in the past are at increased risk for complications in future pregnancies and should be monitored closely.

20. How common is fatty liver of pregnancy? What are the risk factors for developing fatty liver of pregnancy?

Search Date: May 2005

Search Strategy: PubMed, 1988 to 2005, search of "pregnancy AND fatty liver AND prevalence OR incidence OR risk factor." Limited to human studies and English language; 22 citations retrieved. Titles and abstracts scanned, with relevant citations selected. Bibliographies of all citations reviewed. Search of practice guidelines from the American Gastroenterology Association.

Acute fatty liver of pregnancy (AFLP) is a rare complication of pregnancy with an 18% maternal and 23% fetal mortality rate.[109] The incidence is estimated to be 1 in

1000 to 16,000 births.[100,110,111] The vast discrepancy in reported incidence probably reflects an increase in awareness of the disease, increased screening, and availability of specialized care at the institutions being studied.

AFLP occurs in the third trimester of pregnancy. Women with their first pregnancy or with multiple gestations are at increased risk for developing AFLP.[112] Symptoms include nausea and vomiting (70%), right upper quadrant or epigastric pain (50% to 80%), or malaise and anorexia.[113] Within a few weeks, jaundice develops, and it can progress to fulminant hepatic failure. Histologic evaluation has shown a microvesicular fatty infiltrate of the liver.

An association has been recognized between AFLP and long-chain 3-hydroxyacyl-CoA dehydrogenase (LCHAD) deficiency.[114,115] In a study of 24 children with LCHAD deficiency, 62% of their mothers had developed AFLP or the HELLP syndrome while pregnant. It is postulated that the abnormal fatty acid metabolites produced by the fetus homozygous for the trait enter the mother's circulation and cause the disorder. Infants of mothers with AFLP should be screened for fatty acid oxidation disorders.[115]

21. What are the diagnostic tests and treatments for diagnosing fatty liver of pregnancy?

Search Date: May 2005

Search Strategy: PubMed, 1988 to 2005, search of "pregnancy AND fatty liver AND diagnostic OR treatment." Limited to human studies and English language; 43 citations retrieved. Titles and abstracts scanned, with relevant citations selected. Bibliographies of all citations reviewed. Search of practice guidelines from the American Gastroenterology Association.

Unlike HELLP, AFLP represents true hepatic impairment and can lead to liver failure. Laboratory studies show elevated aminotransferase levels, a prolonged prothrombin time, and low fibrinogen concentration. They can also show hypoglycemia and elevated bilirubin.[102]

Treatment consists of immediate delivery of the fetus. There are no long-term sequelae; the liver usually recovers completely.[116]

22. What are the risks associated with diagnostic imaging during pregnancy?

Search Date: May 2005

Search Strategy: PubMed, 1988 to 2005, search of "diagnostic imaging AND safety AND pregnancy." Limited to human studies and English language; 20 citations retrieved. Titles and abstracts scanned, with relevant citations selected. Bibliographies of all citations reviewed. Search of practice guidelines from ACOG and ACR also reviewed. Ovid Medline also searched (diagnostic imaging and pregnancy) and bibliographies reviewed,

Few things provoke more angst in patients and providers than radiologic evaluation of the pregnant patient. Imaging modalities available in pregnancy include ionizing radiation, such as plain radiography, fluoroscopy, angiography, and CT, and nonionizing techniques, such as ultrasound or magnetic resonance imaging (MRI).[117] Although the safety of radiation exposure during pregnancy is a real concern, a missed or delayed diagnosis usually poses a greater risk to the patient and her pregnancy than the risks associated with ionizing radiation.[118] Ionizing radiation (x-rays) is composed of high-energy photons that are capable of damaging DNA and generating free radicals, and all necessary precautions should be taken to minimize exposure.[119,120] Most diagnostic imaging studies are associated with minimal risk, and clinicians and patients' perception of teratogenic risk is higher than the actual risk.[121,122]

There are four categories of fetal risk: intrauterine fetal death, spontaneous and structural malformations, disturbances of growth and development, and mutagenic and carcinogenic effects.[123,124] The frequency of each depends to a large extent on the dose of radiation and the gestational age of the fetus. The preimplantation period (0 to 9 days) is the most vulnerable period for these risks to occur, and the most common fetal malformations caused by high-dose radiation are of the central nervous system, primarily microencephaly and mental retardation.[125] A careful and detailed explanation of the risks and benefits of diagnostic imaging to the patient and family before the exposure is extremely helpful. Radiographic examination during pregnancy requires reassessment of the usual diagnostic algorithms and examination techniques.

The primary goal is to minimize radiation exposure to the embryo or fetus while maintaining a high level of diagnostic accuracy for potential maternal illness. Strategies shown to decrease the dose of ionizing radiation include shielding the abdomen and pelvis when non-abdomino-pelvic structures are being imaged; using a posteroanterior exposure for plain films compared with the traditional anteroposterior exposure, because of the location of the uterus in an anterior pelvic position; limiting the number of views obtained; and limiting the fluoroscopic time.[120,122,126]

The extent to which a patient is exposed to radiation is often expressed as the dose to the skin at the site closest to the radiation beam, described as roentgens or milliroentgens.[123] Fetal dose is always less than maternal dose because of the partial absorption of radiation by maternal tissues overlying the fetus. A more useful calculation for determining maternal and fetal risk is the absorbed dose, which is expressed in two units: radiation absorbed dose (rad) and gray (system international), with 100 rad equaling 1 gray (Table 13-3).[123,124,126]

Table 13-3. Estimated Fetal Exposure from Radiologic Procedures	
Diagnostic Study	**Estimated Radiation (mrad)**
Chest radiography	<1
Helical computed tomography	3-30 (increases with gestational age)
Ventilation lung scan*	1-5
Perfusion lung scan†	6-12
Pulmonary angiography	215-374 (femoral route); <50 (brachial route)

*With technetium 99 sulfur colloid.
†With technetium 99 macroaggregated albumin.
Adapted from Guidelines on diagnosis and management of acute pulmonary embolism. Task Force on Pulmonary Embolism, European Society of Cardiology. Eur Heart J 2000; 21:1301-1336.

All women of childbearing age should be asked whether they could be pregnant at the time of any radiologic examination, and all necessary precautions should be taken to ensure the minimum amount of radiation exposure.[118]

Radiation risks should always be discussed with the patient before the procedure, including an explanation of the background population risk for miscarriage (20%), congenital anomalies (4%), genetic disease (10%), and growth restriction (10%).[117,120] Clinicians should inform patients that a radiation exposure of less than 5 rad is generally considered safe and is not associated with an increased risk of abortion, congenital anomalies, growth restriction, or perinatal mortality.[121] The ACOG has stated that exposure to x-rays during a pregnancy is not an indication for a therapeutic abortion. Women should be counseled that x-ray exposure from a single diagnostic procedure does not result in harmful fetal effects. Consultation with a radiologist is strongly encouraged to plan the optimal study using the least amount of radiation. This is especially useful when multiple diagnostic radiographic procedures are planned. Alternative imaging procedures such as ultrasound and MRI are preferable to those that apply ionizing radiation. However, concern about the possible effects of ionizing radiation should not prevent medically indicated diagnostic procedures. There are no contraindications to ultrasound procedures, including duplex Doppler imaging, and this modality has largely replaced x-ray films as the modality of choice in fetal imaging. MRI is not recommended during the first trimester because safety information during the organogenesis stage of fetal development is limited. The use of radioactive isotopes of iodine is contraindicated for therapeutic use during pregnancy, and although radiopaque and paramagnetic agents are unlikely to cause harm, they should be reserved for cases in which the diagnostic benefit exceeds the potential risk to the fetus.[118]

REFERENCES

1. Centers for Disease Control and Prevention (CDC: Guidelines for vaccinating pregnant women: Recommendations of the Advisory Committee on Immunization Practices (ACIP). Available at http://www.cdc.gov/nip/publications/preg_guide.htm/ Accessed July 2005. IV

2. Centers for Disease Control and Prevention (CDC): General recommendations on immunization: Recommendations of the Advisory Committee on

Immunization Practices (ACIP). MMWR Morb Mortal Wkly Rep 2005;51(RR-2):18-19. **IV**

3. Centers for Disease Control and Prevention (CDC): Prevention of hepatitis A through active or passive immunization: Recommendations of the Advisory Committee on Immunization Practices (ACIP). MMWR Morb Mortal Wkly Rep 1999;48(RR-12):24. **IV**

4. Centers for Disease Control and Prevention (CDC): Prevention and control of influenza: Recommendations of the Advisory Committee on Immunization Practices (ACIP). MMWR Morb Mortal Wkly Rep 2004;53 (RR-6):10. **IV**

5. American College of Obstetricians and Gynecologists (ACOG): Immunization during pregnancy. ACOG committee opinion no. 282. Obstet Gynecol 2003;101:207-212. **IV**

6. Centers for Disease Control and Prevention (CDC): Prevention of pneumococcal disease: Recommendations of the Advisory Committee on Immunization Practices (ACIP). MMWR Morb Mortal Wkly Rep 1997;46 (RR-8):60. **IV**

7. Munoz FM, Englund JA, Cheesman CC, et al: Maternal immunization with pneumococcal polysaccharide vaccine in the third trimester of gestation. Vaccine 2002;20: 826-837. **II**

8. Shahid NS, Steinhoff MC, Hogue SS, et al: Serum, breast milk, and infant antibody after maternal immunization with pneumococcal vaccine. Lancet 1995;346: 1252-1257. **II**

9. Centers for Disease Control and Prevention (CDC: Poliomyelitis Prevention in the United States: Recommendations of the Advisory Committee on Immunization Practices (ACIP). MMWR Morb Mortal Wkly Rep 2000;49(RR-5):14. **IV**

10. Centers for Disease Control and Prevention (CDC): Notice to readers: Revised ACIP recommendation for avoiding pregnancy after receiving a rubella-containing vaccine. MMWR Morb Mortal Wkly Rep 2001; 50:1117. **IV**

11. Centers for Disease Control and Prevention (CDC): Measles, mumps and rubella—Vaccine use and strategies for elimination of measles, rubella, and congenital rubella syndrome and control of mumps: Recommendations of the Advisory Committee on Immunization Practices (ACIP). MMWR Morb Mortal Wkly Rep 1998;47 (RR-8):32-33. **IV**

12. American College of Obstetricians and Gynecologists: Rubella vaccination. ACOG committee opinion no. 281. Obstet Gynecol 2002;100:1417. **IV**

13. Centers for Disease Control and Prevention (CDC): Tetanus and pertussis: Recommendations for vaccine use and other preventive measures: Recommendations of the Advisory Committee on Immunization Practices (ACIP). MMWR Morb Mortal Wkly Rep 1991; 40(RR-10):14. **IV**

14. Centers for Disease Control and Prevention (CDC): Prevention of varicella: Recommendations of the Advisory Committee on Immunization Practices (ACIP). MMWR Morb Mortal Wkly Rep 1996;45(RR-11):19. **IV**

15. Holliman RE: Congenital toxoplasmosis: Prevention, screening and treatment. J Hosp Infect 1995;30(Suppl):179-190. **V**

16. Centers for Disease Control and Prevention (CDC): CDC Recommendations regarding selected conditions affecting women's health. MMWR Morb Mortal Wkly Rep 2000;49:59-68. **IV**

17. Cook AJ, Gilbert RE, Buffolano W, et al: Sources of *Toxoplasma* infection in pregnant women: European multicentre case-control study. BMJ 2000;321: 142-147. **III**

18. Kapperud G, Jenum PA, Stray-Pedersen B: Risk factors for *Toxoplasma gondii* infection in pregnancy. Results of a prospective case-control study in Norway. Am J Epidemiol 1996;144:405-412. **III**

19. Baril L, Ancelle T, Goulet V, et al: Risk factors for *Toxoplasma* infection in pregnancy: A case-control study in France. Scand J Infect Dis 1999;31:305-309. **III**

20. Kravetz JD, Federman DG: Toxoplasmosis in pregnancy. Am J Med 2005;118:212-216. **V**

21. Jenum PA, Stray-Pedersen B, Melby KK, et al: Incidence of *Toxoplasma gondii* infection in 35,940 pregnant women in Norway and pregnancy outcome for infected women. J Clin Microbiol 1998;36:2900-2906. **III**

22. Liesenfeld O, Press C, Montoya JG, et al: False-positive results in immunoglobulin M (IgM) *Toxoplasma* antibody tests and the importance of confirmatory testing: The Platelia Toxo IgM test. J Clin Microbiol 1997;35: 174-178. **III**

23. Szenasi Z, Ozsvar Z, Nagy E, et al: Prevention of congenital toxoplasmosis in Szeged, Hungary. Int J Epidemiol 1997;26:428-235. **III**

24. Ricci M, Pentimalli H, Thaller R, et al: Screening and prevention of congenital toxoplasmosis: An effectiveness study in a population with a high infection rate. J Matern Fetal Med 2003;14:398-403. **III**

25. Wallon M, Liou C, Garner P, Peyron F: Congenital toxoplasmosis: Systematic review of evidence of efficacy of treatment in pregnancy. BMJ 1999;318:1511-1514. **I**

26. Foulon W, Villena I, Stray-Pedersen B, et al: Treatment of toxoplasmosis during pregnancy: Impact on fetal transmission and children's sequelae at one year of age—A multicenter study. Am J Obstet Gynecol 1999; 180:410-415. **III**

27. Gilbert R, Gras L: European multicenter study on congenital toxoplasmosis. Effect of timing and type of treatment on the risk of mother to child transmission of *Toxoplasma gondii*. BJOG 2003;110:112-120. **III**

28. American College of Obstetricians and Gynecologists (ACOG): Perinatal Viral Parasitic Infections. ACOG practice bulletin no. 20. Washington, DC, American College of Obstetricians and Gynecologists, 2000. **IV**

29. Center for Disease Control and Prevention (CDC): Achievements in public health: Elimination of rubella and congenital rubella syndrome—United States, 1969-2004. MMWR Morb Mortal Wkly Rep 2005;54:279-282. **V**

30. Banatvala JE, Brown DG: Rubella. Lancet 2004;363:1127-1137. **V**

31. U.S. Preventive Services Task Force: Screening for Rubella, including Immunization of Adolescents and Adults: Recommendation Statement. Rockville, MD, Agency for Healthcare Research and Quality, 1996. Available at www.ahrq.gov/clinic/uspstf/usprubl.htm **IV**

32. Centers for Disease Control and Prevention (CDC): Control and prevention of rubella: Evaluation and management of suspected outbreaks, rubella in pregnant women, and surveillance for congenital rubella syndrome. MMWR Morb Mortal Wkly Rep 2001;50 (RR-12):17-19. **IV**

33. Cunningham FG, Lucas MJ: Urinary tract infections complicating pregnancy. Baillieres Clin Obstet Gynaecol 1994;8:353-373. **V**

34. Le J, Briggs GG, McKeown A, Bustillo G: Urinary tract infections during pregnancy. Ann Pharmacother 2004;38:1692-1701. **V**

35. Wing DA: Pyelonephritis in pregnancy. Drugs 2001;61:2087-2096. V

36. Smaill F: Antibiotics for asymptomatic bacteriuria in pregnancy. Cochrane Database Syst Rev 2001;(2):CD000490. I

37. American College of Obstetricians and Gynecologists (ACOG): Antimicrobial therapy for obstetric patients. ACOG educational bulletin no. 245. Int J Gynaecol Obstet 1998;64:299-308. IV

38. U.S. Preventive Services Task Force: Screening for Asymptomatic Bacteriuria: Recommendation Statement. Rockville, MD, Agency for Healthcare Research and Quality, February 2004. Available at www.ahrq.gov/clinic/3rduspstf/asymbac/asymbacrs.htm IV

39. Villar J, Widmer M, Lydon-Rochelle MT, et al: Duration of treatment for asymptomatic bacteriuria during pregnancy. Cochrane Database Syst Rev 2000;(2):CD000491. I

40. Stamm WE, Hooton TM: Management of urinary tract infections in adults. N Engl J Med 1993;329:1328-1334. V

41. Vazquez JC, Villar J: Treatments for symptomatic urinary tract infections during pregnancy. Cochrane Database Syst Rev 2003;(4):CD002256. I

42. Millar LK, Wing DA, Paul RH, et al: Outpatient treatment of pyelonephritis in pregnancy: A randomized controlled trial. Obstet Gynecol 1995;86:560-564. II

43. Wing DA, Hendershott CM, DeBuque L, et al: Outpatient treatment of acute pyelonephritis in pregnancy after 24 weeks. Obstet Gynecol 1999;94:683-688. II

44. Duley L. Pre-eclampsia and the hypertensive disorders of pregnancy. Br Med Bull 2003;67:161-176. V

45. Report of the National High Blood Pressure Education Program Working Group on high blood pressure in pregnancy. Am J Obstet Gynecol 2000;183:S1-S22. IV

46. Roberts JM, Pearson G, Cutler J, et al: Summary of the NHLBI Working Group on Research on Hypertension During Pregnancy. Hypertension 2003;41:437-445. V

47. Levine RJ, Hauth JC, Curet LB, et al: Trial of calcium to prevent preeclampsia. N Engl J Med 1997:337:69-76. II

48. Seely EW, Solomon CG: Insulin resistance and its potential role in pregnancy-induced hypertension. J Clin Endocrinol Metab 2003;88:2393-2398. V

49. Sibai BM, Caritis SN: Prevention of preeclampsia with low dose aspirin in healthy, nulliparous women. N Engl J Med 1993;329:1213-1218. II

50. Parazinni F, Bortolus R, Chatenoud L, et al: Risk factors for pregnancy-induced hypertension in women at high risk for the condition. Italian Study of Aspirin in Pregnancy Group. Epidemiology 1996;7:396-308. II

51. Krotz S, Fajardo J, Ghandi S, et al: Hypertensive disease in twin pregnancies: A review. Twin Res 2002;5:8-14. V

52. England LJ, Levine RJ, Qian C, et al: Smoking before pregnancy and risk of gestational hypertension and preeclampsia. Am J Obstet Gynecol 2002;186:1035-1040. II

53. Ward K, Hata A et al: A molecular variant of angiotensinogen associated with preeclampsia. Nat Genet 1993;4:49-61. III

54. Kosmas IP, Tatsioni A, Ioannidis JP: Association of Leiden mutation in factor V gene with hypertension in pregnancy and pre-eclampsia: A meta-analysis. J Hypertens 2003;21:1221-1228. I

55. Chesley LC, Sibai BM: Clinical significance of elevated mean arterial pressure in the second trimester. Am J Obstet Gynecol 1988;159:275-279. V

56. Sibai BM, Lindheimer M, Hauth J, et al: Risk factors for preeclampsia, abruptio placentae, and adverse neonatal outcomes among women with chronic hypertension. N Engl J Med 1998;339:667-671. III

57. Ferrer RL, Sibai BM, Mulrow CD, et al: Management of mild chronic hypertension during pregnancy: A review. Obstet Gynecol 2000;96:849-860. I

58. McCowan LM, Buist RG, North RA, Gamble G: Perinatal morbidity in chronic hypertension. Br J Obstet Gynaecol 1996;103:123-129. III

59. American College of Obstetricians and Gynecologists (ACOG): ACOG practice bulletin. Chronic hypertension in pregnancy. Obstet Gynecol 2001;98(Suppl):177-185. IV

60. Sibai BM, Mabie WC, Shamsa F, et al: A comparison of no medication versus methyldopa or labetalol in chronic hypertension during pregnancy. Am J Obstet Gynecol 1990;162:960-966. II

61. Magee LA, Ornstein MP, von Dadelszen P: Fortnightly review: Management of hypertension in pregnancy. BMJ 1999;318:1332-1336. I

62. von Dadelszen P, Ornstein MP, Bull SB, et al: Fall in mean arterial pressure and fetal growth restriction in pregnancy hypertension: A meta-analysis. Lancet 2000;355:87-92. **I**

63. Montan S, Anandakumar C, Arulkumaran S, et al: Effects of methyldopa on uteroplacental and fetal hemodynamics in pregnancy-induced hypertension. Am J Obstet Gynecol 1993;168:152-156. **III**

64. Magee LA, Elran E, Bull SB, et al: Risks and benefits of beta-receptor blockers for pregnancy hypertension: overview of the randomized trials. Eu J Obstet Gynecol Reprod Biol 2000;88:15-26. **I**

65. Collins R, Yusuf S, Peto R. Overview of randomized trials of diuretics in pregnancy. Br Med J 1985; 290:17-23. **I**

66. Sibai BM, Grossman RA, Grossman HG: Effects of diuretics on plasma volume in pregnancies with long-term hypertension. Am J Obstet Gynecol 1984;150:831-835. **III**

67. Gruppo di Studio Ipertensione in Gravidanza: Nifedipine versus expectant management in mild to moderate hypertension in pregnancy. Br J Obstet Gynaecol 1998;105:718-722. **II**

68. Hanssens M, Keirse MJ, Vankelecom F, Van Assche FA: Fetal and neonatal effects of treatment with angiotensin-converting enzyme inhibitors in pregnancy. Obstet Gynecol 1991;78:128-135. **I**

69. Alwan S, Polifka JE, Friedman JM: Angiotensin II receptor antagonist treatment during pregnancy. Birth Defects Res A Clin Mol Teratol 2005;73:123-130. **I**

70. Sibai BM, el-Nazer A, Gonzalez-Ruiz A: Severe preeclampsia-eclampsia in young primigravid women: Subsequent pregnancy outcome and remote prognosis. Am J Obstet Gynecol 1986;155:1011-1016. **III**

71. Hannaford P, Ferry S, Hirsch S: Cardiovascular sequelae of toxemia of pregnancy. Heart 1997;77:154-158. **III**

72. Gherman RB, Goodwin TM, Leung B, et al: Incidence, clinical characteristics, and timing of objectively diagnosed venous thromboembolism during pregnancy. Obstet Gynecol 1999;94:730-734. **III**

73. Soomro RM, Bucur IJ, Noorani S: Cumulative incidence of venous thromboembolism during pregnancy and puerperium: A hospital-based study. Angiology 2002;53:429-434. **III**

74. Gherman RB, Goodwin TM, Leung B, et al: Incidence, clinical characteristics, and timing of objectively diagnosed venous thromboembolism during pregnancy. Obstet Gynecol 1999;94:730-734. III

75. McColl M, Ramsay JE, Tait RC, et al: Risk factors for pregnancy associated venous thromboembolism. Thromb Haemost 1997;78:1183-1188. III

76. Simpson EL, Lawrenson RA, Nightingale AL, Farmer RD: Venous thromboembolism in pregnancy and the puerperium: Incidence and additional risk factors from a London perinatal database. BJOG 2001;108:56-60. III

77. Zotz RB, Gerhardt A, Scarf RE: Prediction, prevention, and treatment of venous thromboembolic disease in pregnancy. Sem Thromb Hemost 2003;29:143-153. V

78. Chan WS, Ray JG, Murray S, et al: Suspected pulmonary embolism in pregnancy: Clinical presentation, results of lung scanning, and subsequent maternal and pediatric outcomes. Arch Intern Med 2002;162:1170-1175. III

79. Bates SM, Ginsberg JS: How we manage venous thromboembolism during pregnancy. Blood 2002;100:3470-3478. V

80. American College of Obstetricians and Gynecologists (ACOG): ACOG practice bulletin: Thromboembolism in pregnancy. Int J Gynecol Obstet 2000;75:203-212. IV

81. Kearon C: Diagnosis of pulmonary embolism. J Can Med Assoc 2003;168:183-194. IV

82. Quiroz R, Kucher N, Zou KH, et al: Clinical validity of a negative computed tomography scan in patients with suspected pulmonary embolism: A systematic review. JAMA 2005;293:2012-2017. I

83. Chan WS, Ray JG, Murry S, et al: Suspected pulmonary embolism in pregnancy: Clinical presentation, results of lung scanning, and subsequent maternal and pediatric outcomes. Arch Intern Med 2002;162:1170-1175. III

84. Hull RD, Raskob GE: Serial impedance plethysmography in pregnant patients with clinically suspected deep-vein thrombosis. Clinical validity of negative findings. Ann Intern Med 1990;112:663-667. III

85. Ray JG, Chan WS: Deep vein thrombosis during pregnancy and the puerperium: A meta-analysis of the period of risk and the leg of presentation. Obstet Gynecol Surv 1999;54:265-271. I

86. Gherman RB, Goodwin TM, et al: Incidence, clinical characteristics, and timing of objectively diagnosed

venous thromboembolism during pregnancy. Obstet Gynecol 1999;94:730-734. III

87. Ginsberg JS, Kowalchuk G, Hirsh J, et al: Heparin therapy during pregnancy. Risks to the fetus and mother. Arch Intern Med 1989;149:2233-2236. III

88. Sanson BJ, Lensing AW, Prins MH, et al: Safety of low molecular weight heparin in pregnancy: A systematic review. Thromb Haemost 1999;81:668-672. I

89. Wong V, Cheng CH, Chan KC: Fetal and neonatal outcome of exposure to anticoagulants during pregnancy. Am J Med Genet 1993;45:17-21. III

90. Monreal M, Lafoz E, Olive A, et al: Comparison of subcutaneous unfractionated heparin with a low molecular weight heparin (Fragmin) in patients with venous thromboembolism and contraindications to coumarin. Thromb Haemost 1994;71:7-11. II

91. Warkentin TE, Levine MN, Hirsh J, et al: Heparin induced thrombocytopenia in patients treated with low-molecular-weight heparin or unfractionated heparin. N Engl J Med 1995;332:1330-1335. II

92. Barbour LA, for the American College of Obstetricians and Gynecologists (ACOG) Committee on Practice Bulletins: ACOG practice bulletin: Thromboembolism in pregnancy. Int J Gynecol Obstet 2001;75:203-212. IV

93. Bates SM, Greer IA, Hirsh J, Ginsberg JS: Use of antithrombotic agents during pregnancy. Chest 2004;126;627S-644S. IV

94. Greer IA: Prevention and management of venous thromboembolism in pregnancy. Clin Chest Med 2003;24:123-137. V

95. Grandone E, Margaglione M, Coaizzo D, et al: Genetic susceptibility to pregnancy related venous thromboembolism: Roles of factor V Leiden, prothrombin G20210A, and methylenetetrahydrofolate reductase C677T mutations. Am J Obstet Gynecol 1998:179:1324-1328. III

96. Gerhardt A, Scharf RE, Beckmann MW, et al: Prothrombin and factor V mutations in women with a history of thrombosis during pregnancy and the puerperium. N Eng J Med 2000;342:374-80. III

97. Dizon-Townson D: Pregnancy-related venous thromboembolism. Clin Obstet Gynecol 2002; 45:363-368. V

98. Brill-Edwards P, Ginsberg JS, Gent M, et al: Safety of withholding heparin in pregnant women with a history

of venous thromboembolism. Recurrence of Clot in This Pregnancy Study Group. N Engl J Med 2000;343: 1439-1444. III

99. Sibai B, Ramadan M, Usta I, et al: Maternal morbidity and mortality in 442 pregnancies with hemolysis, elevated liver enzymes, and low platelets (HELLP syndrome). Am J Obstet Gynecol 1993;169: 1000-1006. III

100. Ch'ng C, Morgan M, Hainsworth I, Kingham J: Prospective study of liver dysfunction in pregnancy in Southwest Wales. Gut 2002;51:876-880. III

101. Sibai B: Diagnosis, controversies, and management of the syndrome of hemolysis, elevated liver enzymes and low platelet count. Obstet Gynecol 2004;103: 981-991. V

102. Riely C: Liver disease in the pregnant patient. Am J Gastroenterol 1999;94:1728-1732. IV

103. Matchaba P, Moodley J: Corticosteroids for HELLP syndrome in pregnancy. Cochrane Database Syst Rev 2002;(4):CD002076. I

104. Sibai B, Ramadan M, Usta I, et al: Maternal morbidity and mortality in 442 pregnancies with hemolysis, elevated liver enzymes, and low platelets (HELLP syndrome). Am J Obstet Gynecol 1993;169:1000-1006. III

105. Gul A, Cebeci A, Aslan H, et al: Perinatal outcomes in severe preeclampsia-eclampsia with and with out HELLP syndrome. Gynecol Obstet Invest 2005; 59:113-118. III

106. Sibai B, Ramadan M, Chari R, Friedman S: Pregnancies complicated by HELLP syndrome: Subsequent pregnancy outcome and long term prognosis. Am J Obstet Gynecol 1995;172:125-129. VI

107. Sullivan C, Magann E, Perry K, et al: The recurrence risk of the syndrome of hemolysis elevated liver enzymes, and low platelets (HELLP) in subsequent gestations. Am J Obstet Gynecol 1994;171:940-943. III

108. Chames M, Haddad B, Barton J, et al: Subsequent pregnancy outcome in women with a history of HELLP syndrome at ≤ 28 weeks of gestation. Am J Obstet Gynecol 2003;188:1504-1508. VI

109. Kaplan M: Acute fatty liver of pregnancy. N Engl J Med 1985;313:367-370. V

110. Castro M, Fassett M, Reynolds T, et al: Reversible peripartum liver failure: A new perspective on the diagnosis, treatment, and cause of acute fatty liver of

pregnancy based on 28 consecutive cases. Am J Obstet Gynecol 1999;181:389-395. VI

111. Reyes H, Sandoval L, Wainstein A, et al: Acute fatty liver of pregnancy: A clinical study of 12 episodes in 11 patients. Gut 1994;35:101-106. VI

112. Knox T, Olans L: Liver disease in pregnancy. N Engl J Med 1996;335:569-576. V

113. Rolfes D, Ishak K: Acute fatty liver of pregnancy: A clinicopathologic study of 35 cases. Hepatology 1985;1149-1158. VI

114. Wilcken B, Kin-Chuen L, Hammond J et al: Pregnancy and fetal long-chain 3-hydroxyacyl coenzyme A dehydrogenase deficiency. Lancet 1993;341:407-408. VI

115. Ibdah J, Bennett M, Rinaldo P, et al: A fetal fatty-acid oxidation disorder as a cause of liver disease in pregnant women. N Engl J Med 1999;340: 1723-1731. III

116. Riely C, Latham P, Romero R, Duffy T: Acute fatty liver of pregnancy: A reassessment based on observations in nine patients. Ann Intern Med 1987;106: 703-706. VI

117. Winer-Muram H: Diagnostic imaging in obstetrics and gynecology: New developments. Curr Opin Obstet Gynecol 1999;11:421-425. V

118. American College of Obstetricians and Gynecologists (ACOG): ACOG Committee opinion no. 299: Guidelines for diagnostic imaging during pregnancy. Obstet Gynecol 2004;104:647. IV

119. Mettler FA, Upton AC: Medical Effects of Ionizing Radiation, 2nd ed. Philadelphia, WB Saunders, 1995. V

120. Bentur Y: Ionizing and nonionizing radiation in pregnancy. In Maternal-Fetal Toxicology, 2nd ed. New York, Marcel Dekker, 1994, p 515. V

121. Ratnapalan S, Bona N, Chandra K, Koren G: Physicians' perceptions of teratogenic risk associated with radiography and CT during early pregnancy. AJR Am J Roentgenol 2004;182:1107-1109. III

122. Yamazaki JN, Schull WJ: Perinatal loss and neurological abnormalities among children of the atomic bomb. Nagasaki and Hiroshima revisited 1949 to 1989 [see comments]. JAMA 1990:264:605-609. III

123. National Council on Radiation Protection and Measurements: Medical radiation exposure of pregnant and potentially pregnant women. Report no. 54. Washington, DC, 1977. IV

124. Bentur Y, Horlatsch N, Koren G: Exposure to ionizing radiation during pregnancy: Perception of teratogenic risk and outcome. Teratology 1991;43:109-112. III

125. Stewart A, Kneale GW: Radiation dose effects in relation to obstetric x-rays and childhood cancers. Lancet 1970;1:1185-1188. III

126. Diethelm L, Xu H: Diagnostic imaging of the lung during pregnancy. Clin Obstet Gynecol 1996; 39:36-55. V

Index